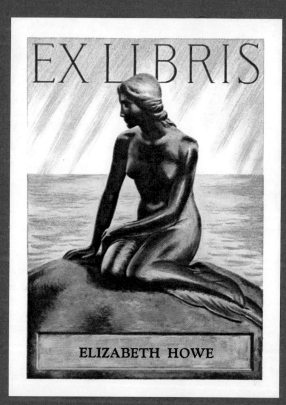

EX LIBRIS

ELIZABETH HOWE

Love
Needs
Care

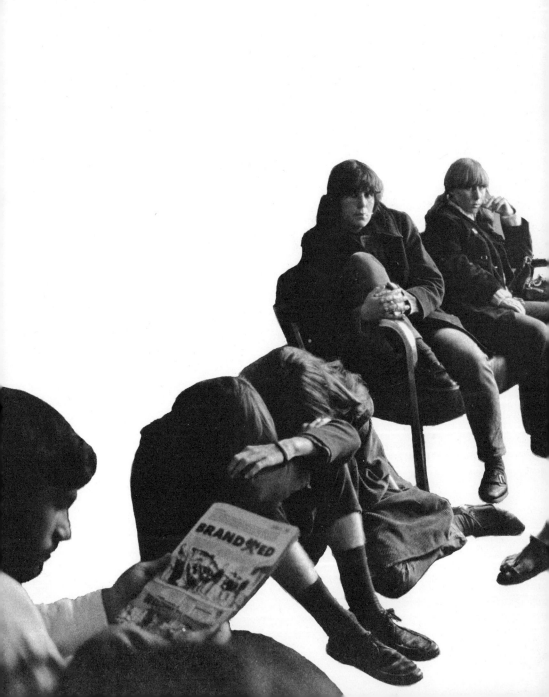

Love
Needs
Care

A history of San Francisco's
Haight-Ashbury Free Medical
Clinic and its pioneer role in
treating drug-abuse problems

By David E. Smith, M.D. and John Luce

Little, Brown and Company · Boston · Toronto

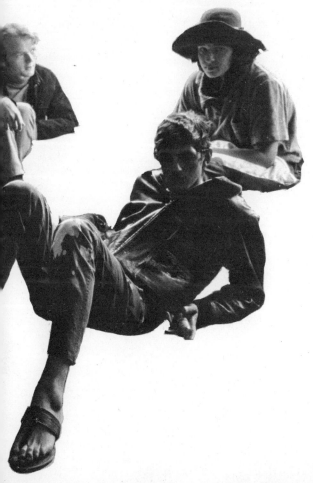

LIBRARY OF CONGRESS CATALOG NO. 77-121434
TO 5/71

FIRST EDITION

The authors gratefully acknowledge permission to quote from the following sources:
Lines quoted from "Burnt Norton" in **Four Quartets** by T. S. Eliot are reprinted by
permission of Harcourt, Brace Jovanovich, Inc. Copyright 1943 by T. S. Eliot.
"White Rabbit" by Grace Slick, Copyright 1966 by Irving Music, Inc. & Copperpenny
Music Publishing Company (BMI); and "The Long Road" by Joe Kooken, Copyright
1967, 1970 by Irving Music, Inc. & Copperpenny Music Publishing Company (BMI) are
used by permission of the publisher.
A portion of this book originally appeared in slightly different form in an
Esquire Magazine article by John Luce.

Published simultaneously in Canada by Little, Brown & Company (Canada) Limited

PRINTED IN THE UNITED STATES OF AMERICA

Dedication

This book is dedicated to the many people — and particularly to the patients — who have made the Haight-Ashbury Free Medical Clinic a reality.

Rejection: The process or fact of regarding something as worthless or throwing it away . . .
The Encyclopedia of Mental Health

Nurturance: The providing of food, shelter, care and narcissistic supplies . . .
The Encyclopedia of Mental Health

Time present and time past
Are both perhaps present in time future,
And time future contained in time past.
If all time is eternally present
All time is unredeemable.

T. S. Eliot, "Burnt Norton," **Four Quartets**

Acknowledgments

Our lives are communal; hundreds of people have helped the Haight-Ashbury Free Medical Clinic and contributed to this book. Space limitations prevent us from thanking all of them, but we would like to express our appreciation to several who have afforded us their talents and experiences and stimulated our efforts. In addition to those mentioned in the text, they include:

Dean Marvin Anderson, Dr. Michael Arlen, Atlantis, Abra and Skhy, Mrs. Charles Aubrey, Paul Barrata, Nan and Howie Becker, Maggie Bedford, John Berggruen, Donovan Bess, Pam Blum, Claudia Border, Dr. Peter Bourne, Norm Bouton, Nancy Brown, Phoebe Bryan, Dr. Robert Burns, Joan and Chuck Bushey, Mrs. Lynne Caine, Ruth Campbell, Robert Campos, Lou and Nancy Caputo, Dr. Gene Carmody, Dr. Linda Cleaver, Dr. Seymour Cohen, Karen Crescio, Don and Sharon deZordo, Nancy Dorr, Kitty Drescher, Dr. Stu Frank, Bob Frazier, Judy Freidman, Dr. Morton Garfield, Dr. Martin Gershman, Martin Goldman, Sara Greenman, Mrs. Richard Guinn, Holly Halse, Mrs. Owen Halse, Dr. Robert Hank, Art Harper, Dr. Michael Hart, Bill Hatch, Charles Hepler, Tom and Sally Hickey, Dr. Linda Hilles, Richard Hongisto, Lois Hullman, Joy, Michael and Mary Kasper, Dr. Phyllis Kempner, Robert Kimball, Dr. John Kramer, Rich and Jean Krasno, Dr. Jack Lange, Ken Lee, Dr. Philip Lee, Mike and Flicka Leibert, George and Lillie Leonard, Mrs. Mildred Liffler, Geoff Link, Leo Litwak, Si Lowinsky, Mary Pat McKinney and the members of Youth Projects, Patti McWilliams and the staff of Immediate Psychiatric Aid and Referral Service, Frances Moffat, Debby Moxham, Frank Muncey, Dan Munn, Mike Murphy, Pat and Gail Murphy, Dr. Shelby Nankin, Marlys Nelson, Dave Newlin, Kenneth Parker, Tom and Nancy Parker, Kathy Parrish, Mike Payette, Penny Perlman, John and Julia Poppy, Aileen Regan, Bill Resner, Trudi Reynolds, Dr. Christy Robb, Dr. Larry Rose, Dr. Shelly Rosen, Rudy Schleif, Dr. Kurt Schlesinger, Rock Scully, Dr. Robert Shapps, Robert Sherrill, Mrs. Marion Shrimpton, Margaret Shyppertt, Dr. Hyman Silver, Tad Slocum, Bill Starr, David Steinhart, Alan Stone, Georgia Taft, Annie Taylor, Bill Thompson, Myra Thompson, Jack and Vicky Tomlinson, Bill and Wendy Turnbull, Mary Turner, Dr. Robert Van Bruggen, DeWitt Wallace, Wendy Watriss, John Wasserman, Dr. Charles Weill, Dr. Harvey Weinburg, Arthur Weiner, Gene and Connie Williams, and Mrs. Gail Woolaway.

We would also like to thank the several authors we have drawn on most heavily. They are: Roger Smith, "The Marketplace of Speed," unpublished manuscript; Drs. Frederick Meyers, Ernest Jawetz and Alan Goldfien of *Review of Medical Pharmacology*, Lange Medical Publications; Drs. Henry Brainerd, Sheldon Margen and Milton Chattan of *Current Diagnosis and Treatment*, Lange Medical Publications; and Drs. Louis Goodman and Alfred Gilman of *The Pharmacological Basis of Therapeutics*, Macmillan. These latter texts are used as standard references at the Haight-

Ashbury Free Medical Clinic. We would also like to thank Franklin Watts, Inc., publishers of *The Encyclopedia of Mental Health,* for their permission to use several definitions from the encyclopedia's glossary. And we would like to thank Dr. Joel Fort for his editorial help and long-standing personal and professional assistance. We highly recommend his book, *The Pleasure Seekers: The Drug Crisis, Youth and Society,* Bobbs-Merrill.

In addition, we wish to thank Jim Marshall, Michael Alexander, and especially Elaine Mayes for providing us with the photographs for this book. Miss Mayes's portraits, a dozen of which are in the permanent collections of the Metropolitan Museum and the Museum of Modern Art in New York City, are in our judgment the most compelling ever taken in the Haight-Ashbury. She, Jim and Michael live in San Francisco and have been loyal friends of the Clinic.

Finally, our deepest gratitude goes to Fred Belliveau, General Manager of the Medical Book Division of Little, Brown and Company, and to Harry Sions, Senior Editor of Little, Brown and editor of this book. Mr. Belliveau took an early interest in the Clinic and in our project. Mr. Sions has guided our efforts, given us his enthusiasm and affection, and contributed immeasurably to *Love Needs Care.*

Special Acknowledgment

Although many people have helped with this book, one person deserves special mention. This is Dr. Ernest A. Dernburg, former psychiatric director of the Haight-Ashbury Free Medical Clinic, who is now on the staff of Mt. Zion Hospital and in private practice in San Francisco. In addition to sharing his knowledge of the Haight-Ashbury with us, Dr. Dernburg has provided us with a psychoanalytic orientation that enriches the book. Dr. Dernburg is not listed on the cover or on our title page, but he should be considered a coauthor. His understanding of young people, drug abuse and the hippie modality will find a fuller expression in a companion volume to *Love Needs Care* the three of us are preparing.

David E. Smith, M.D.
John Luce

San Francisco, California
September, 1970

Contents

Acknowledgments   vii

Part I: A Case of Terminal Euphoria   1

Part II: The New Community   73

Part III: Summer of Love   149

Part IV: After Love Has Gone   211

Part V: Epitaph   301

Bibliography   371

Glossary   379

Appendices   391

Photographs by
Elaine Mayes, Jim Marshall
and Michael Alexander

Part I

A Case
of Terminal
Euphoria

There is a feeling of Eternity in youth
which makes amends for everything. To
be young is to be as one of the Immortal Gods.

William Hazlitt, ''The Feeling of Immortality in Youth''

Now that my ladder's gone,
I must lie down where all ladders start,
In the foul rag-and-bone shop of the heart.

W. B. Yeats, ''The Circus Animals' Desertion''

I seen a lot of people with tombstones in their eyes.
If they don't get the hard stuff, you know they're gonna die.

Hoyt Axton, ''The Pusher''

Desolation Row

In the fall of 1968, San Francisco's Haight-Ashbury district looked like a disaster area. Most of the Victorian houses, flats and apartment buildings lying in the Flatlands between the Panhandle of Golden Gate Park and the northern slope of Mt. Sutro had deteriorated badly, and many property owners had boarded over their windows and blocked their doorways with heavy iron bars. The original residents of the Haight were hiding, in a self-imposed internment. "We're frightened," said one sixty-year-old member of the Neighborhood Council. "The Haight-Ashbury has become a violent teen-age slum. The streets aren't safe; rats romp in the Panhandle; the neighborhood gets more run-down every day. The only thing that'll save this place is a massive dose of federal aid."

Nowhere was the aid more needed than on Haight Street, the strip of stores which runs east to west through the Flatlands. The street was once a prosperous shopping area, but it had so degenerated by the fall of 1968 that the storefronts were covered with steel grates and sheets of plywood, and the sidewalks were littered with dog droppings, cigarette butts and broken glass. According to the owner of a small realty agency on the corner of Haight and Stanyan, over fifty grocers, druggists, and other straight merchants had moved off Haight Street since the 1967 Summer of Love; property values had fallen twenty percent in the same period, and none of the remaining businessmen could find buyers for their stores. The Safeway Supermarket at Haight and Schrader had closed in August after being shoplifted out of ten-thousand-dollars worth of merchandise in three months. "The only people making money on Haight Street now sell cheap wine or dope," the realtor said. "Our former customers are all gone. There's nothing left of the old community anymore."

Nothing was left of the Haight-Ashbury's new hippie community in the fall of 1968, either. There were no paisley-painted buses on Haight Street, no flower children parading the sidewalks, no tribal gatherings, no H.I.P. — Haight Independent Proprietors — stores. Almost all of the long-haired merchants had followed their straight counterparts out of the district; the Print Mint at Haight and Clayton stood vacant; the Psychedelic Shop across the street was closed. The Straight Theatre at Haight and Cole, a neighborhood movie palace outfitted with a dance floor in 1967, was now struggling to survive on B-grade reruns. The owner of Mnasidika's was trying to sell her boutique and leave the area. "The Haight is dead," she said. "It's lonely out here on Desolation Row."

This shop owner also reported that the heroes of the new community had abandoned it. Allen Ginsberg was in New York recuperating from an automobile accident. Dr. Timothy Leary was promoting *High Priest,* his autobiography, and lecturing at the Berkeley Free University on psychedelic anthropology. Dr. Richard Alpert had become a high priest himself, the Baba Ram Dass of an Indian spiritual society, and was scheduled as a guru-in-residence at the Esalen Institute next year. Neil Cassady, the protagonist of Jack Kerouac's *On the Road,* had died in February on a railroad track in Mexico from an overdose of barbiturates and alcohol. Many of the Merry Pranksters had gone their separate ways, and the city was off limits to author Ken Kesey, who was sitting out a three-year probation for possession of marijuana on his brother's farm in Springfield, Oregon.

Furthermore, none of the rock musicians or other artists who once inhabited the Haight-Ashbury were still around. The Grateful Dead had vacated their communal house in the district. Janis Joplin had been evicted from her apartment near the Panhandle and quit Big Brother and the Holding Company to start her own band. Quicksilver Messenger Service and the Charlatans were undergoing internal changes; Grace Slick and the crew of Jefferson Airplane had become celebrities and moved from the Haight to wealthier neighborhoods across town. Alton Kelly, Rick Griffin and their fellow poster artists were living in other parts of the city. Allen Cohen had disbanded the *Haight-Ashbury Oracle* and left the area for parts unknown.

Also missing were the quasi-political figures who once exerted influence in the new community. Ron and Jay Thelin, founders of the Psychedelic Shop, still drifted in and out of the district occasionally, but they were hostile and refused to be interviewed. Arthur Lisch had come back to town to disrupt the American Psychological Association convention in September and then left for Mexico, along with several of the original Diggers. And although a few young people using the Digger name were running a free bakery and housing office out of the basement of All Saints' Episcopal Church on Waller Street, Father Leon Harris there considered them an insignificant minority. "For all intents and purposes," he said, "the peaceful hippies we once saw in the Haight-Ashbury have disappeared."

They had started disappearing over a year earlier, when worldwide publicity brought a more disturbed population to the Haight and the city escalated its undeclared war on the new community. Many of the long-haired adolescents the public considered hip had left Haight Street and were hanging out on Telegraph Avenue in Berkeley or on Grant Avenue in San Francisco's North Beach district. Some of the summer hippies who once played in the Haight-Ashbury had either returned home or reenrolled in school. Others had moved to the Mission district and other parts of the city, to Sausalito and Mill Valley in Marin County, to Berkeley and Big Sur or to the rural communes operating throughout northern California.

A few hundred were still trapped in the Haight, but they took what they hoped was mescaline, LSD and other hallucinogens indoors and stayed as far away from Haight Street as possible. When they had to go there, to cash welfare checks or shop with food stamps at the one remaining supermarket, they never went at night or walked alone. "It's too dangerous for me," said a twenty-year-old expectant mother named Jackie, who ran away from a middle-class home in Detroit during the summer of 1967 and then became a staff member of the Haight-Ashbury Free Medical Clinic; "Haight Street used to be groovy. I could get high just being there. But I don't know anybody on the street today. The only hippies left around here are people like me who are committed to the Clinic, the kids who've switched from LSD to other drugs, and the spiritual types who still take acid and think they can save this godforsaken place. Believe me, they don't have a chance. Since I've been here, the Haight-Ashbury's become the roughest part of town."

The New Population

The new population that had moved into the district and taken over Haight Street like an occupying army was responsible for this roughness. This population was made up of as many kinds of people as had ever frequented the Haight before. It was also a transient population which fluctuated daily in consistency and size. However, the number of street people found on Haight could be approximated at five thousand on any given weekend afternoon. And they could be arbitrarily divided into several groups, according to how they looked and lived and what drugs they used.

The first group included occasional visitors. Some were tourists who drove through to gawk at hippies, journalists who came to write obituaries about the psychedelic movement, and social scientists who came to study deviance. Others were AWOL soldiers and draft-evaders searching for sanctuary, or students, servicemen and businessmen dropping by the district to pick up girls and purchase psychoactive chemicals. These people sometimes failed to score with the few females who hung out on the street, but they had no trouble finding drugs. According to Matthew O'Connor, supervising agent for the State Bureau of Narcotics in northern California, "You could buy every toxic substance known to man in the Haight during the fall of 1968. Shopping there for drugs was like choosing your dinner at a smorgasbord."

A second group which sampled from this smorgasbord was interested mainly in alcohol. It consisted of grizzled white and black winos, who dressed in rags and looked as though they belonged on a more traditional type of skid row, and American Indians, many right off reservations, who wore the inexpensive clothes they bought with government allotments when first arriving in town. These Indians could become belligerent when drinking, but they usually huddled in protective clumps on the street corners and kept out of other people's way. The other alcoholics preferred to congregate in front of the liquor stores on Haight Street, where they spent their days sleeping in the gutters and slugging down wine.

Another group that often gathered in front of the liquor stores was made up of young blacks, many of whom lived in the Haight-Ashbury Flatlands or in the Fillmore ghetto nearby. Although a few of these Negroes wore African dashikis and natural hairstyles to indicate their involvement with Black Power, most dressed in high-collared shirts and pegged trousers and pomaded their hair to form fierce-looking prides. These Negroes were called street spades by many young white residents. They supported themselves primarily by stealing and by selling such drugs as marijuana, barbiturates, heroin and cocaine. Some also took these drugs to achieve a blissful somnolence. Others drank alcohol and became assaultive and mean.

The same meanness could be seen in a fourth group on the street, which consisted of young whites in their late teens and early twenties. Like their black counterparts, most of these youths had criminal records in San Francisco and other cities and were known in the Haight only by aliases and nicknames. They were uneducated and lacking any religious or mystical interest, and had traveled from across the country to exploit the flower children they assumed were still living there. Some had grown long hair and assimilated the hip jargon and ethic in the process, but they resembled true hippies in no real physical, philosophic or psychological way. These young people were tough and aggressive. Instead of beads and bright costumes, they wore ankle chains, leather jackets and coarse, heavy clothes. Instead of ornate buses, they drove beat-up motorcycles and hot rods. Although they used many drugs on occasion, they dismissed the hallucinogens as child's play and preferred to intoxify themselves with opiates, barbiturates and amphetamines.

Dr. Ernest Dernburg, psychiatric director of the Haight-Ashbury Free Medical Clinic, called these people hoodies to emphasize their dissimilarity from the beats and hippies who once inhabited the Haight-Ashbury. He described them diagnostically as psychopaths, the same kind seen in the city's Tenderloin district for years. Unlike the beats and hippies, the hoodies who hung out on Haight Street neither withdrew from threatening circumstances nor valued introspection. They were unable to delay gratification, and usually acted upon any impulse. They had little compassion, warmth or mature sense of conscience. When they hurt somebody or did something others might consider morally wrong, they felt not guilt but fear.

Dr. Dernburg attributed this response of fear to the hoodies' poor superego development. Most of those who allowed themselves to be interviewed and/or treated at the Psychiatric Section of the Clinic had been constantly exposed to illicit sexual activity and violence in their homes and never had responsible parents or parental figures with whom to identify. The hoodies' mothers were apparently depressed, impetuous women who resented their children and deprived them of proper guidance and understanding. Their fathers were often rigid, distant and punitive men who beat their children regularly. In some cases, the hoodies had no fathers and were never disciplined. In others, they were continually bullied by their mothers' many boyfriends.

Because they came from such environments, these young people felt cheated by life. They also either failed to internalize the controls necessary to direct their energy into socially acceptable channels or developed punitive consciences which they could escape only by impulsiveness. Whatever their particular family situations, the hoodies never gained emotional restraints to govern their antisocial behavior. They therefore acted out externally what others might try to deal with internally, and set up confrontations with other people instead of confronting themselves. In the vernacular of the Haight, they were always running games.

These games were usually dangerous, for the hoodies made their living mainly by criminal means. Some were called cattle rustlers because they stole food and merchandise from the few stores left on Haight Street and then sold these goods to their companions. Others were sidewalk commandos, who frequently quit the street to burgle whatever private residences they could in the adjacent area. But most manufactured drugs or sold them on Haight Street. Many of these dealers held up their customers if they failed to close a sale, or burned their confederates by selling them impure chemicals. The tougher ones even robbed or ripped off other dealers and raided those places where drugs were manufactured. They then became known as rip-off artists and were universally feared.

The hoodies also took drugs, but they were generally too cagey to become physically addicted to or psychologically dependent on them. Instead, they employed certain chemicals to alter their moods or sold them to gain financial profit and gather followers. Next to the recognition they received as accomplished rip-off artists, these young people derived their greatest satisfaction from being regarded as successful dealers. Because they seemed so street-wise and criminally knowledgeable, the more prosperous psychopaths were held in awe by those younger and less shrewd adolescents in the Haight-Ashbury who bought their products and wanted desperately to participate in their supposed power. They fed off the adoration of these followers and used them to gratify their needs.

These needs varied, but almost all of the hoodies capitalized on their fans to obtain feelings of mastery and self-esteem. Although they prided themselves on their independence, the hoodies required constant reassurance that they were projecting unflinching images. To achieve this, some of them stalked the Haight with vicious German shepherds and Doberman pinschers to collect stares. Others organized gang rapes, called themselves members of the Mafia, and carried guns and knives, promising to use these weapons on anyone who hassled them. A few even played cops-and-robbers games, in which they would flaunt their private arsenals in front of police officers whenever their admirers were around.

Dr. Dernburg observed that the hoodies seemed to gain great excitement from these activities, an excitement which obviously paralleled that of their early lives. Even more obvious to him was the feeling of power the young people achieved. He believed that the hoodies played games with policemen primarily because they could not police themselves; in effect, they tried to trick their own, externalized, consciences. They were able to check their impulsiveness only when they set out to flirt with the police or to avenge themselves on people who had burned them. Although they lacked mature consciences, their ego functions and reality testing were not greatly impaired. Thus, they were adept at mastering other people and their environment. This was fortunate for the hoodies, for they needed to feel in control.

Control was also essential to a fifth group in the Haight-Ashbury. It consisted of Hell's Angels, Gypsy Jokers and members of other outlaw motorcycle gangs. Many of these bikers actually lived outside of the district, yet they still roared through regularly on their gleaming Harley-Davidsons and could often be seen on Haight Street, eating pills like candy and roughing up passersby. The bikers were generally older than the hoodies. They dressed in grease-encrusted Levi's, T-shirts and jean jackets emblazoned with swastikas, club patches, which they called colors, and other motor paraphernalia.

The gang members were intensely proud of their colors and would defend one another to the death against overwhelming odds. They were also less crafty in their criminal behavior than the hoodies, less subtle in playing with the police, less discriminating in their drug choices and more eager to engage in such suicidal practices as screaming around turns on their choppers at ninety miles an hour. Almost all of the bikers had gone over the high side of a turn at least once, and they placed no value on human life, including their own. The patches on their jackets identified them as "One Percenters," "Born To Lose."

Because of their behavioral differences from the hoodies, Dr. Dernburg classified the bikers as borderline psychotics, or psychotic characters. Most of them seemed to come from homes that were similar to, yet much more emotionally overloaded than those of the hoodies. Their mothers were not only depressed and impulsive in many cases, but also so deficient in their ego-boundary formation that they could not readily distinguish between their own feelings and sensations and those which they perceived in the outside world. As a result, the bikers also had great difficulty in determining the validity of their perceptions and externalized much of their anger and hostility. This externalization led them to react with uncontrollable fury at the slightest hint of provocation, even if they caused the provocation themselves.

Furthermore, while the hoodies used drugs primarily to heighten their courage and to help manipulate their environment, the bikers employed them to feel in control of themselves. They might have become frightened by their confused thinking and by their social impotence if they did not create distracting chemical challenges. For example, they would inject or swallow any kind of drug just to prove that its pharmacological effects could neither stun nor confuse them significantly. At the same time, they loved to live on a razor-thin edge, to turn reality into an obstacle course for their Harley-Davidsons, to see if they could go over the high side and come back alive. In these instances, they seemed to be projecting their internal chaos onto the external world, chaos which they could then master as they did chemicals, to assure themselves that they were in charge of their psychological processes. This made the bikers so dangerous that they often destroyed other people. But they were far more likely to destroy themselves.

Although such self-destructiveness was certainly associated with the bikers, it was even more synonymous with another group found in the Haight-Ashbury. This group was probably the largest and was made up of overtly psychotic young people who had either come into the district since the

Summer of Love or had lived there long before the hippies arrived. These people resembled the hoodies somewhat in appearance, but their clothes were often older, dirtier and more threadbare. Furthermore, although they were as antisocial as both the hoodies and the bikers, they were much more passive, disoriented and confused. They emulated the tougher psychopaths and psychotic characters, tried to be crafty, carried guns and knives and sometimes qualified as sidewalk commandos. Yet they were usually too disorganized to scheme effectively and had such poor reality-testing capabilities that they were easily and often victimized.

Like the hoodies, these seriously disturbed young people generally supported themselves by hustling, stealing and dealing drugs and greatly enjoyed the presitge of their profession. But they derived less pleasure from selling chemicals to others than from taking the compounds themselves. Some of them had learned to employ certain drugs for their specific pharmacological properties. Others were multiple and habitual abusers who took different chemicals when their first choices were not available. Many were physically addicted to the drugs. Most were psychologically dependent on them for their self-esteem.

The abuse patterns of these psychotics were apparently dictated by their early environments. Most of them came from fatherless homes in which they were deprived of affection and nurturance. Their mothers were often severely anxious, depressed and disturbed women who failed to establish guidelines for their children, assaulted them with their own disappointment, rage and sexual frustration, and could not relate with any feelings resembling warmth or affection. Because of this, the young people were anxious, depressed, disturbed and unable to relate themselves. Many had been so overpowered by intrusive stimuli that they could not tolerate the presence of other people. Like the alcoholics on Haight Street, they apparently needed toxic chemicals to regulate such stimuli and to anesthetize their physiological and psychological pain.

Dr. Dernburg felt that others in this group took drugs primarily to fill their inner voids. These young people experienced extreme emptiness and overwhelming oral longings, which they translated into drug abuse, among other ways. By using toxic chemicals, they could suppress drives that otherwise might have motivated them to assuage their hunger and to seek sexual release. Whatever particular compounds they preferred, they wanted to achieve a state of nonfrustration in which they would not have to rely on other people or on their environment for gratification or narcissistic supplies.

This effort was most obvious in those who ingested drugs intravenously. These young people considered chemicals a source of nourishment; some even reported in utero fantasies to Dr. Dernburg, in which they imagined feeding themselves by injecting drugs into their bloodstreams. Others said that the compounds gave them orgasms, which were enhanced if they jacked off or regulated the pressure in their needles. They might fix up together and inject chemicals into companions of the opposite sex, but they generally substituted such practices for sexual intercourse. Even when they did ball with one another, theirs was usually a form of mutual masturbation, with little shared tenderness or love.

When these people took drugs that altered their moods rather than their mental functioning, they were probably using the chemicals to come to grips with the emotionally inconsistent situations which they had encountered in their early lives. As children, these psychotic young people apparently could not control the up and down atmosphere of their homes. Most ran away during early adolescence, but remained dominated by their early experiences. In the Haight, however, they could take substances singly and in combination to go up and down at will. The psychotic young people liked to think that they could govern their moods by deciding how, when, where and with what they would become intoxicated. This gave them a feeling of active mastery over their anxiety and depression — emotions which in fact they could not control.

A similar attempt at self-regulation was evident in those who induced toxic psychoses with mind-altering hallucinogenic chemicals in order to deny their own mental dysfunctioning. Like the bikers and the earlier hippies who abused LSD, they insisted that the compounds they consumed were responsible for making them and the world seem so bizarre. Some of them appeared to sense their own insanity from time to time, but they quickly took more drugs and thereby disguised the true cause of their confusion. To simplify the matter: they disturbed themselves with chemicals in order to avoid realizing how disturbed they already were.

Another pattern in the psychotics' drug abuse related to the ever-present issue of control. Although the hoodies in the Haight-Ashbury could conquer other people and the bikers could overcome their self-imposed challenges, the psychotics could do neither. So they tried to master drugs by taking repeated high doses that would kill most human beings. Whereas the tougher young people on Haight Street could brag about their sexual conquests and criminal successes, the more disturbed ones could claim only that they had taken every chemical imaginable and still survived. Theirs was a pathetic attempt to gain recognition, but an understandable one. And some of these confused people were actually admired.

Such admiration stemmed from a final group found in the Haight during the fall of 1968. It was composed primarily of school dropouts and runaways in their early teens. These adolescents were naïve and impressionable. Like their contemporaries in other subcultural settings, they had come to the Haight-Ashbury with no money, expecting to be cared for in hippie communes and planning to test themselves by experimenting with drugs. Most wanted love and understanding as well as stimulation. When they did not find it, they usually started living on the street, where they could not fend for themselves.

Part of the problem was that the new arrivals had almost no source of financial support. Many tried to panhandle spare change from the visitors on Haight Street or peddled copies of *Love Street,* the *Haight-Ashbury Tribune* and the *Haight-Ashbury Maverick, Oracle* imitations designed for tourists with pictures of phony flower children in Kama Sutra poses on the cover and ads for dildoes and erotic films inside. But there was too little money and too much competition on the street for either begging or vending to be profitable. Because of this, some of the young people had to pose for pictures used in the tourist papers or participate in the making of stag films. Others were forced to work the meatrack by becoming male or female prostitutes or find employment as topless dancers and waitresses on Broadway Street in the North Beach district across town. A few were eligible for welfare or wise enough to go home.

But most had no decent homes to return to or had burned too many bridges behind them in coming to the Haight. They were therefore committed to the district, and had to try either to maintain a semblance of self-sufficiency or attach themselves to older people for protection. As a result, the new arrivals were soon involved in drug dealing, cattle rustling and other forms of criminal activity and had to assume aliases, signifying their severance from society. They then increased their experimentation with chemicals to impress their heroes and to share in their alleged potency. Yet all they really shared were the drugs and a disease-ridden and potentially fatal life-style.

What particular path the new arrivals took naturally depended more than anything else on their personalities. But also relevant was the availability and the pharmacological properties of the chemicals they used. If these adolescents had stayed at home or come to the district a year or so earlier, they might have begun their drug experimentation with marijuana and/or LSD and progressed no further. Yet since these chemicals were no longer preferred in the Haight-Ashbury, they became involved with drugs which exerted a much more powerful effect on their physical and psychological functioning. The most popular and readily available of them during the fall of 1968 were amphetamines.

Instant Self-Esteem

The amphetamines which set the drug tone of the Haight are known to most people as diet or pep pills. They are classified pharmacologically as nonselective central nervous system stimulants because they can excite all areas of the nervous system. The amphetamines are related to a group of compounds called sympathomimetic amines for their adrenalinelike effect on the body. The amphetamine molecule, alpha-methylphenylethylamine, is common to all amphetatmines and to amphetamine equivalents, drugs that are chemically different from amphetamines but have approximately the same pharmacological properties.

The amphetamines were synthesized in Germany early in the twentieth century and were first used as substitutes for ephedrine, a substance which has been employed extensively in the treatment of asthma. They are produced at present in many forms, the most common of which are methamphetamine hydrochloride, amphetamine sulfate and dextroamphetamine sulfate. These are manufactured by several large pharmaceutical companies and are marketed under such trade names as Methedrine and Desoxyn, Benzedrine and Dexedrine, respectively. Methamphetamine is also mixed with the barbiturate phenobarbital and marketed as Desbutal. Similarly, a combination of dextroamphetamine and amobarbital is sold under the trade name Dexamyl. Two amphetamine equivalents, phenmetrazine and methylphenidate, are marketed as Preludin and Ritalin. These drugs are all sold in tablet form on a prescription basis. In addition, methamphetamine is available in some states in ampules of injectable liquid bearing the trade names Desoxyn and Methedrine.

Like all psychoactive agents, the amphetamines exert certain effects on both the peripheral and the central nervous systems. The peripheral actions of the compounds include an increase in blood pressure, a dilation of the pupils, a constriction of the blood vessels on such mucosal surfaces as the lips and the lining of the nose, a relaxation and dilation of the bronchial muscles of the respiratory tract, a relaxation or a spasmodic contraction of the gastrointestinal tract and a secretion of sparse, thick saliva. The drugs' dilating action on the bronchial passages explains their former use in treating hay fever and asthma.

Although these peripheral actions are both marked and potentially therapeutic, amphetamines are generally employed today only for their more profound stimulative effects on the central nervous system. Of these, the three most pronounced actions are the suppression of appetite, the elevation of mood and the warding off of fatigue. The former property is used medically in the control of weight, while the second is employed in the treatment of some forms of psychological depression.

Amphetamines are also used in the treatment of certain hyperactive neurologically impaired children and as a major part of the treatment of narcolepsy, a relatively rare condition which is characterized by an uncontrollable desire to sleep. Finally, physicians have been known to prescribe amphetamines to athletes, students, and truck drivers who desire wakefulness. But since these chemicals have a high abuse potential, informed doctors now recommend safer stimulants or the caffeine available in coffee, No-Doz and comparable over-the-counter medications.

Physicians often administer amphetamines in tablet form and advise that the drugs be taken in single five-to-fifteen milligram doses daily. Desoxyn and Methedrine ampules were also once prescribed for such purposes, but many doctors now believe that these injectable ampules should be prohibited. They are not available on a prescription basis in California, for in 1963, the state attorney general's office urged the pharmaceutical companies responsible for their manufacture to remove their products voluntarily from the market.

This action was taken by the state to prevent people from becoming dependent on amphetamines because they were injecting high doses of Methedrine and Desoxyn to achieve the euphoric state of enhanced energy, well being and self-confidence which accompanies the drugs' central effects. Medical records compiled in the early 1960's revealed that some of these people were former military personnel who had begun taking the compounds for medical or tactical reasons and then became habituated to them. Others were housewives and businessmen who used amphetamines for weight control or as antidepressants until they began employing the drugs to produce euphoria.

At the same time, it was learned that several doctors in the San Francisco Bay area were prescribing the chemicals to opiate addicts both to make a profit and because they considered amphetamines less harmful than heroin. These physicians knew that the stimulants caused little addiction and few withdrawal symptoms, although they were not aware of the other consequences of abuse. They also reasoned that the addicts might lead more productive lives if they could obtain pharmaceutical amphetamines at one-sixth the cost of underground narcotics. The addicts were helped by this action in some cases, for by obtaining amphetamines legally and cheaply they did not have to resort to criminal action to support their habits. But in other cases, they began selling the ampules on the black market or using them in combination with heroin. It was primarily because of this that the attorney general's office tried to inhibit the drugs' consumption.

This act may have been well intentioned, but it only forced the addicts to find new chemical sources. Furthermore, since amphetamine abuse was never limited to the drugs' injectable form, or to the underground, it continued to mount beyond the attorney general's wildest expectations. Although amphetamines are now classified as dangerous drugs under state and federal law, Dr. Joel Fort, founder and former director of the San Francisco Center for Special Problems, reports that over one hundred and fifty-three thousand pounds of the compounds were obtained through doctors' prescriptions alone during 1968 in the United States. The American pharmaceutical industry advertises the drugs as panaceas for fatigue, boredom, depression and practically all other human problems, while physicians indiscriminately dispense them to their patients. As a result of these and other factors, millions of people today ingest amphetamines to induce euphoria and thereby achieve what they have been led to expect is instant self-esteem.

In doing so, these people run a serious risk of incurring adverse reactions. According to Dr. Frederick Meyers, professor of pharmacology at the University of California Medical Center and former research director of the Haight-Ashbury Free Medical Clinic, even low-dose amphetamine consumption can cause tremulousness, anxiety, drying of the mouth, alteration of sleep habits and other unpleasant effects. It may also lead to an increased awareness of heart function, which can be compounded by tachycardia, a rapid, forceful pounding that stems from extreme cardiovascular stimulation.

Tachycardia also shows up in cases of acute amphetamine toxicity due to intentional or accidental overdosage. Although no fatalities have been recorded as a direct result of high-dose consumption, it commonly produces restlessness, hypertension, extreme anxiety, impaired judgment, hyperventilation (a state of excessively rapid breathing), hallucinations and possible psychosis. Sedatives may be profitably employed in treating acute toxicity, but patients may require isolation and reassurance that they are not suffering heart attacks or losing their sanity.

More serious, and increasingly common in this country, is chronic amphetamine toxicity. The chemicals are not addictive in small doses, but people who take larger amounts do experience extreme psychological dependence and may even suffer mild physical withdrawal symptoms when deprived of the drugs. Such dependence is complicated by the fact that as the body develops a tolerance to amphetamines, increasingly higher doses are required to maintain their effects. Prolonged high-dose amphetamine consumption often results in physical deterioration and in a toxic psychosis characterized by perceptual alterations, visual and auditory hallucinations, severe depression and a state that resembles paranoid schizophrenia. It may also lead to organic brain damage and personality change, as studies of amphetamine abusers in Japan seem to reveal.

Another probable result of high-dose consumption is violent behavior. Studies performed on laboratory rats at the University of California Medical Center by Drs. David E. Smith, Charles Hine, Eugene Schoenfeld and Charles Fischer have shown that grouping the animals and injecting them with amphetamines quadruples the toxicity of the drugs and significantly lowers the median lethal dose. These animals become inordinately aggressive and assaultive when they are caged together and turn upon one another with unexpected savagery. Their violent behavior is probably intensified by confinement, for it is strikingly similar to that observed in amphetamine abusers who consume the drugs in crowded atmospheres.

Such behavioral parallels are not conclusive, and it has yet to be determined whether amphetamines modify the personality primarily by biochemically altering the central nervous system or by reinforcing or precipitating long-term psychological tendencies.

It is known that abuse of amphetamines is not limited to a single socioeconomic level in our society, as that of opiates traditionally has been. Dr. Meyers, for one, argues that people from all walks of life who initially experiment with amphetamines or employ them for therapeutic purposes often increase the doses of the drugs and begin taking them habitually in a cyclical pattern, alternating between depression and chemically induced euphoria.

Speed Kills

The same cyclical pattern was common to the young people who abused amphetamines in the Haight-Ashbury. But since they came from lower-income backgrounds and lived outside the law, these individuals were less likely to employ pharmaceutical amphetamines than their counterparts in middle-class society. And they did not call the drugs amphetamines, but speed.

Speed is a street name for amphetamines and any number of substances that provide the same central stimulation. According to Roger Smith, the criminologist who directed the Amphetamine Research Project housed in the Haight-Ashbury Free Medical Clinic during the fall of 1968, the term probably originated in the early 1950's with servicemen stationed in Korea and Japan who brought back to this country the practice of mixing amphetamines with heroin. This resulted because of the shortage and prohibitive expense of cocaine, the more traditional stimulant component of the speedball.

Those Bay Area doctors later named by the attorney general's office then began prescribing Methedrine and Desoxyn ampules to opiate addicts, at which point San Francisco became a national center of the speed scene. Although generally looked down on by heroin aficionados for being too uncool to maintain, or control, their behavior, amphetamine abusers continued to proliferate in the city. When the state requested the removal of methamphetamine ampules from the market in 1963, abusers constituted a large fringe element in San Francisco's Haight-Ashbury, Tenderloin, Mission and North Beach areas.

By 1968 the scene had been extended to incorporate younger and more amateurish abusers, while its local center had shifted geographically to the Haight. The young people there lacked the kinds of experience which characterized the early ampule users and had therefore developed a spree pattern of abuse. They had also created a marketplace that added a new dimension to the original Methedrine and Desoxyn scene. In addition, while the words "speed" and "Methedrine" were once used synonymously in the Bay Area underground, young people in the Haight-Ashbury and elsewhere had begun applying the term "speed" to any stimulant that would bring them up, just as they were using the word "downer" to describe alcohol, opiates, barbiturates and all other depressants. Speed was also referred to on Haight Street as "splash," "grease," "uppers," "rhythm," "crank," "meth" and "crystal," the latter three terms applying particularly to a powdered form of methamphetamine.

As far as Roger Smith could determine, very little of the speed in the Haight was of pharmaceutical quality. Some came into the district either from forged prescriptions or drugstore robberies; other amphetamines were channeled into the area from Mexico, where dealers obtained the chemicals en masse from American drug companies. But most of the speed was manufactured by local cooks, amateur or semiprofessional chemists who operated out of clandestine laboratories and often stamped counterfeit brand names on their products.

The first such laboratory was set up in the Bay Area around 1963, Smith believed, in anticipation of the withdrawal of Methedrine and Desoxyn ampules from the pharmaceutical market. By 1968, between five and ten labs, most of them established in secluded neighborhoods outside the district, were each supplying it with from ten to twenty-five pounds of speed per week, in addition to impure LSD. Small laboratories in kitchens and in bathrooms throughout the Haight-Ashbury were also contributing their share to the local amphetamine supply.

The cooks who made speed generally obtained their raw materials from more professional criminals, who either stole the chemicals or ordered them directly from wholesale houses. Once the speed was prepared, it was passed through a few upper-echelon distributors or sold directly to ounce dealers. They in turn marketed the drugs to low-level nickel (five dollar) and dime (ten dollar) bag dealers, who also sold other compounds throughout the Haight.

Since all the people involved in this network cut the drugs with additives and raised their prices, a pound of speed costing one hundred dollars to cook was worth well over thirty-two hundred dollars when it reached the street. It was also adulterated with other chemicals. Although the street dealers invariably denied this and praised the purity of their crystal, what they advertised as genuine U.S.P. quality methamphetamine on Haight Street usually contained ether to heighten its flash effects and often turned out to be little more than quinine, baking powder, monosodium glutamate (Accent), photo developer or insecticide.

In spite of this fact, and because much of the available acid was also adulterated, many people living in the Haight-Ashbury during the fall of 1968 would take almost anything purported to be amphetamine to get high. New arrivals in the district were occasionally introduced to speed orally, but they and the older abusers more frequently injected the drugs directly into the bloodstream. After gathering in crystal palaces, filthy flats and apartments once used as communes by the hippies, they often shot up to fifteen hundred milligrams of what they hoped was amphetamine to experience an orgasmic rush or flash as the drug hit their central nervous systems. Then, buoyed by feelings of self-confidence and temporarily insulated from their anxiety and depression, the young people would stay wired and jacked up for hours. Some would rap, or talk excitedly and incoherently, to anyone in their vicinity. Others would become physically hyperactive and begin knick-knacking, or fingering and walking off with whatever objects they touched. Many would merely freak out for the amusement of their so-called friends.

Such instances of acute toxicity were particularly common among those younger adolescents in the Haight who were inexperienced about speed's pharmacological effects. When they took amphetamines in massive doses and in crowded environments, they often became anxious, excitable and paranoid as they started to feel stimulated. Many of them gradually managed to come down from the chemicals if they were given sedatives or calmed by their companions. But others who had overdosed began hyperventilating and suffered extreme tachycardia, mucosal dryness and muscle cramping. They screamed that their hearts and brains were burning and presented a clinical picture referred to at the Clinic as overamping.

Overamping was actually quite rare during the fall of 1968, for chronic amphetamine toxicity far surpassed the acute form in the Haight. Roger Smith also felt that since a well-defined stimulative drug subculture had been established in the district, most of those young people who became acutely toxic survived their freak outs and quickly learned what to expect from speed. After being educated by their companions, they either rejected the drugs or became recognized as habitual speed freaks who had settled on amphetamines as their chosen chemicals.

The adolescents may have somewhat mastered speed by this point, but they had not graduated past all drug problems. Indeed, the more often they took amphetamines, the more often their rhapsodic highs evolved into toxic psychoses or were followed by reaction phases and depressions as the compounds' effects wore off. These depressions could be so agonizing and filled with self-doubt that they had to shoot more speed to get high again. They would then repeat this up-and-down cycle until they launched into prolonged runs, or binges lasting as long as ten or twelve days.

The young people ate little more than ice cream and candy bars during these binges. They also deprived themselves of REM sleep, a state of rapid eye movements in which dreaming occurs. REM sleep seems to be vital for psychological stability, and people going without it in the course of laboratory experiments or while trying to set endurance records often experience hallucinosis and personality disorders. Few of the speed freaks competed to see who among them could stay awake the longest, but most became progressively more confused as their binges were extended. By the end of their runs, many of them looked like zombies from lack of sleep — and because they were shooting as much as seven thousand milligrams of speed in several doses per day.

The speed freaks eventually crashed, or collapsed from exhaustion, and would often sleep for forty-eight straight hours. They then woke up, only to experience even deeper depression as well as the paranoid-schizophrenic psychoses characteristic of chronic amphetamine toxicity. They suffered terrifying hallucinations, mistook their friends for police officers, and lashed out with murderous rage at any real or imagined intrusion. Some of them started new runs at this point to escape their depressions, or injected barbiturates to induce sleep. Others had to be segregated and restrained before they could do physical harm, especially if they were going up or coming down in crowded atmospheres.

Although these instances of violence were often precipitated and/or heightened by the pharmacological effects of amphetamine, they naturally differed according to the personalities of the young people involved. The hoodies, for example, rarely went on long drug binges or became seriously disoriented, primarily because they wanted to prove that they could control themselves. Instead, they took speed to enhance their self-confidence, particularly if they had just been burned or ripped off by confederates, and went hunting with their dogs and their weapons for those who had humiliated them.

The more psychotic youths also created a serious menace, yet their violence was of a more random kind. The thinking of these young people was always disorganized, but they became inordinately disturbed and paranoid when they were strung-out on speed. If they then shot barbiturates to come down from extended runs, they were likely to become assaultive as well. When taken in combination, the drugs seemed to produce a toxic state of confusion which could prompt the disturbed individuals to confront those other adolescents who so frequently bullied them. As one speed freak told Roger Smith, "barbs make you want to get out on the street and start kicking ass. Speed gives you the energy to get up and do it."

The same person, whose nickname is Fleas, described to Smith how the combination of amphetamines and barbiturates could lead to bizarre incidents of mistaken identity.

It happens by accident when they're all jacked up and have been for say a week, maybe two or three weeks, and somebody burns them. They may go crash for a day or two to get their heads together, and when they get up and shoot barbs they don't remember much what the person looked like, just that he burned them. Then they go running around with guns under their jackets and they run up behind someone and say, "That looks like him — long blond hair — we got you" and then, "Sorry, wrong one," and they go on to the next guy with long blond hair and stop him. And maybe this guy isn't even the real one, but they're so strung out he may get shot anyway.

I know another kid who always freaks out on speed and barbs. He's a very nice person but when he gets all jacked up and he's also doing reds (Seconal) then he's in trouble, because pretty soon he's got a shotgun and everybody else has got a shotgun, or so he thinks. I've seen him out, in front of the freeway entrance west of the Haight, herding the hitchhikers away because he's so paranoid on them. At four o'clock in the afternoon, with a full-length shotgun,

he's screaming, "Move on — you can't stand there — move on!" That's the way
he gets when he's mixing barbs and speed.

Fleas also agreed that new arrivals to the district contributed their share
of impulsive crime. Roger Smith felt the majority of these incidents occurred in group situations where the young people consumed speed. While
congregating in the dilapidated residences occupied by older and more habitual abusers, for example, the young adolescents often became tense and
excitable not only because they were inexperienced about the drugs they
were taking but also because their courage was on the line.

If their passions were then ignited by some emotional spark, such as the
presence of a persistent knick-knacker, the arrival of a suspected rip-off
artist, or the appearance of a spaced out and sexually available girl, the
novice speed freaks could become torn between their wish for peer group
approval and whatever sense of conscience they possessed. As a result, they
sometimes exploded into sudden savagery to release their accumulated tension and could end up assaulting the knick-knacker or the supposed thief,
or raping and/or torturing the hapless girl. Roger Smith and those Clinic
physicians who were familiar with such turnouts and gang bangs explained
to the police, yet did not excuse, the events in terms of the precipitous
impulsiveness of the adolescents and the behavioral sink aspects of the district. But the police wanted no explanation. As far as they were concerned,
the young people behaved like rats in a cage.

"A Law-Enforcement Nightmare"

This attitude was not held by all policemen, and some of the one hundred and
eight patrolmen from the Park Police Station at Stanyan and Waller who worked
the Haight did differentiate between the
various kinds of people there. Yet others
considered all drug abusers animals and
treated them accordingly. This was particularly the case with younger and
newer recruits, who knew none of the speed freaks and other abusers personally and had little love for the Haight-Ashbury. These recruits often
overreacted to the new population when they and their fellow patrolmen
made regular sweeps of Haight Street in squad cars and paddy wagons
during the fall of 1968. They beat up the street people, busted new arrivals
to the district, and indiscriminately hauled them off to jail.

The police became unusually nervous and often redoubled their punitive
efforts against the young people on weekends, when the Haight filled up

with visitors. They also carried two-way radios linking them with the city's Tactical Squad, an allegedly elite corps of two-hundred-pound-plus bruisers trained in hand-to-hand combat and riot control. The thirty-eight man squad was available for major disturbances throughout San Francisco and had already been called into the Haight twice that year to stomp out — or start, as many people thought — rioting, rock-throwing and fires. Although they were praised by Mayor Joseph Alioto, some of its members seemed to be as sadistic and impulsive as the people they were paid to help control.

In spite of this, neither the Tactical Squad nor the patrolmen and narcotics agents assigned to the Haight-Ashbury had any significant deterring effect on its adolescent population. In fact, the police probably provoked as much violence by their repressive tactics as they hoped to prevent. The narcs sometimes pressured the young people they caught selling chemicals into informing on their confederates, but most of these snitches were identified by the dealers before they could do them much harm. When the police could catch the known peddlers they often threatened to plant drugs on them and arrest them if they would not voluntarily leave town. Yet these and other extreme measures seemed only to act like a negative filter in the Haight, screening out the nonviolent hippies and the healthier criminals and leaving the blacks and the more desperate drug abusers behind.

Furthermore, the narcotics agents were rarely able to locate the larger laboratories which supplied the Haight-Ashbury, and the cooks who manufactured chemicals within the district regularly moved their labs. The young people they sold drugs to were usually "veterans of wars elsewhere," as a lieutenant at Park Station described them.

They are kids who've gone from one scene to another and picked up plenty of savvy in the process. They know the schedules of our patrolmen and the identities of many of the undercover agents in the Haight and pass their knowledge on to these new arrivals, who often become criminals themselves.

These kids have turned the Haight-Ashbury into a law-enforcement nightmare. During the first half of this year alone, eighteen murders, fifty-eight rapes, three hundred and seventy robberies, two hundred and four assaults and over sixteen hundred cases of burglary were reported at this station. The figures for this fall are already that high and should be much higher, since many of the victims were criminals themselves and would never report the damage done to them. The murder rate increases every day; three of our most recent ones occurred in one week, and drug dealers were involved in at least two of the fatal crimes.

But this is nothing. We get some incidents out here you simply wouldn't believe. A few weeks, ago, my men picked up an eighteen-year-old kid and his girl friend on Haight Street selling military explosives out of a shopping bag.

We get these people standing in the middle of the street shooting at anything that moves. We hear all the time about runaway girls coming to the area with no place to stay who get picked up by Negroes or bike riders on the street, locked in closets and raped for days at a time. Gang bangs and turnouts occur all the time, and burns are so common we should really list them in a separate category.

It's hopeless. There are too many kids, too many ineffective laws and too much dope for us to control. The Haight-Ashbury is now recognized as the spawning ground for multiple and habitual drug abuse for the entire nation. The quantities of narcotics and dangerous drugs confiscated in, say, New York are greater than they are in this district, but that's to be expected, since the traffic there is run by organized crime. Here, most of your criminals are comparative amateurs, excepting the more competent ones who supply them. They have created the toughest law-enforcement problem we have ever known.

Public Health: A License for Suicide

They had also created one of the most difficult health problems in the history of San Francisco. Many of the young people in the Haight were not only overtly or potentially psychotic but physically ravaged as well. The bikers often broke their arms and legs by falling off motorcycles, while some of the dealers were so frequently beaten up they seemed to spend most of their lives in plaster casts. Others frequently exhibited gunshot wounds, suppurating abrasions, knife and razor slashes and similar traumatic injuries — all caused by violence.

Even more visible was the violence they did to themselves. Because they were continually stoned on drugs, the adolescents who hung out on Haight Street often overexerted themselves and failed to notice as they mangled and infected their feet by walking through broken glass and animal excrement. Furthermore, since the chemicals they used insulated them from pain, they often overlooked the physical deterioration which resulted from their prolonged drug binges. When combined with their poor eating habits, this general debility left many of the young people continually malnourished and extremely susceptible to infectious disease. Some of them suffered protein, mineral and vitamin deficiencies which had heretofore been observed only in chronic alcoholics. A few had even progressed in their emaciation to the point of kwashiorkor, a nutrition-deficiency syndrome which usually occurs in weaning infants in underdeveloped areas.

Treatment for kwashiorkor consists of the administration of milk and high-protein diets. Vitamin and mineral supplements may also be indicated, along with transfusions and antibiotics to curb concomitant infections. The

American public was perhaps most aware of the need for such measures in Biafra, where thousands of children were dying daily during the fall of 1968. But high-protein diets were also required for a number of young people in the Haight-Ashbury. Like the children in Biafra, they were beyond the reach of most relief agencies and at war with a government. They simply would not eat while they were using speed.

The street people also experienced a wide variety of dental problems because of their poor diets and improper hygiene. Halitosis, tooth discoloration, caries, dental pulp infections, periapical abcesses and trench mouth were widespread among the drug abusers, and some had gone so long without treatment that they also exhibited periodontal disease. This condition results from the presence of food particles and bacteria which lie between the teeth and gums, causing an inflammation and the formation of pus through a process known as pyorrhea. If this continues unchecked, the involved teeth will become loose, while accumulated pus may lead to acute swelling and pain.

Local cleansing, drainage and the application of such oxygenating mouth rinses as hydrogen peroxide can reverse these symptoms and allow for further corrective dentistry. But many speed freaks would neither use dentists nor spend what little money they had for hydrogen peroxide. Although they could not stand the slightest pressure on their mouths, they let their gums bleed and their teeth rot with decay.

Because the young people shared drugs and needles and shot up in crowded and unsanitary environments, they were also exposed to an incredible amount of contagion. Many of them had upper-respiratory-tract and eye, ear, nose and throat infections and were constantly wheezing, coughing, sneezing, weeping and dripping from the nose. In addition to common colds and the secondary complications of influenza, these infections ran the gamut from pharyngitis, laryngitis and tonsillitis to allergic rhinitis or hay fever, sinusitis and bronchial asthma.

Most common of all were acute and chronic bronchitis. Bronchitis is caused by numerous bacterial and viral strains and often accompanies other general infections. It is characterized by a mild or severe congestion of the bronchial tract which leads to coughing, wheezing and the production of a thick sputum. In certain cases, the congestion may result in a slight impairment of breathing. In others, it can become serious enough to cause pneumonia and subsequent mortality.

Treatment of both the acute and chronic forms of bronchitis should include a mandatory convalescence, a curtailment of smoking, and the administration of agents to relieve coughing, along with antibiotics and antihistamine drugs to reduce bronchial irritation. Such medications were especially called for in the Haight, where the young residents used marijuana and tobacco cigarettes which had a strong bronchial irritating effect. Indeed, marijuana-aggravated bronchitis had emerged as a prevalent problem in the district. Some young people who chain-smoked marijuana were known to have been afflicted for over twenty months with the disease. In addition, an average of from one to three people per week showed signs of acute pneumonia. Yet most tried to mask their symptoms with toxic chemicals until they collapsed on Haight Street and had to be carted away.

Upper-respiratory-tract infections and secondary complications were the most widespread adolescent health problems in the Haight, but they were followed closely in number by infections of the skin. Few young people in the district bathed regularly, if at all, and their poor hygiene, improper diets, cramped living conditions and emotional agitation all aggravated their dermatological problems. Among these difficulties were acne vulgaris, which causes painful pustules on the face, back and shoulders and may result in residual scarring if not cleansed and combated with antibiotics; impetigo, a contagious staphylococcal infection that is spread by scratching with dirty fingernails and requires antibiotic ointment; and contact dermatitis and pyoderma, both of which can be curbed or prevented by washing the skin with antibacterial detergents.

In addition to these infections, some of the amphetamine abusers developed abcesses of the subcutical fossae and a diffuse skin infection called cellulitis from using dirty needles and adulterated drugs. Others missed their veins while shooting up or ruptured them by injecting undissolvable chemicals which clogged their needles. The speed freaks' lips often became cracked from the drugs' constricting effect on mucosal surfaces. And they frequently gouged their faces by picking at so-called crank bugs, imaginary insects they felt crawling under their skin.

A few also had relatively rare skin problems like erythema nodosum, which is characterized by exceedingly painful red nodules on the legs and is related to such systemic illnesses as rheumatic fever and to allergic drug reactions. Many sustained eczema and other allergies, while a surprisingly large number contracted such fungal infections as tinea corporis, or body ringworm, from the animals and humans they slept with. Ringworm can be treated with special soaps, but the young people usually let the disease go untreated and constantly reinfected themselves.

Two other problems they picked up from their bedmates in the Haight-Ashbury were scabies and pediculosis, the crabs. Both are parasitic infestations of the scalp, trunk and/or pubic areas that usually result from sleeping and having sexual relations with an infected person. Scabies is caused by a female mite that burrows between the layers of the skin and deposits her eggs. Vesicles housing the mite and her eggs then appear on the skin surface and develop into pustules and an itchy rash. Pediculosis is caused by the tiny bites of the crab louse, which generally buries its head in the follicles of the pubic hair and attaches its body to the hair itself. Because the parasites are quite hardy, patients who are infested with them sometimes must have their bodies shaved and require repeated applications of topical insecticide for pediculosis and antiparasitic lotions like Kwell for scabies. Such medications were in great demand in the Haight, for most of the young people there were personally familiar with the crabs.

Many were also familiar with the runs. These generally resulted from several types of gastrointestinal disturbance, including ulcers, chronic ulcerative colitis, viral infections, influenza, food poisoning and bacillary dysentery, an inflammation of the intestine which is manifested by fever, chills, cramping and diarrhea with blood and mucus in the stools. Dysentery is usually treated with broad-spectrum antibiotics; patients should also be isolated and all body discharges and bed linens should be carefully disinfected. Such disinfection was virtually impossible in the Haight-Ashbury. Because of this, many individuals suffered from the disease.

Another problem they experienced was the clap, or gonorrhea, the most common form of venereal disease in the district. Gonorrhea is caused by gonococcal bacteria that grow in the mucous membranes of the genitourinary tract and may spread occasionally to other parts of the body, particularly the joints and eyes. The disease is almost always contracted during sexual intercourse with an infected person, and although the bacteria usually restrict their attack to the genital and urinary regions, the rectum may be infected by extension from the genitals or from anal intercourse.

The diagnosis of gonorrhea is usually made by microscopic examination of a smear of urethral or cervical discharge, but since this test is not reliable many venereal disease clinics rightly insist on the immediate treatment of anyone displaying gonorrheal symptoms. Treatment consists of the administration of high doses of penicillin intramuscularly for up to ten consecutive days or of high doses of other antibiotics every six hours over a comparable period. Proper treatment should also include the administration of antibiotics to any and all people exposed to gonorrhea to prevent further spread of the disease.

Such proper treatment is not always available or accomplished, and gonorrhea ranks as the number-one reportable communicable disease in this country as a result. There is more gonorrhea in America than in any other part of the world at present except southeast Asia, where many American servicemen are stationed. These servicemen have brought several penicillin-resistant strains of bacteria back to this country, and the rate of gonorrheal infection has risen astronomically in recent years.

This has been particularly true in such California port cities as San Francisco and Los Angeles. California accounted for 63,783 out of the 432,388 cases of gonorrhea reported in the United States during 1968, while almost one out of every ten residents of the state between fifteen and twenty-five years of age had VD. Such precise statistics were hard to come by in the Haight, where young people and servicemen were constantly in motion and where illnesses were reported no more accurately than was crime. But it was safe to assume that approximately seventy-five percent of the young residents were exposed to or at one time afflicted with the disease.

Other infections that caused problems in the Haight-Ashbury were non-specific urethritis, vaginitis, cervicitis and other infectious diseases of the genitourinary tract. Also common was trichomoniasis, which is caused by a minute one-celled parasite, *Trichomonas vaginalis*. This organism may infect the mucous membrance of the vagina or the penis and reveals its presence by producing an intense burning and itching and a white or yellowish discharge. The infection is most often transmitted during sexual intercourse. Although it has been difficult to control trichomoniasis in the past, it can now be treated very effectively with a new and expensive drug called Flagyl.

More difficult to treat are "venereal warts" or condyloma accuminata. These are warty growths which are believed to be caused by a virus and often appear together with other forms of venereal disease. They are seen more frequently in women than in men and may be present anywhere on the vulva or the vagina. Treatment for them includes the application of a liquid known as Podophyllin. They seem to appear most often in women who bathe infrequently, display profuse vaginal discharge, and engage in promiscuous sexual activity.

All forms of such activity were found in the Haight during the fall of 1968, including rape. This fact naturally explained the high incidence of venereal disease and presence of "venereal warts" and other genital infections which are rather rare in the general population. But in spite of their prevalence, these disorders could not be considered the most crippling adolescent health problems in the district. Nor did they set its health tone. This was established by serum hepatitis, because drug abuse, more often than sex, was the basis of the street people's life-style.

Hepatitis is caused by a virus which infects and destroys liver cells, resulting in a loss of the functioning capacity of the liver and causing nausea, vomiting, fever, jaundice, emotional instability, severe abdominal pain and alterations in stool and urine color. The disease has been believed to occur either in an infectious or a serum form. Serum hepatitis is transmitted through transfusions of infected blood or plasma or by the use of unsterilized needles and other medical equipment. The virus enters the bloodstream directly and is revealed in prominent symptoms after a few months. This form of hepatitis has an extremely long carrier state, lasting from five years to life. No known drugs are effective against the virus, regardless of its mode of transmission. For this reason, the disease is extremely difficult to control.

Controlling serum hepatitis was impossible in the Haight-Ashbury. The illness, spread primarily by dirty needles, caused more suffering during the fall of 1968 than all other types of adolescent health problems combined. Most of the resident speed freaks had contracted hepatitis at least once, and some with previous cases seemed to reinfect their livers with every new injection of speed. Jaundiced eyes and faces were a common sight on Haight Street, almost as common as the burns there. In fact, hepatitis had reached epidemic proportions in the Haight by this point, and the few doctors at Park Emergency Hospital at Frederick and Waller could not check the spread of the disease through the district any better than the police could curb the crime.

Furthermore, these physicians seemed unwilling to attempt to solve this and other local health problems. Like many policemen, the public health officials who manned the tiny and inadequately equipped facility looked on the young people in the Haight-Ashbury as subhuman beings. When drug abusers came to Park Emergency for help, the doctors there sometimes assaulted them with sermons or reported them to the police. The receptionists often told needy adolescents to take their sickness elsewhere. The ambulance drivers frequently "forgot" calls for emergency assistance. They and the other staff members apparently believed that the best way to handle health problems in the Haight was to stand back and let its younger residents destroy themselves.

Given this attitude, it was hardly surprising that the young people were just as frightened of public health officials as they were of policemen. Some would sooner risk death than seek aid at Park Emergency and were both psychologically unwilling and financially unable to go to San Francisco General Hospital or Mission Emergency Hospital, a mile away. Most simply lived with their symptoms, doctored themselves with home remedies or narcotized themselves with toxic drugs, kept black-market tranquilizers handy when they expected to freak out, and administered heroin, barbiturates or other downers when they became too strung-out on speed.

The young people refused to consult private physicians, who they assumed would overcharge them and hand them over to the law. Because they were uneducated about medical matters and lacked a nonrepressive source of public health information, they listened only to the witch doctors, drug dealers and few remaining gurus who prowled the Haight, prescribing either macrobiotic diets or their own chemical products for practically every physical and psychological ill.

A few of the young people were receptive to responsible opinion and anxious to be treated, especially the sicker speed freaks and those new arrivals who had recently made the Haight-Ashbury their home. But they had nowhere to go for help. Huckleberry's for Runaways, a residential center set up by the Reverend Larry Beggs during the Summer of Love, had suspended operations in the Haight by October of 1968 and had moved to a more benign location in the Sunset District to avoid police harassment. Al Rinker's Switchboard, once a vital nerve center of the new community and the model for hundreds of similar facilities across the country, was operating under a severe financial deficit. The Mendocino Drug Abuse Program and Family were still open, and Dr. Harry Wilmer was running his Youth Drug Unit at the Langley-Porter Neuropsychiatric Institute of the University of California. But Mendocino was over two hours away from the city, and Dr. Wilmer's rehabilitation program was limited to twenty participants at a time.

Professor Leonard Wolf, who once helped the hippies, had also left the district after his Happening House was disbanded. Father Harris and Howard Rochford remained to offer free and sound advice at All Saints' Episcopal and Hamilton Methodist churches, yet they could hardly deal with all the disturbed adolescents who flocked to them. Other than the San Francisco Center for Special Problems, the only organization which might have helped these young people was the Haight-Ashbury Free Medical Clinic. But, during the fall of 1968, the Clinic was virtually closed.

The Clinic: An Alternative in Ruins

The doors to its Medical Section at 558 Clayton Street had been shut since Labor Day, when the Clinic and a local foundation sponsored a financially disastrous fund-raising festival at the Palace of Fine Arts in the Marina district across town. The facility had been operating on a budget of five thousand dollars a month prior to the four-day event, and its organizers needed to raise enough money to launch new projects and to maintain both their Medical Section at the corner of Haight and Clayton and the Psychiatric and Publications sections housed in the Clinic annex at 409 Clayton

Street a block away. They chose the Palace as the setting for the festival because it could hold fifteen thousand people at one sitting and had never been used for such a purpose. With John Handy, the Steve Miller Band and other local jazz and rock groups and light-show artists volunteering their services, the organizers hoped to present a successful sequel to the International Pop Festival held one and a half years earlier in Monterey.

But they never anticipated the city's reaction to their plan. After arguing for months to obtain use of the Palace of Fine Arts from the San Francisco Recreation and Park Commission, the organizers were saddled with permit requirements and security provisions that made profits from the festival all but impossible. The commission then almost canceled the event in deference to homeowners living near the Palace who objected to "long-haired criminals cluttering up our area." The organizers countered by introducing statements of support from many public leaders who had visited the Clinic, and the commission eventually sanctioned the festival. But it imposed a restrictive occupancy level and a substantial rent on the Palace, something it had never done before.

The organizers appealed these conditions to Mayor Alioto, who had publicly praised their work in the past. Yet the mayor was against the festival for political reasons and, rumor had it, because his family owned property in the Marina area. Whatever his motivation, he did his best to scuttle the event. Word then spread that the festival would not be held, and some performers bowed out because of the uncertainty of the affair, while others said that they had never committed themselves to the Clinic's business manager, Jerry Read. Read believed that the benefit would still be a success. But when it was finally given, only fifteen hundred people, most of them adults, attended the first two shows. They were lost in the cavernous Fine Arts building and almost outnumbered by the security guards. By the end of the Labor Day weekend, the Clinic had lost twenty thousand dollars.

After paying some of these expenses out of their own pockets, the organizers suspended medical operations in the Haight-Ashbury and allocated what was left of their resources to the Annex at 409 Clayton Street. The staff members then posted a sign on the doorway to 558 Clayton Street and passed word through the district that it was closed. Even so, the front steps were crowded night and day with sick and shivering adolescents, as they had been since the Clinic first opened at the start of the Summer of Love.

Inside, the dance-concert posters, bright paint and psychedelic art which lent an air of acceptance to the fourteen-room former dentist's office spoke of life and occasional gaiety. But there was little life or gaiety left in the facility. Once the main hallway at the top of the stairs had been jammed with young people; no one occupied the space at present. The five examining rooms where casually attired physicians once saw patients were empty and quiet as tombs. The other rooms and the corridors that veined the Medical Section were also silent, save for the steps of volunteer watchmen who patrolled the halls.

Off one of these passageways, cases of antibiotics, antibacterial detergents, vaginal suppositories, Kwell lotion and other medications collected dust in the Clinic pharmacy. A sterilizer, centrifuge and microscope used to prepare and analyze blood, urine and genital discharge samples remained idle in the laboratory at the far end of the office, while boxes of bandages, tongue depressors, stethoscopes and medical equipment sat under Day-Glo drawings on a faded couch in the waiting room. Nearby, a donated refrigerator chilled badly needed ampules of penicillin. And in the reception room stood cabinets that contained over thirty thousand patient histories and served only as sad reminders of what might have been.

Equally saddening was the scene at 409 Clayton Street, which had been turned into an emergency receiving unit during the interim. The Episcopal Peace Center on the first floor of this ancient, pale blue Victorian home was intended to be a tranquil refuge, but it was packed during the fall of 1968 with patients in every imaginable form of dress and undress. Some of the young people were wrapped in blankets, their anguished faces barely visible behind blood-soaked bandages. Others, wearing diaphanous gowns and Salvation Army discards, were huddled together, trying to stay warm.

The Reverend Lyle Grosjean, the Episcopal minister who supervised the center, once had the opportunity to circulate among the people who used 409 House. Yet he was now working overtime in his small office behind the kitchen to counsel youths with draft, welfare and spiritual problems. His shop area in back of the basement downstairs was also busy, but instead of peace crosses and other handiworks, its tables and benches were occupied with young people who had collapsed from amphetamine-induced exhaustion. Meanwhile, center staff members were exhausting themselves in the reading and meditation room, where they served coffee, made conversation, and attempted to comfort the patients waiting to get upstairs.

There, in large and sparsely furnished rooms, usually reserved for counseling, Dr. Richard Gleason, Dr. Alan Matzger and a few other doctors from 558 Clayton Street were attempting to treat the Haight's health problems. A makeshift Gynecological and Obstetric Section had also been established on the second deck, and a half-dozen weary physicians wearing sports shirts were treating young women with VD. Working with them were a dozen younger interns and residents, many of whom had originally come to the district to study drug abuse and related disease.

The students were afforded an excellent opportunity, for every illness in the Haight-Ashbury was paraded before them. Shy hippie mothers with malnourished babies, frantic speed freaks with swollen abcesses, surly bikers with broken arms and frightened twelve-year-old runaways with bloated stomachs all sought help in the area which usually housed only the Psychiatric Section. The interns and residents may have received an education, but their faces showed more empathy than scientific detachment. They also revealed a certain hopelessness, for the doctors were too swamped with patients to be medically effective. They also knew that they would soon run out of supplies.

Because of this shortage, the physicians were actually treating fewer young people than they were turning away. A referral service had been set up near the second-floor landing, where Carter Mehl, Delores Craton, Renée Sargent, the pregnant girl named Jackie and other paramedical staff members from the Medical Section were sending as many patients as possible to the city's Veneral Disease Clinic at 33 Hunt Street, to the Hepatitis Section and the Oral Surgery Unit at San Francisco General, to Mission Emergency Hospital, to the Center for Special Problems and to such private facilities as the Pediatrics Department of the University of California Medical Center.

Other volunteers were also on hand to make referrals, while staff members who usually manned the Publications Section on the third floor at 409 Clayton Street were chauffeuring patients to Planned Parenthood for contraceptives and birth-control information. The staff members and volunteers were able to find some form of treatment for over one hundred young people on most days during the fall of 1968. Yet they could not be certain that those helped would keep their appointments. Neither could they begin to touch all the sickness that stalked the streets outside.

Nor could they guarantee that their patients would be properly treated if they did keep their appointments. The Clinic's referral service was one of the most active in the city, but many public facilities to which it directed young people provided only nominal care. Long-haired individuals were frequently denied treatment at General Hospital and Mission Emergency. The Center for Special Problems and the city's VD Clinic were staffed by liberal physicians, yet they were only open on an eight-to-five basis. And although the Hepatitis Unit at San Francisco General would often accept young people during these hours, it treated only the most serious cases. Instead of practicing preventive medicine, the staff doctors forced some patients who were not sick enough to return to the streets and spread their disease.

Because of these factors, the Clinic volunteers had to accept all those who came to them. This was appropriate, for they were as young and vulnerable as the patients they wanted to heal. Some lived in the Haight and were therefore familiar with its health problems. Others had experienced the problems themselves. All were antagonized by San Francisco's repressive attitude towards youth and alienated by the cold and emotionally antiseptic atmosphere of most medical settings. They were more effective than most straight people in preventing and treating illness and drug abuse because they and their patients looked, spoke, and often felt the same way.

Trina Merriman, the warm twenty-two-year-old who administered the second-floor area of the Annex, was such a person. She had been a resident of the Haight-Ashbury and a Clinic patient since the Summer of Love, when she assisted Dr. Dernburg and Stuart Loomis in the founding of the Psychiatric Section. Miss Merriman wore beads and sandals and was neither rattled nor repulsed by even the most disturbed patients. When young people came to her to make appointments, she talked in their language and never tried to substitute forms and procedures for personal contact. Instead, she waited quietly, discussing rock music and other subjects with the patients until they found the courage to ask for help. Then, if space was available, she sat with them until a psychiatrist or counselor could see them in one of the counseling rooms.

Little space was available during the fall of 1968, but some psychiatric work was being conducted in the midst of the chaos. Dr. Dernburg and others were seeing their long-term hippie patients on the second floor and were also trying to handle as many emergency cases as the crowded conditions permitted. Yet they were all discouraged by the bedlam at the Annex. "I thought 409 House was created to be a calm center," a psychiatrist shouted over the roar around him one evening. "Hell, it's so confusing here now we might as well be working in the middle of an air raid."

As always, most of the confusion was caused by drug abusers of all sorts, who streamed into the Annex for detoxification. On some afternoons, burly hoodies numbed by barbiturates would stumble up to the second deck and harass Miss Merriman. On other evenings, bleary-eyed and unshaved middle-aged alcoholics would slump against the walls and mumble obscenities or try to pass their wine bottles to the better-scrubbed young people sitting nearby. And even more frequently, all present would be assaulted by people freaking out on speed.

The Clinic physicians did their best to segregate the amphetamine abusers and help them down with quiet words and emotional support. But many of their patients were too disturbed to understand words and were liable to become violent at any moment. Their agitation, combined with the noise and congestion in the Psychiatric Section, made the type of verbal detoxification employed in treating adverse LSD reactions in the early days of the Clinic all but impossible.

Because of this, the doctors administered Librium and other sedatives to pacify acutely toxic people, along with such antipsychotic tranquilizers as Thorazine to those suffering the paranoia and hallucinosis characterisic of chronic toxicity. When all else failed, they used a donated Peugeot station wagon in place of public ambulances to transport patients either to the psychiatric wards or Mt. Zion Hospital or to the Immediate Psychiatric and Referral Service at San Francisco General, where Dr. Arthur Carfagni, a member of the Clinic's Executive Committee and the one public health official who supported the facility, offered hospitalization and occasional care.

One final effort to remove young people from the Haight-Ashbury was being made by Stuart Loomis, a forty-eight-year-old associate professor of education at San Francisco State College, who was conducting his counseling classes at 409 House because of the strike crippling that school. As the Clinic's chief psychologist, Professor Loomis was responsible for a great deal of crisis intervention at the Annex during the fall of 1968. He and his students were also working with Robert Laws and other volunteer attorneys to obtain admissions for patients to the Langley-Porter Youth Drug Unit and to Mendocino State Hospital. In October alone, they managed to place over two dozen people in these and other facilities.

But in spite of such efforts, the chaos and lack of real segregation at 409 Clayton Street precipitated a number of explosive situations. On one evening, for example, Professor Loomis had to prevent a fourteen-year-old girl from jumping out the front window because she thought a fellow patient was trying to kill her. Two of his students were also forced to tackle a boy who pulled a gun and ran screaming down the hall in pursuit of someone who he said had once sold him adulterated drugs. This patient quieted down eventually, but the students were busy by then with a potential suicide.

"It gets worse every day," Professor Loomis insisted. "The Clinic is probably the only organization in this city that can exert a positive influence on these young people. We are nonjudgmental toward what the Establishment dismisses as deviance. We approach patients in their own environment and on their own terms. We respect their difficulties — and our services are free. Yet even when the Medical Section was operating we could not cope with all the drug-abuse problems in this district. Now, even if we get help, we still face an uncertain future. None of us has a solution for the Haight at the present time."

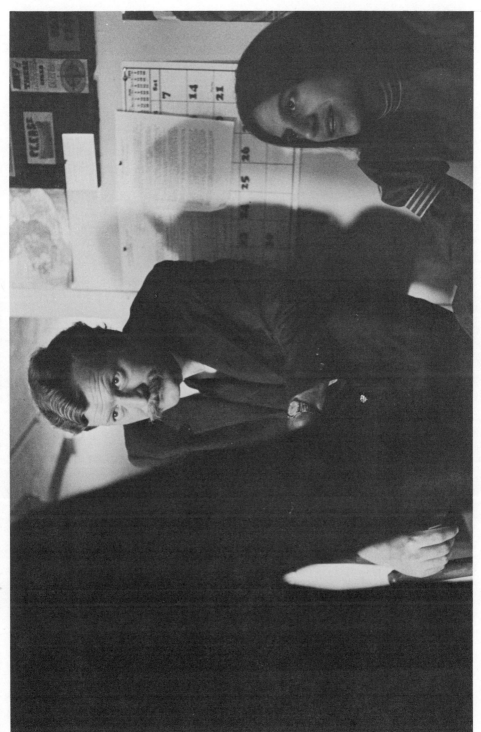

409 Clayton Street: Roger Smith and Gail Sadalla of the Amphetamine Research Project.

(Elaine Mayes)

The Drug Treatment Program

The only person who thought he had an answer was Roger Smith. The thirty-one-year-old criminologist had been employed as a street-gang worker in Chicago, an administrator of a drug-abuse center for black adolescents at the East Oakland Parish and a federal probation officer prior to January of 1968, when Dr. David Smith and Dr. Frederick Meyers secured a thirty-seven-thousand dollar grant from the National Institute of Mental Health to study speed in the Haight-Ashbury. Dr. Meyers, who became principal investigator in charge of the funds, then invited Roger Smith to direct the Amphetamine Research Project. Smith, who saw the academic and personal value of the study, "took off my gray-flannel suit and my wing-tip shoes and grew a moustache. Soon, the kids on Haight Street were calling me the Friendly Fed and asking me to help them with the law."

Roger Smith did volunteer work at the Medical Section during the spring of 1968 and came to know and to counsel many of the regular patients, including Charlie Manson and his infamous family. In May, when the Amphetamine Research Project was finally funded, he converted the front basement of 409 Clayton Street into an office, hired a San Francisco State graduate named Gail Sadalla as his assistant, and began interviewing young residents of the Haight on their drug practices. Smith continued his research into the summer, while his office gradually grew into a social center comparable to that supervised by Father Grosjean in the back of the basement and on the first floor upstairs. It might have remained that way had not several of the sicker speed freaks he was interviewing begged him for medical help and refused to leave the Annex until he found them a safe place in San Francisco to stay.

Roger Smith knew that shelter and medical attention were necessary if the young people were to survive. But the grant which funded his project was designated for research alone and could not be applied towards treatment. So, in July, he took it upon himself to establish an emergency aid program. Although he and his wife, Carol, were already involved with Charlie Manson and his family, they found space for several speed freaks in their Tiburon home. Smith next moved his office into the back of the basement of 409 House and transformed the front room into a detoxification area where patients could come down in relative seclusion. He then secured the assistance of physicians from the Medical Section on a standby basis and arranged to refer young people to Dr. Meyers.

Although he had resigned from his position as research director of the Clinic by this point, Dr. Meyers had never lost interest in the Haight-Ashbury. In fact, he treated dozens of speed freaks in his offices at the Medical Center on Parnassus Street during the summer of 1968 and also worked in the basement of 409 Clayton when his schedule permitted. In one three-hour period, he and Roger Smith handled fifteen people, including ten with adverse drug reactions, two with gunshot wounds and three who had been mauled during a gang bang.

Word soon spread through the Haight-Ashbury about their efforts, and the Amphetamine Research Project evolved into an independent medical service with its own group of regular patients. As it did, Smith decided to expand his program and create an alternative to the drug abusers' lifestyle. He first raised several thousand dollars from private sources, including the physicians at the Psychiatric Section, moved his detoxification activities to an apartment near the Annex, and rented a flat outside the district where a half-dozen adolescents could live. He then asked a thirty-six-year-old Lutheran minister named John Frykman to work out of the Amphetamine Research Project office and supervise what was becoming its communal family.

Father Frykman was a stocky, bearded individual who had worked with Smith at the East Oakland Parish and shared his belief that drug abusers should be helped in their own environment rather than at distant hospitals. In August of 1968, he moved a desk into the front of the basement, recruited several volunteers, and won the speed freaks' approval. He then set up an employment service and instituted variations of the encounter group and sensitivity-training techniques developed at Synanon, the Esalen Institute and the Langley-Porter Youth Drug Unit to bring his family closer together. It remained intact after the Palace of Fine Arts fiasco, when he and Roger Smith started looking for larger donations with which to rent more flats in the Haight. They were concluding negotiations with two foundations by late October and had succeeded in getting over thirteen young people off the streets and off amphetamines.

Roger Smith phased out of these activities after October to resume his research, leaving John Frykman in charge of the Drug Treatment Program. Father Frykman was hard pressed to handle all the adolescents who hung out in his basement office and was sorely taxed when the flat he was super-

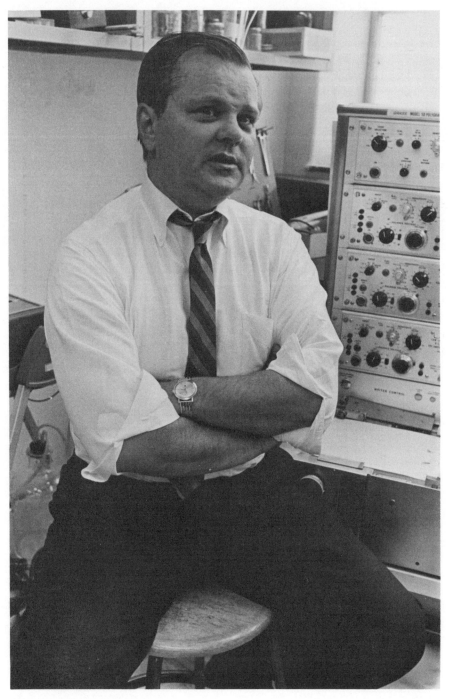

The University of California Medical Center: former clinic research director Dr. Frederick Meyers.

(Elaine Mayes)

vising outside the Haight-Ashbury was torn apart by fights among its young residents. But he managed to house two young people with his volunteers and somehow kept the rest of his family together. This led Smith to say that, "So far the program has been relatively successful. With help, it may prove to be an answer to some of the district's needs."

Yet in spite of his optimism, Roger Smith had come to several sobering conclusions while studying the Haight and its speed marketplace. Although the report he was preparing for Dr. Meyers was not complete, Smith had already determined that many of the confirmed abusers in the district were destroying themselves. He also knew that adolescents innocent about intoxication were still arriving daily and turning into habitual abusers much faster than the police or the public realized. And he suspected that competition in chemical consumption was becoming a new ethic in the Haight-Ashbury, totally replacing the hippie philosophy of love.

Smith felt that the sense of status in the Haight was more twisted than anything he had yet experienced. Most members of the straight world, he believed, considered excellence in socially acceptable fields to be of the highest possible value and rewarded it accordingly. In the ghettos where he had worked, the young blacks could not succeed like their white counterparts, yet they did gain some distinction out of being the best hustlers. The same was true of the more psychopathic youths in the Haight-Ashbury, who built reputations by being successful dealers or rip-off artists. But the same mechanism did not apply to the more disturbed individuals; their values were so warped that they turned what others might regard as totally negative identities into positive ones. Many speed freaks, for example, tried to be degenerate. They took every drug available to see how freaked out they could become.

Another obvious feature of new amphetamine abusers was their lack of community orientation. Smith felt that the bohemians and hippies who once inhabited the Haight had a sense of community, as well as a form of philosophic solidarity. They also had a eupsychic do-your-thing ethic and a love philosophy that held them together and reinforced the peaceful aspects of their behavior. But that ethic was taken to its logical, destructive extreme by the new population. The love philosophy was exploited, and the sense of community vanished during the summer of 1967, while those individuals who gave the district its illusive solidarity drifted or were driven out, to be replaced by others, interested primarily in speed. Smith described the change in the district in pessimistic tones.

These new kids are among the most hopeless I've ever seen. They are also responsible for developing a different kind of drug-taking than you find in the ghetto. There, where heroin, alcohol and barbiturates are king, the kids use chemicals to block out reality and kill their pain, but they maintain some sense of fraternity, if not an esprit de corps. Here there is no fraternity; the only spirit is that of young people who compete in terms of their drug consumption. In my research so far, I've interviewed some fourteen- and fifteen-year-olds who are frightened to death of doctors and want to spend the rest of their lives shooting amphetamines. These kids and some of the older, more confused ones can't establish their identities by being tough; as a matter of fact, they can hardly take care of themselves. So, they do just the opposite: they try to get as sick as they can.

One of the more psychotic kids, named Randy, who hangs around the office calls this new ethic "Terminal Euphoria," a chemically induced state of well-being that is totally destructive. Randy knows the damage drugs cause; in fact, he knows more about them than most physicians do. Yet he still shoots up every day and boasts about how many needles he's used, how much garbage he's shot into his veins. The only way this poor guy can prove he's somebody is to take doses that would kill anyone else. He's felt like a freak all his life; his mother treated him that way, and society confirms the point whenever an article about speed freaks is printed in the paper. Randy takes it all personally, but instead of letting the criticism penetrate his defenses he turns it into an attribute, calls himself the most frightening freak in the Haight-Ashbury and seems damned proud of it. Now, Randy doesn't speak for everyone in the Haight, yet he does represent the essence of the new ethic and the natural result of really doing one's thing. Believe me, status here has come to mean being the furthest out, the sickest, the biggest freak around.

A Case of Terminal Euphoria

Randy, the boy Roger Smith referred to, was also called Dr. Zoom, Mumbles or George Beasley in the Haight-Ashbury. He was known as a walking epidemic and had been a regular patient at the Medical Section for months before it closed. At the moment, Randy's health problems ranged from acne, abcesses, skin infections and serum hepatitis to the chronic depression, adverse drug reactions and suicidal impulses that regularly brought him to Dr. Dernburg.

Randy was quite popular with the physicians, most of whom had treated him at one time or another and had come to appreciate his puppy-dog manner. He leaned on the doctors for emotional support and would frequently report his drug exploits or rattle off his current symptoms, trying to attract an audience by saying "look how sick I am." Indeed, Randy was a human guinea pig and a perpetual patient for one good reason: he could relate to people in no other way.

Randy had found several parent surrogates during his involvement with the Clinic, one of whom was Head Nurse Peggy Sankot. But since Miss Sankot and many other staff members had left the district, Roger Smith was now his favorite. The two first met the night Robert F. Kennedy was assassinated, when Dr. Arthur Carfagni asked Smith to drive Randy to Napa State Hospital, where he had been committed by the court. Randy escaped from the facility and almost beat Roger Smith back to the Amphetamine Research Project. Smith took a parental interest in him and tried to get him into several other state hospitals and rehabilitation programs, but Randy either ran away or was discharged by physicians who did not know what to do with him.

Finally, Roger Smith began using him as a sort of consultant to recruit other amphetamine abusers for interviews and treatment. He also let him talk with the journalists and social scientists who dropped by 409 Clayton Street periodically. Randy spent most of the fall of 1968 in the basement office, coming down from drugs, crashing on the couch, talking shop with the young people who came to be interviewed, advising Father Frykman on his Drug Treatment Program, and boasting about his chemical consumption to whomever would listen. "I am the Amphetamine Research Project," he told John Luce, who was writing an article about him and the Clinic for *Esquire.* "Hell, I've done more speed research in the last ten years than anyone."

Speed was Randy's drug of choice, but he also drank alcohol and shot or swallowed anything he could get his hands on except LSD, which he sold on Haight Street in so-called variety packs also containing heroin, Dexedrine, Seconal, STP and various compounds alleged to be THC, the active ingredient in marijuana. His supply came from friendly cooks who invited him into their labs occasionally to test new batches and gave him samples as a reward. Randy's pockets were usually loaded with drugs, and when he was not too stoned, he read the *Physicians' Desk Reference,* studying the compounds and dreaming up new concoctions to make himself more weird. "I like to mix my poison," he said. "It's stupid to stay too long in one bag."

Violence also fit into Randy's bag, and he often found room for a four-inch knife and a twenty-two caliber automatic — "superpistol," he called it — in his frayed pea jacket. These, he insisted, were necessary for his protection and would be used on anyone who tried to burn him. Randy talked a great deal about how tough he was and proudly displayed the scars he had picked up street fighting. Yet, for all his traumatic injuries and his talk, Randy was more often sinned against than sinning; he could hardly hold his own in the Haight-Ashbury and invariably arrived at the Annex with some new horror story of his collisions with the world. "One big hassle," he said of his life in a characteristic burst of candor; "One day I get rolled in the park, the next day the whole fucking police department is down on me. Nothing but crap, and I've been through it all before."

Randy's ordeal started in San Bernardino, California, twenty-three years ago, the day he was born. His father left town a week later. When he was eight years old, he moved with his alcoholic mother to Stockton, fifty miles east of San Francisco. When he was thirteen, they attended a party together where Randy took some of his mother's prescription diet pills for the first time. He enjoyed the drugs; they sped up his system and helped him forget his mother, a sexually starved and impulsive woman who apparently took out all her frustrations on him. One year later, he left home after learning to use amphetamines to heighten his courage and overcome his depression.

I just couldn't take my old lady. She's get loaded and start in on me and I'd be loaded too and pretty soon we'd really be at it. I was getting big then, big enough to hit her back when she started swinging. Finally she started coming on like some whore and it got so bad I just couldn't stay there anymore.

So I cut out, made it to New York, got adopted by some junkies on the lower East Side and pretty soon I was hooked on heroin. Joined the navy, got ahold of some codeine, and spent time in a couple hospitals and jails. Four or five apartments and maybe fifty hotel rooms later I'm in North Beach here in San Francisco strung out on morphine. Played beatnik for a while on Grant Avenue until the tourists and cops came and I followed the gang out here.

Weren't too many people around when I came in, just the beats and a few junkies and speeders I knew from the Beach. Then the place started to fill up with artists and college kids. Pretty soon it broke superpsychedelic, everyone eating acid and getting away with it. All that love crap, street full of fucking hippies until the press and the tourists and the cops and the dealers came and then the speed and good dope arrived. Nothing left but freaks and gangsters today. It's like a speed-freak heaven, like a dope-fiend Bowery.

I should know, I been there, I know what it's like. I been everywhere, man, I've seen it all. Over the years I've shot more shit, stuck more spikes in my arm than any man alive. I'll shoot up two grams of speed just to be doing something, like me and this spade junkie got a bottle of Desoxyn once and shot the whole hundred just to see what'd happen.

Usually, though, I just shoot three-quarters of a gram, like when I'm on a long run, fixing up every four or five hours or so. My longest was eighteen days once, just sitting in one room with a guy fixing up around the clock, what a time. My biggest hit ever an eighth of an ounce, pure methamphetamine, none of this crap you pick up on the street, some kind of record in the Haight-

Ashbury. I shot up and started walking right out of the place I was in and wandered around dreaming the world all red and yellow till I wound up in the park somewhere. Then I came back to the Haight and shot up a gram or so from those dime bags I was selling and kept the run going.

It's weird, speed, the flash takes over your mind, keeps it from scheming on you. It's like an explosion in your skull, like a monster bomb in your whole body, warm like fire. Your head gets so big you can't imagine how big it is, then you get into a trance, spaced out, making plans. I get into this megalomaniac bag about five days into a run. I'll build monstrous castles in my head, all the far-out things I'm going to do, the money I'm going to make, like I'll be sitting behind the wheel of my Rolls Royce with six chicks, have two speed labs going at once, a heroin refining plant and my own private airplane. I'll be running the Mafia, in charge until I start to come down, my mind collapses, the girders fall apart and I realize none of this stuff exists and none of it's going to exist and it's like you pull the bottom out of my brain. I feel empty and suicidal in about five hours.

Other drugs I feel different. I can't handle acid anymore, took some, even shot some back in the hippie days but it screws my head up now. I got pretty wiped out my last few runs on speed too so I been shooting barbiturates, lots of reds and some heroin to get down. I dig barbs; they really knock you on your ass. It's like somebody attacking your stomach and your head at the same time. But my body starts to hurt so much and my mind I get insane. I go on monster barb runs and everybody in the Haight-Ashbury gets freaked out when I'm around. I'm so paranoid, such a maniac, people know I'm capable of anything when I'm stoned and carrying my superpistol so they leave me alone.

You need a rod; this is a mean place, everybody running games on you. I was ripped off for a half-ounce of speed couple of days ago, expected the bastard to pay me but he pulled a knife. Another time I can't remember too well I had ten bucks trying to buy a forty-five from one of these big dope-dealing cats in the park when the dude sticks it in my face and takes my dough. Then I was talking yesterday with some guy on Haight Street, this cat I was dealing acid with, and one of those street spades comes up and crashes him on the head with a bottle. Shit, I didn't want trouble, I just walked away.

I mean the place is so crazy. Freaky things happen to me like I'll be walking around stoned, minding my own business and I run into all kinds of weird people. Like where I've been staying, in this crystal palace, the Jeffrey Haight Hotel right on Haight Street, people just falling apart all over the place freaking, running around naked and shooting up and screaming and the cops breaking down the door and beating the shit out of you. It's like a black-and-white flash, everybody screaming around, nobody in control.

Still, I sorta dig the hassle. I mean it's exciting, plenty of action. Sex, too, if you want it, but I haven't had a hard on in so long, it's just dope for me. When you're in the middle, everything strange, you know how good you're gonna feel when you fix up again. I like being on the street, scheming to stay alive. People'll come up and say, "Randy, can you get me ten pounds of speed?" and you know, I feel kinda big for ten minutes. Then when I get a monster pile of speed or barbs sitting right there in front of me all piled up and wondering how it's gonna be, all that beautiful dope. That's real pleasure, all that shit, knowing it's mine.

It's not a bad life, at least I ain't become a vegetable like some of the freaks out here. Roger and Ernie say I can't keep this up too much longer and they're supposed to know but I'm not dead yet. Speed kills is true, no bullshit, I know it but I get more weird without drugs than with them. I'm just one of those people who's got to get high. When I'm not stoned I feel incomplete; when I'm not selling on the street I get bored.

Speed is part of my body chemistry, something I gotta have. I tried to quit, been in lots of programs, but they don't do any good, first thing they want you to do is get a job. I mean how could you dig washing dishes and sweeping floors after you've seen all the action I'm seen? Hell, I get spaced out the minute I get back on the street. Put me in a hospital and soon as I'm out I'll be shooting up again.

I'm a freak, see? A needle freak, a speed freak, a dope freak — read about me in the paper, man. I been in a couple down-to-the-death dope contests with dudes before, taking shit till I can't see, but I've lived through. I've lived through a lot, shot more shit into my arms than any man alive and I'm just twenty-three. So I die. So big deal. Everybody's gotta die. Look at the Haight, all these teenyboppers walking around, little twelve-year-old kids out of their fucking skulls, acting like they got more cool than anybody in the Haight-Ashbury. Well, I tell you all they got is Terminal Euphoria. Hell, the whole place has got it. I tell you, I may be dying, but the Haight is dying, too.

Diagnosis Confirmed

Randy's diagnosis was hardly professional, but it squared nonetheless with that of Dr. Dernburg. Although he had long considered the Haight-Ashbury a destructive environment, Dr. Dernburg had once been hopeful about the people who comprised its new community. He had made significant inroads in understanding what he called the hippie modality, and Alan, Jackie and his other long-term hip patients had profited considerably from intensive, analytically oriented psychotherapy.

But Dr. Dernburg could not say the same for the new population. Few blacks, hoodies or bikers ever asked him for treatment, and the more disturbed individuals living in the Haight were too unable to tolerate frustration and too enmeshed in drugs and in their daily crises to be reached by therapy. Randy, for one, needed not only chemical stimulation but also the excitement associated with dealing speed. It would take years of care in a private psychiatric hospital to wean Randy from drugs and give him something else to live for. All Dr. Dernburg could do was ease his suffering and try to keep him from committing suicide.

Dr. Dernburg felt that the entire Clinic was subject to similar limitation. Although he believed that the new Drug Treatment Program might prove to be therapeutic for some of the younger and more malleable adolescents in the district, he had little faith in group treatment methods and suspected that Father Frykman could keep his patients off drugs only by placing them on the staff. This in itself had a certain value and was an important key to the Clinic's success. But like the wound-cleansing normally done at the Medical Section, it seemed to him to be only a form of psychological first aid.

Furthermore, such possibly incomplete treatment did not call for Dr. Dernburg's specialty. Although he considered Professor Loomis's one-to-one counseling approach applicable to the Haight, he felt that it was no longer the place for individual depth psychotherapy. Dr. Dernburg had accomplished little treatment and received no recognition during the fall period; most of his hip patients had left the district by this time, and he was spending so much time detoxifying some speed freaks and preventing others from attacking him that he had almost no energy left for healing. He had anticipated this situation after the riots in July of 1968, when he first considered quitting the Psychiatric Section and seeing his regular patients at his private office. Although he had stayed in the Haight-Ashbury through the closing of 558 Clayton Street, he now decided to leave the district after the end of the year.

Other organizers and staff members had left earlier. Along with Dr. Meyers and head nurse Peggy Sankot, the Clinic had lost Alan Rose, administrator of the Medical Section for several months, who had gone home in June after he became involved with Charlie Manson's family. Jerry Read, whose grandiose visions and personal ambitions contributed to the Palace of Fine Arts fiasco, had been asked to resign from his position as business manager in September. Most of the long-time Clinic physicians had resumed their private practices following the July riots, founded adolescent health centers or joined Dr. Bertram Meyer at the Black Man's Free Clinic in the Fillmore ghetto. Of the organizers who were present during the summer of 1967, only Medical Director Dr. David Smith, Administrative Director Donald Reddick, Dr. William Nesbitt, President of Youth Projects, and Stuart Loomis were determined to open the Medical Section again.

The main reason for their determination related to the needs of their patients. All were as pessimistic as Dr. Dernburg about the Haight-Ash-bury, particularly because they suspected that amphetamine abuse had peaked in the district and feared that its young residents might switch to addictive alcohol, barbiturates and opiates in place of speed. This fear had been reinforced by Dr. Herbert Freudenberger, a New York psychoanalyst who studied the Clinic while attending the American Psychological As-sociation convention and predicted that the Haight would soon turn into a depressant-dominated ghetto like Harlem, rather than a speed-based slum. The organizers respected Dr. Freudenberger's forecast. But although they interpreted it as a death sentence, they felt a strong loyalty to the district and could not leave their patients to die.

At the same time, they were also concerned about the beats, hippies, and summer hippies who still sought treatment at 558 Clayton Street. Most of them lived outside the Haight-Ashbury at this point, but many continued to view the Clinic as their only source of medication and health informa-tion. Several doctors and staff members from the Medical Section had be-gun to visit and study the hippie communes in northern California and southern Oregon before the fall closing, and they needed a home base to operate from. The organizers were also interested in developing a way to deliver medical services to the urban and rural residents. Thus, they needed a base of operations too.

Furthermore, Dr. Smith wanted the Clinic to maintain its symbolic function. Although he had finally realized that the new community was past history, he still felt that the Medical Section stood for a new concept in medicine and health-care delivery now needed in America more than ever before. Dr. Smith did not agree with those who thought that the Clinic had outlived its usefulness, for he valued 409 and 558 Clayton Street as facili-ties which trained young physicians in San Francisco, inspired others in distant cities, and helped establish his reputation. All this would be impos-sible if either one were permanently closed.

At stake was not only the Clinic's role on the West Coast but also its special position in American society. The Medical Section had managed to treat twenty thousand people during 1968, approximately one-half of whom came for more than one visit, by earning the trust of its patients and by functioning in America's first white teen-age slum. It had also produced original research on adolescent health problems and had innovated a num-ber of techniques in drug-abuse treatment. Young people across the country respected the Clinic and subscribed to its *Journal of Psychedelic Drugs*. Private physicians and public health officials used the facility as a reference, as did legislators in Sacramento and Washington.

The organizers had less influence on these legislators than they might

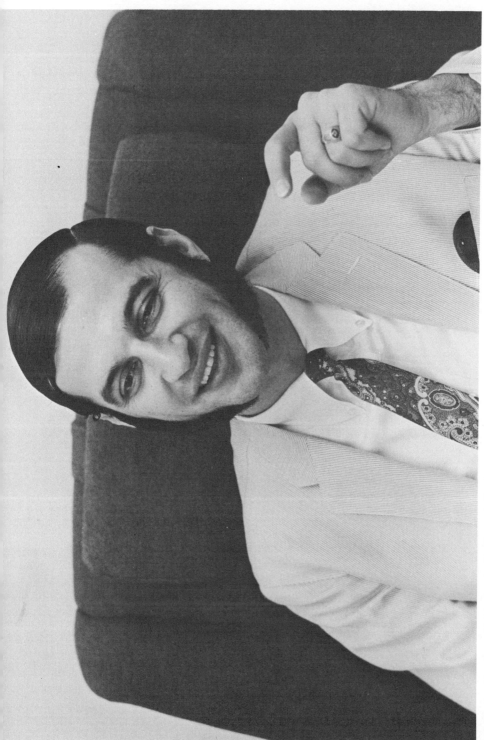

409 Clayton Street: psychiatric director Dr. Ernest A. Dernburg.

(Elaine Mayes)

have wished, but they were in a position of leadership in the countrywide free clinic movement they had helped start during the 1967 Summer of Love. Physicians in Seattle, Boston, Los Angeles, Portland, Honolulu and over twenty other cities and college communities had established centers modeled after the Medical and Psychiatric sections since the Clinic was founded, and the organizers were now considering the creation of a National Free Clinic Council to coordinate their activities. Because they felt a sense of responsibility towards these other facilities, they never questioned whether or not theirs should reopen. Their only concern was how to raise enough money after the Palace of Fine Arts benefit to begin operating again.

One possibility was the San Francisco Board of Supervisors, which was studying a proposal for the regional drug rehabilitation centers based on the Smith-Frykman model. The city had first heard about their work in early October, when Dr. Smith described the Drug Treatment Program at a panel discussion of amphetamine abuse sponsored by the Haight-Ashbury Neighborhood Council. Supervising Agent Matthew O'Connor of the State Bureau of Narcotics and the head of the San Francisco Narcotics Detail were present at the meeting, and both agreed on the need for regional centers in the Haight and in other parts of California. The liberal members of the Neighborhood Council also endorsed the Clinic program, then passed a resolution urging support for it from the Board of Supervisors.

Several supervisors were receptive to the resolution, and one member of the board spoke of the Drug Treatment Program as if it were his own. But other supervisors seemed reluctant to throw their weight behind any effort advanced by such an unofficial agency as the Clinic. Instead, they invited Dr. Smith to present his views at a public hearing and then consulted with Dr. James Stubblebine, director of Mental Health Services for the Public Health Department, who had never supported the Clinic. Dr. Stubblebine subsequently announced that his staff had come up with a master drug-abuse plan for the entire city — a plan that is still lacking today. At this point, the supervisors asked him to help the Clinic and other private facilities. But Dr. Stubblebine never acted on their request. By December 1968, a skeleton abuse proposal which his staff authored was safely buried in a supervisors' committee. The organizers assumed that it was intended for oblivion in the first place and began looking for private support, as they had so often done.

But they had a hard time finding help. Although amphetamine abuse was a relatively recent phenomenon in San Francisco, the Haight-Ashbury was such an old problem that many people who had previously aided the

Clinic had gone on to new causes. Physicians, staff members and volunteers were extremely difficult to recruit, for although some supporters had enjoyed helping the new community, they could not relate to the new population. The organizers had relied on dance-concert benefits for the past year, yet they now seemed a dubious source of revenue. And without the city's endorsement, they were hesitant to approach large foundations or the federal government for funds.

They were also being called upon to defend their activities in the Haight far more than usual, for many accused the Clinic of complicity in the district's destruction. Although this position was held throughout the country, it was particularly popular among those local merchants and homeowners who believed that 409 and 558 Clayton Street had encouraged drug abuse and disease by being permissive towards their patients. These older residents were opposed to any allocation of city funds for a health center in the Haight-Ashbury and were instead urging the Board of Supervisors to pass a law prohibiting street people from loitering on "their" sidewalks. They saw no justification for the Clinic and did not think its patients were worth being saved.

The organizers thought differently. They could not help but be revulsed by the condition of the young people they treated, but they did consider them human beings. They also knew that drug abuse had increased after the closing of the Medical Section, contrary to the arguments of the Clinic's detractors, and they felt that society could not afford to write off any one group because it might someday forget to draw the line regarding who was expendable. The people who worked at the Medical and Psychiatric sections were not judges but healers. They believed that the Haight had become a repository for unwanted people from across the nation, a garbage can into which society had dumped its most diseased members. But they felt that society had a duty to provide an equal opportunity of health services. And they conceived of the Clinic as a symbol of the traditional moral neutrality of medicine.

Although this tradition was followed no more frequently in 1968 than it is today, it was respected by some. As a result, new doctors stepped forward to aid the facility, while several dedicated young people offered to fill administrative roles. In early December, Dr. Smith secured a pledge of ten thousand dollars from Norman Stone, a local artist who had already donated thirty thousand dollars to the Clinic. And he was awarded a ten-thousand dollar state subsidy for a marijuana study which could be conducted in collaboration with the Medical Section.

In addition, the Clinic received grants of twenty-five hundred dollars from the San Francisco Foundation and ten thousand dollars from the

Mary Crocker Trust. Roger Smith and Father Frykman then secured six-teen thousand dollars for the Drug Treatment Program from the Luke B. Hancock Trust and the Aquinas Fund. By January 1, 1969, the organizers were satisfied with their financial condition. Six days later, David Smith and Don Reddick held an early-afternoon press conference arranged by John Luce to announce how the money would be used.

The Eye of the Hurricane

January seventh was a cold and gloomy day in the city, and the Flatlands were blanketed with a damp, bone-chilling fog. An emotional shadow also hung over the Haight-Ashbury, for a nineteen-year-old girl had been brutally raped and murdered in the district two days after Christmas. She was Ann Jiminez, who had weighed over two hundred pounds when she left her mother in the state of Washington over Thanksgiving and headed for the Haight, hoping to find hippies there. Miss Jiminez seemed friendly and eager for affection, a girl who knew her told the *San Francisco Examiner*. "Yet she never really fit in here; she wanted to swing with the crowd, but she didn't know how."

Miss Jiminez lost twenty-five pounds after three weeks in the Haight-Ashbury, but she was not accepted anywhere in the district except at 409 House. On her way to the Annex one evening, she drifted into a crystal palace at 1480 Waller Street, four blocks away. There, she was accused of either knick-knacking or intentionally stealing a pair of boots. She was then beaten, forced to have oral and anal sex with six bikers while three girls looked on, had her hair clipped off, her body shaved — and was left to die with obscenities scrawled on her body in lipstick. One of the girls who attended the orgy justified it to the police in terms of "motor ethics." "No one usually gets hurt bad at a turnout," she said. "It's very difficult for a person who's not motor to understand."

The San Francisco coroner could not understand the ethics, but he did determine that Miss Jiminez died of a massive blood clot, probably because she had been kicked in the head by a boy who was trying to revive her. The police from Park Station produced her nine companions a few days later and charged them with murder. They also swept Haight Street several times the following week, forcing the people who hung out there indoors. But most of the speed freaks were back on the street by January seventh, and almost a dozen young people in tattered jackets and burly overcoats were sitting on the front steps at 409 Clayton when the press arrived to hear the Clinic organizers outline their future plans.

Reddick and Dr. Smith said that they planned to create a multiservice center in the Haight. The state funds could not be applied toward treatment, but they would allow 558 Clayton Street to start an in vivo marijuana study with the assistance of Carter Mehl. Mehl, Delores Craton, Renée Sargent, Jackie and other young people would also oversee the other activities at the Medical Section. They would schedule doctors and nurses to treat physical health problems and to administer medication and emotional support in detoxifying those patients not using speed.

The more severe amphetamine reactions would be segregated and treated in the Annex. 409 Clayton Street would also continue to house Roger Smith's Amphetamine Research Project, Father Grosjean's Episcopal Peace Center and Father Frykman's Drug Treatment Program. Father Frykman would be in charge of two flats near the Annex where patients would live communally and participate in group therapy. These young people would then have access to counseling at the Psychiatric Section, which would be supervised in the future by Stuart Loomis. Professor Loomis would also try to get them into the few available state rehabilitation programs, thereby maintaining a link between the Haight-Ashbury and the outside world.

The organizers concluded by stressing the importance of this connection. The district they served had long been a barometer of change in drug preferences among adolescents, and they had found that abuse patterns which began there reached other areas within a short time. Young people were still dropping out of society at an unprecedented rate; amphetamine, barbiturate, opiate and hallucinogenic abuse was steadily increasing in every state; and drug-related health problems would continue to plague the nation. No single part of the country had deteriorated as badly or as rapidly as the Haight. But the district was only the eye of the national hurricane. America was creating new Haight-Ashburys every day.

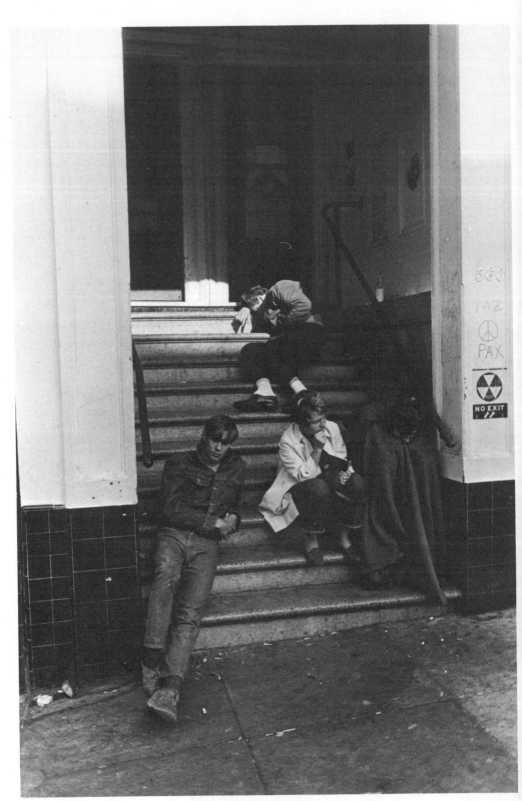

558 Clayton Street: the Clinic's Medical Section . . . closed.
(Michael Alexander)

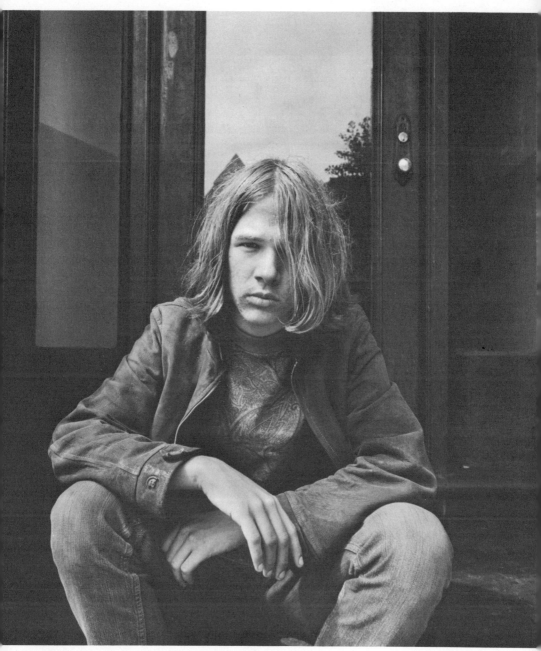

Masonic Street: Charlie — "You can't let your past get to you."
(Elaine Mayes)

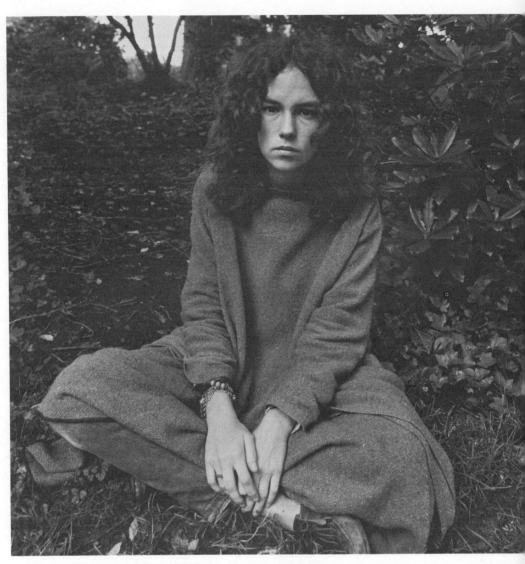

Golden Gate Park: Kathleen — "Om."
(Elaine Mayes)

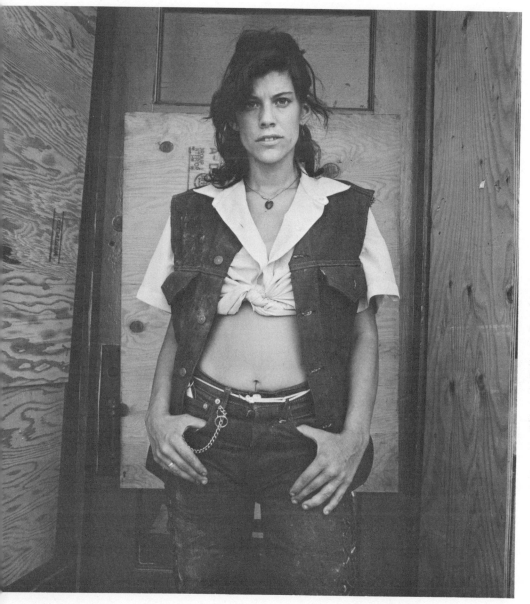

Haight Street: Sparky — "Kids want to be bikers. They turn twenty-one, and they try for the good groups. I'm a loner right now; usually I ride with the 69ers out of Connecticut. But I thought I'd come back and look up my friends."
(Elaine Mayes)

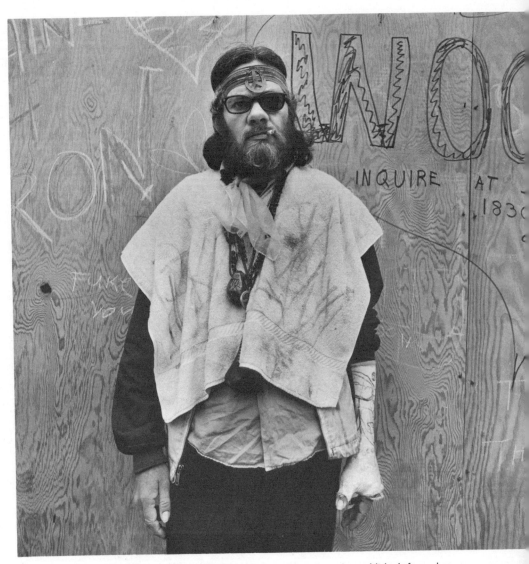

Haight Street: John — "I've been waiting for my picture to be published for a long time. I'm very happy."
(Elaine Mayes)

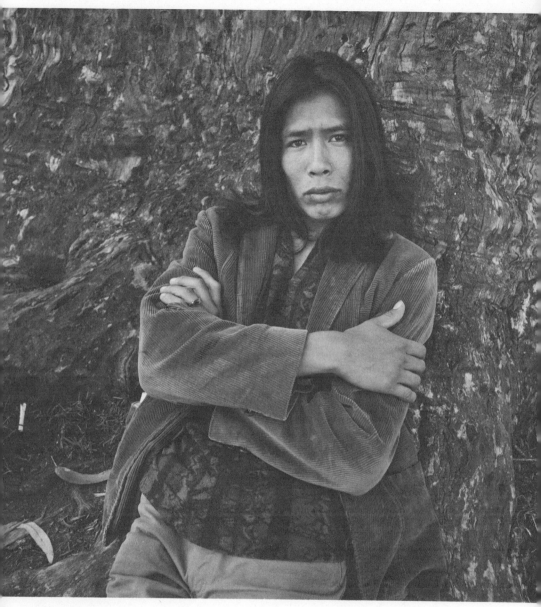

The Panhandle: Eugene — "Love has left here and the days are all alike."
(Elaine Mayes)

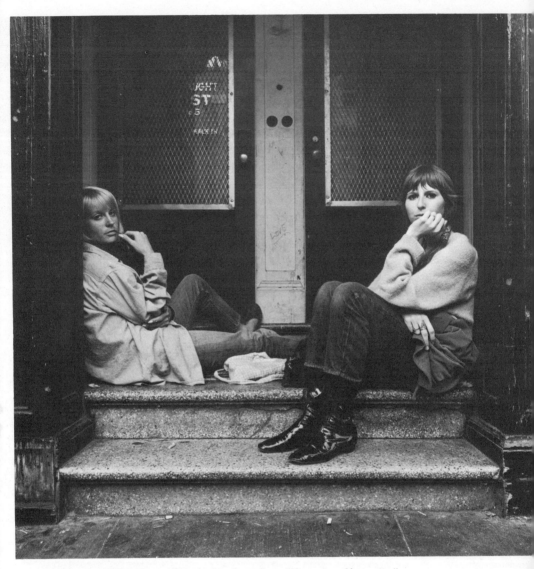

Haight Street: Christine and Kay, the Iron Butterfly — "The crying of humanity."
(Elaine Mayes)

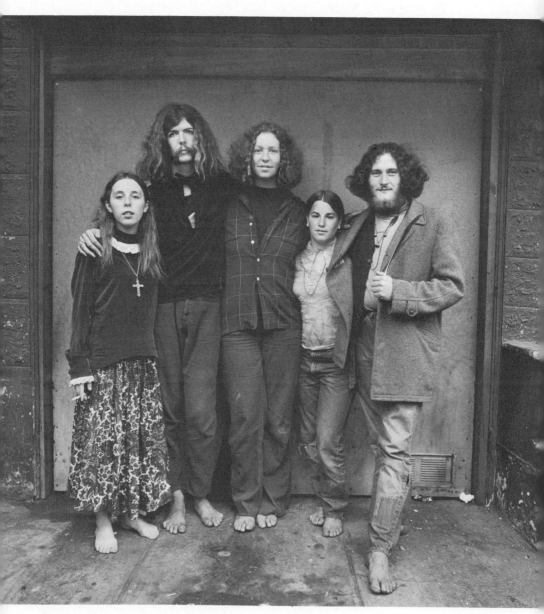

Clayton Street: Pamela, Dennis, Joan, Aileen, Ralph — "Home."

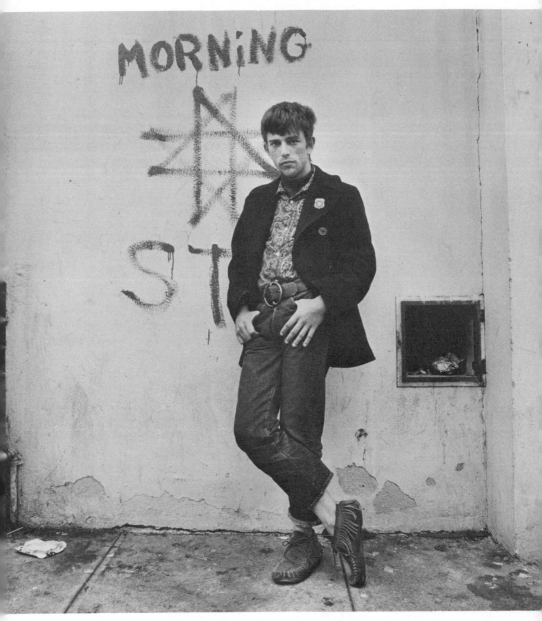

Cole Street: Joe — "Had nothing yesterday . . . got nothing today."

(Elaine Mayes)

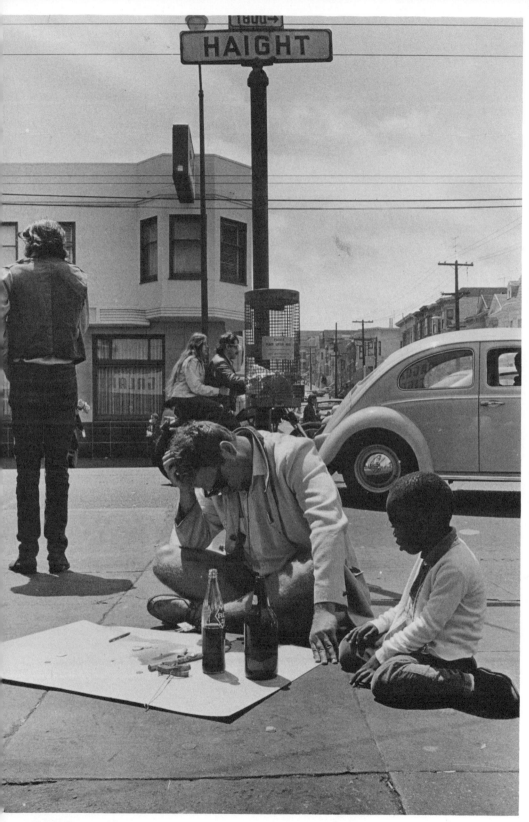

Haight Street: acid art.
(Elaine Mayes)

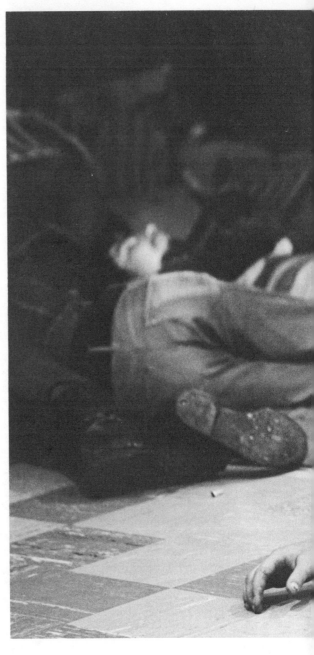

Haight Street: crashing on the floor
of the Print Mint.
(Elaine Mayes)

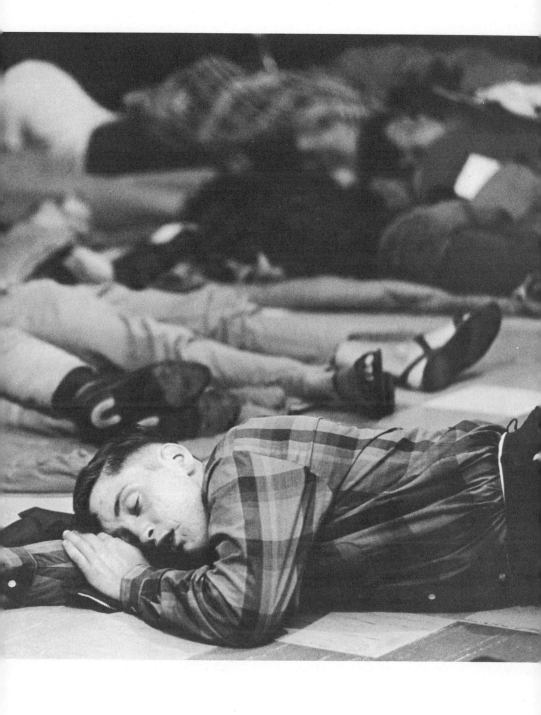

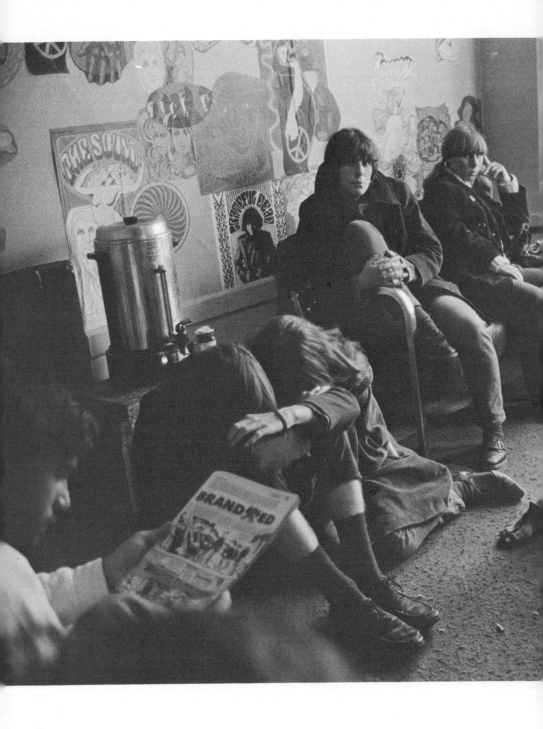

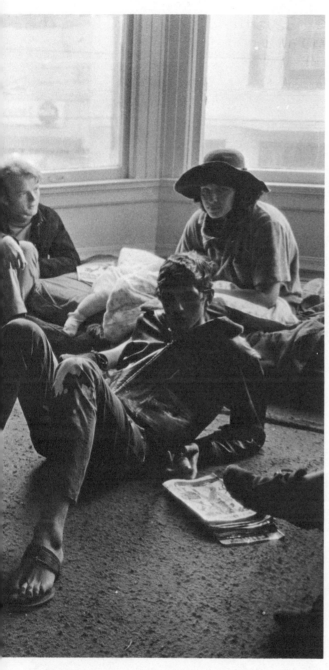

558 Clayton Street: the waiting room.
(Elaine Mayes)

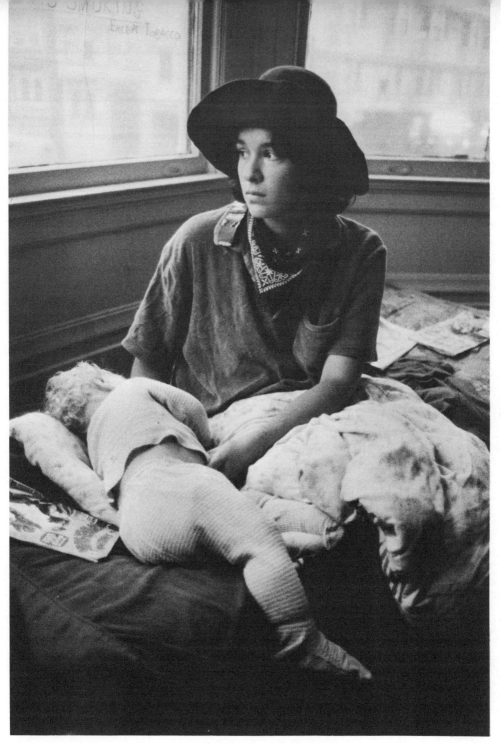

558 Clayton Street: Nature Girl — "We all come, I guess, looking for love."
(Elaine Mayes)

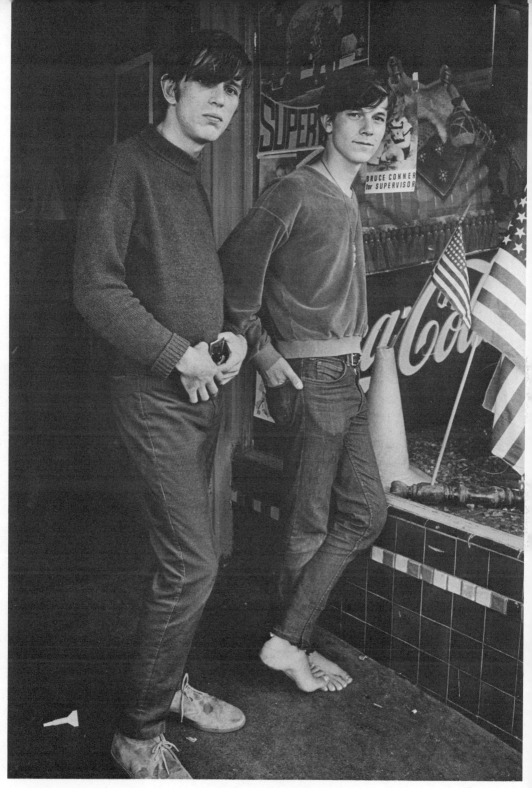

Haight Street: Joe and companion during the Summer of Love.
(Elaine Mayes)

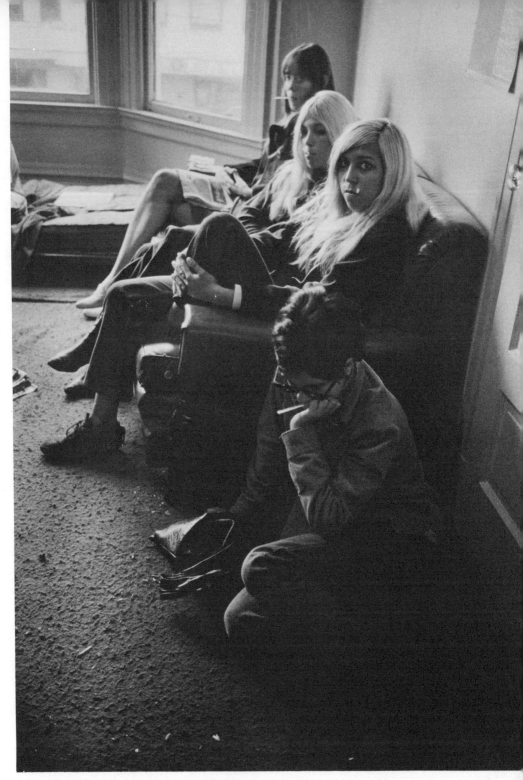

558 Clayton Street: measles.
(Elaine Mayes)

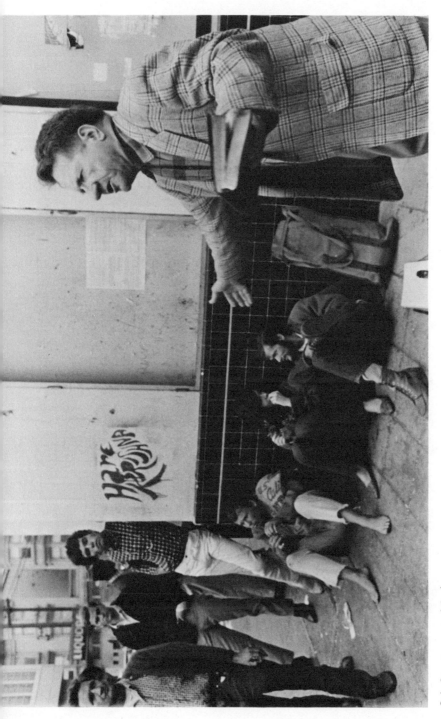

Cole Street: a man of God.
(Michael Alexander)

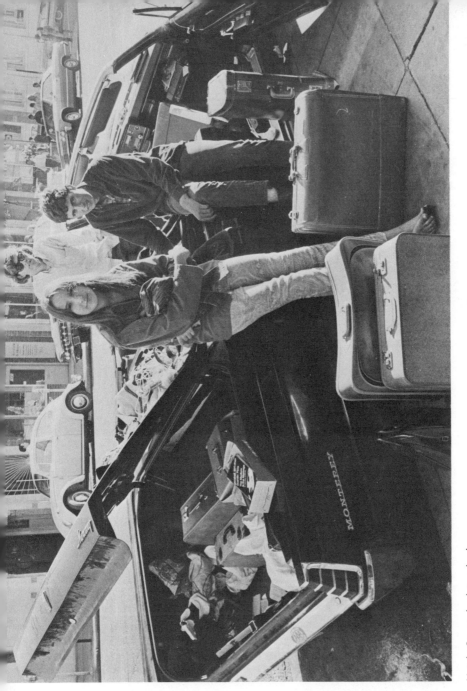

Haight Street: back to school.
(Michael Alexander)

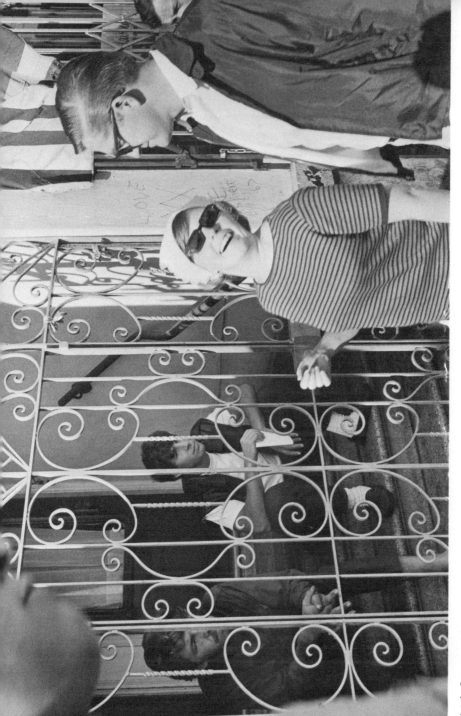

Haight Street: rats in a cage.
(Michael Alexander)

Part II

The

New

Community

The wolf also shall dwell with the
lamb, and the leopard shall lie down with
the kid . . .

Isaiah 11:6

One pill makes you larger
And one pill makes you small
And the ones that mother gives you
Don't do anything at all.

Grace Slick, Jefferson Airplane, "White Rabbit"

I saw the best minds of my generation
destroyed by madness, starving hysterical
naked . . .

Allen Ginsberg, "Howl"

From Old Community to Bohemian Colony

The complete breakdown of the Haight-Ashbury took nearly a century, but the district was a repository for unwanted people long before Randy and the new population arrived. It began as an exclusive community ninety years ago, when some of San Francisco's first families erected ornate Victorian houses on Mt. Sutro and envisioned a few shops and services on the Flatlands below. Their vision lasted until the 1900's, at which point two policemen had to be stationed at Stanyan and Waller to ease the congestion on Haight Street. Ten years later, when the Haight Theatre rose at the corner of Haight and Cole, the Haight had become one of the busiest middle-class white neighborhoods in town.

It continued growing that way until the 1940's, when San Francisco's building codes were relaxed to provide housing for workers in the war industries. Homeowners in the Haight-Ashbury who had been hurt by the depression converted their property into flats and apartments as a result, and lower-income whites came into the district for the first time. They were followed after the war by pensioners, east Europeans and Orientals. In the early 1950's the Redevelopment Agency razed much of the city's Western Addition in the name of urban renewal, leaving the black families living there with nowhere to go but the Fillmore ghetto or the Flatlands near Haight Street. They started migrating into the Haight and many white families began moving away.

When the races were evenly mixed, two groups stepped forward to curb the white exodus. The first included local homeowners and merchants who blamed San Francisco for forcing the Negroes into their area; the second, attorneys, ministers, professors from San Francisco State College and physicans at the University of California Medical Center who wanted the Haight-Ashbury to be a model integrated community. In 1958 this group organized the Haight-Ashbury Neighborhood Council and formed a temporary alliance with the homeowners and merchants. They then fought a city plan to turn the Panhandle into a freeway and petitioned the Redevelopment Agency not to tear down their Victorians.

Although both efforts proved successful, neither the Neighborhood Council nor the merchants and homeowners could prevent the Haight from gradually evolving into a ghetto. But they did forestall it for at least twenty years, and the fight against an outside enemy united them. "We suddenly regained our feeling of community," Robert Laws, former council president and legal counsel to the Haight-Ashbury Free Medical Clinic, recalled. "People started their own renewal work, and the older homeowners decided it was their duty to accept minorities that needed housing here. The Haight-Ashbury became identified as the most cosmopolitan neighborhood in town."

This reputation initially delighted the residents, but they soon realized it was attracting minorities they had not counted on. Shortly after the Neighborhood Council was formed, a number of homosexuals whom the merchants objected to moved into the Flatlands, purchased shops on Haight Street and bid unsuccessfully for the old Haight Theatre. Then, in the early 1960's, rising rents, police harassment and the throngs of tourists, thrill-seekers and hoodlums on Grant Avenue squeezed many young whites out of the North Beach district two miles away. They started looking for space in the Haight, and landlords there saw they could make more money renting their property to young people willing to put up with poor conditions than to retired people or to black families. For this reason, a small subculture took root in the Flatlands and spread slowly up the slope of Mt. Sutro. By 1963 the Haight-Ashbury was the center of a small and unpublicized bohemian colony.

Not all of the colony's members were young white bohemians. Some were older alcoholics and younger multiple drug abusers like Randy who had moved over from North Beach. Others were Negroes who enjoyed the cosmopolitan atmosphere in the Haight. Although a few of these blacks were psychologically similar to those later seen in the district, most were musicians, civil rights activists or intellectuals who were held in high regard by the majority of the colony.

This majority was made up of young whites in their middle and late twenties, many of whom were superficially identifiable by their inexpensive and colorless costumes. They were known as beats or beatniks, a word coined by *San Francisco Chronicle* columnist Herb Caen. Most were poets, painters, writers, musicians, actors in the city's small theater groups, school dropouts or students at the San Francisco Art Institute or the state college. They usually lived alone or as married and unmarried couples. They supported themselves primarily through the sale of their work, with loans from their friends, with welfare, or by taking odd jobs.

The bohemians generally came from middle-class homes, but they believed in voluntary poverty and lived a low-income life-style. Their pads were usually drab dwellings, for they spent little money on themselves. Some were artists who could not afford luxuries. Others only played with art and used poverty to emphasize their disinterest in material goods and their disdain for the values of the middle class. Most were preoccupied with philosophy, esthetics and/or personal problems. They preferred peace and quiet to the furious pace of most American cities, considered San Francisco a small town and regarded the Haight-Ashbury as a sanctuary. They kept to themselves and met only when they walked in the park, shopped on Haight Street, or gathered to make the scene.

When they did come together, the beats usually congregated in one another's pads. There, they shared drugs, listened to and played music, talked over their problems or argued about intellectual subjects. Many of them were well read, and most were at least familiar with the existential works of Norman Mailer, Allen Ginsberg, Jack Kerouac and other bohemian writers, some of whom lived in the Haight or visited it from time to time. The beats were fond of listening to these writers and discussing their artistic merits. They also took pleasure in sophisticated gripe sessions, at which anyone could read his poetry or lecture about the deplorable state of the world.

Such carping was characteristic of the bohemians, for most were intense and introspective people who were critical of society. Although many were physically passive, they were quite verbally aggressive and seemed to channel their impulsivity into onslaughts aimed at the outside world. At the same time, they were warmer within the confines of their own colony, for they lived by firm, if unwritten and unconscious, rules. Most were extremely protective of one another and permissive towards criminal behavior, sexual experimentation, drug abuse and psychological problems, including those which sprang from their own ranks as well as those exhibited by others. They let each member of their colony lead his own private search for artistic expression and spiritual understanding.

Dr. Francis Rigney and L. Douglas Smith, who conducted a sociological and psychological study of North Beach in the late 1950's, found that these searches were probably efforts to overcome the unrelatedness which the young people experienced. Dr. Ernest Dernburg, a war refugee from Nazi Germany who considered himself bohemian by temperament and treated and/or interviewed several contemporaries from the Haight-Ashbury in

1963 and 1964 while a psychiatric resident at Mt. Zion Hospital, came to a similar conclusion. Although a few of his patients were overtly psychotic, most seemed to be psychologically intact individuals, with strict and punitive superegos, who could function adequately in all areas but their interpersonal relations. Because of this, Dr. Dernburg described them as schizoid personalities, emotional loners who manifested certain exaggerated hangups or neurotic symptoms that made them eccentric, often charmingly so.

The beats may have been charming, but their hang-ups caused them considerable agony. A few were so emotionally dammed up that they suffered nervous exhaustion. Some experienced chronic anxiety and depression and were ridden with a hostility that poisoned their relationships. Others had compulsive and obsessional problems that crippled their artistic production and forced them to medicate themselves with tranquilizers and toxic drugs. Most suffered an affective numbness which made them appear physically cold. The coolness they showed outsiders was really a manifestation of their inability to relate to other human beings.

This inability apparently stemmed from their backgrounds. Some of Dr. Dernburg's patients said that they had overprotective mothers who never allowed them to be self-assertive but instead treated them as extensions of themselves. As children they were continually threatened by maternal dominance and became afraid of any intimacy and involvement. Because few of them left home as precipitously as many young hippies were later to do, they apparently managed to keep maturing psychologically in several ways but also had to construct defenses to prevent other people from intruding on them. They became intellectually competent, for example, and could use verbal and symbolic modalities — words and abstract concepts — to communicate. Yet they were unable to relate on an emotional level no matter how hard they tried.

Others experienced the same difficulty, but their early lives were distinguished less by maternal overstimulation than by parental neglect and abandonment. These children were left with baby sitters and books or had to fend entirely for themselves when their fathers worked and their mothers socialized. They were forced to move as their parents switched jobs and were therefore unable to develop lasting friendships. School further diluted their family life, while the conflicting viewpoints they were exposed to only confused them. Their already fragile identities were weakened as a result, and they never grew to trust other people. Nor did they learn how to meet the demands of others or to feel at ease in highly structured social situations. They moved to the Haight to escape demands and competition, to find love, and to forge some sort of group identity. But they remained fearful of being rejected and had to develop complex defense mechanisms to deal with the world.

Words were one such defense, for with them the bohemians could hold back others and maintain the interpersonal distance they required. Art was another — and an effort at communication as well. By expressing themselves at their gatherings, they could partially overcome the loneliness they experienced. They could also express their emotions and disturbed thinking freely through art and feel more comfortable in relating to an anonymous audience rather than to one person at a time.

A third defense they used was denial. Dr. Dernburg felt that many beats were extremely dependent people who had transferred their unresolved dependence on their parents into a dependence on others like themselves. But they denied this and asserted independence by their costumes. They knew they would repel others by growing beards and wearing old clothes and they often acknowledged that such provocation served a conscious offensive function. Yet it also served several unconscious defensive functions. The bohemians gained a great deal of attention by their dress, an attention which many of them never received in their homes. And they achieved a certain self-protection, for by thinking they were being snubbed for what they looked like, they may have avoided facing the possibility that they could be rejected for who they were.

This fear of rejection was evident in their attitude toward health matters. As artists, most of the beats were suspicious of science and modern medicine and often advanced a health code which resembled Christian Science in its emphasis on the ability of willpower to heal the body. They also distrusted physicians and condemned psychiatrists for allegedly forcing their patients to accept reality and thereby upholding the status quo. Yet many were obsessively health conscious. They kept abreast of current medical information, observed proper sanitation in their residences, and rarely permitted overcrowding. Because they feared the disapproval of doctors, they would go to Park Emergency or leave the Haight to consult public and private physicians only if severe illness pre-empted their self-reliant creed.

When this occurred, the bohemians were often snubbed because of their looks and behavior. This aggravated their isolation and prompted them to retreat further within themselves. It also intensified their most common defense mechanism, that of projection. After returning to gripe sessions in the Haight-Ashbury from their forays, the young people would compare notes and then launch into blanket indictments of society until they were projecting all their feelings outward, away from their colony and onto the outside world.

According to Dr. Dernburg, this allowed some of them to locate their internal anguish externally and to find the source of all their problems in society. Many of his patients externalized their confusion, isolation and anger and therefore saw the world as a frightening, empty and hostile place without realizing the personal as well as social origin of these perceptions. Gripe sessions assured them that their observations were valid, for they could match them with those of their companions. The meetings also helped to unify them against external enemies and thus prevented them from fighting too vociferously among themselves.

Projection may therefore have been vital for their psychological survival. Because of their backgrounds, many of the beats had complex identity proglems and negative self-images. But by criticizing others and endowing them with their own unwanted aspects, they could gain a sense of superiority which compensated for their inferiority feelings. They considered themselves different, yet they did not recognize their alienation as a deficiency and instead turned it into a positive virtue, even an ideal. The more they projected their own hostility and other unwanted feelings onto outsiders, the more they clung to one another and thereby "found'" themselves. Thus, alienation served a defensive function within their colony. It also acted as an adhesive to keep the colony together.

This alienation took many forms, but in general the bohemians said that ours is a repressive society. They were unable or unwilling to admit to their own rigidity and therefore saw social restraints everywhere. They were especially angered by people like their once liberal parents who had struggled through the depression and become bourgeois. These squares, they insisted, were Babbitts stamped from the same mold. They had sacrificed art and natural values for the sake of technology and commercial progress. They sold out to gain security, spent their lives chasing success, and took only ulcers to the grave.

This bothered the beats, for they did not see life as a progression towards distant goals. In fact, many thought that death and the possibility of nuclear destruction made planning for the future impossible. Because of this — and because they could neither tolerate frustration nor bind their anxiety — they lived for today. They also devalued rationality and esteemed emotionality more than the life of the mind. They wanted to become psychologically primitive, to open themselves to sensory stimulation and deep feeling and to function on a simpler, less sophisticated and more spontaneous level. Real living for them meant an often frantic search for experience and enlightenment. Real wisdom, they believed, came from spiritual illumination rather than analytic deduction. It required only a complete immersion in the Here and Now.

Now

Now-ness was both an existential and a transcendental ideal to the bohemians. They envisioned it as a Divine Madness, an ecstatic state in which one not only plunged into life and savored its essence, but also merged his consciousness with the cosmos, broke through the veil of so-called ordinary reality, and rose above the loneliness, the limitations and the pain of individuality. Now-ness to them was a direct perception of life through the senses. It promised emotional freedom, an end to social and sexual repression, and the dawning of a Golden Age.

Professor Daniel Bell has characterized this concept of Now-ness as eupsychic because it reflects "a kind of utopian thinking oriented towards the release of psychic impulses rather than the restructuring of social arrangements." Norman Mailer, who apotheosized the beats in 1957, called them Hipsters and compared their anarchic ideal of instant disinhibition and psychic release to "philosophic psychopathy." Mailer claimed that the Hipsters were interested in codifying the suppositions on which their inner universes were constructed. Their personal and social goal was "to accept the terms of death, to live with death as immediate danger, to divorce oneself from society, to exist without roots, to set out on that uncharted journey into the self."

Whether the life is criminal or not, the decision is to encourage the psychopath in oneself, to explore that domain of experience where security is boredom and therefore sickness, where one exists in the present, in that enormous present which is without past or future, memory or planned intent, the life where a man must go until he is beat. . . . One is Hip or is Square (the alternative which each generation coming into American life is beginning to feel), one is a rebel or one conforms. . . .

What is consequent therefore is the divorce of man from his values, the liberation of the self from the superego of society. The only Hip morality (but of course it is an ever-present morality) is to do what one feels whenever and wherever it is possible, and — this is how the war of the Hip and the Square begins — to be engaged in one primal battle: to open the limits of the possible for oneself alone because that is one's need. Yet in widening the arena of the possible, one widens it reciprocally for others as well, so that the nihilistic fulfillment of each man's desire contains its antithesis of human cooperation.

If the ethic reduces to Know Thyself and Be Thyself, what makes it radically different from Socratic moderation with its stern conservative respect for the experience of the past is that the Hip ethic is immoderate, childlike in its adoration of the present — the nihilism of Hip proposed as its final tendency that every social restraint and category be removed, and the affirmation implicit in this proposal is that man would then prove to be more creative than murderous and would not destroy himself.*

This, then, was the eupsychic ethic to which the bohemians in the Haight-Ashbury and other centers subscribed: a bold ethic, but one riddled with irony. Although Norman Mailer may have seen himself as a psychopath, most of the people he was speaking for were no more capable of arbitrarily becoming psychopathic than most people are. They spent much more time dreaming about the "enormous present" than ever inhabiting it. Because of their crippling inhibitions, they could rarely escape their own superegos, let alone the "superego of society." And they could not "open the limits of the possible," for little was possible for them.

Nevertheless, they tried. The beats were generally unwilling and/or unable to work through their hang-ups in psychotherapy, but they did adopt and adapt therapies of their own. Some thought they could dissolve their defenses in alcohol or become liberated by joining the Sexual Freedom League, which was located in a coffeehouse near Haight Street. Others sat on their intellectual talents and became craftsmen, attempting to find life not in words, but in their hands. Still others practiced yoga, meditated at the San Francisco Zen Buddhism Center to achieve satori, a state of so-called serenity, or pored through Hindu theology. A few even followed Allen Ginsberg to the Far East in search of enlightenment and looked on the sages of India as heroes.

Other heroes lived closer to home. Chief among them were bohemian writers and the people they worshiped: self-proclaimed supermen like Neil Cassady, who served as the prototype for Dean Moriarity in Jack Kerouac's *On the Road*. The beats glamorized the Hell's Angels and other outlaws who were coming into fashion in California because they lived life on the edge and seemed twice as large. Some even admired older alcoholics and

* Norman Mailer, *The White Negro* (San Francisco: City Lights Books, 1961), pp. 2–3, 15.

younger drug abusers, whose chemical consumption they construed as a form of existential rebellion.

But their universal hero was the American Negro. Many bohemians saw black people as natural primitives who suffered through life and gained soul in the process. Each had his own idea of what soul was, but in composite it appeared to embrace emotional exuberance, sexual prowess and the comradeship they assumed Negroes acquired by sharing a common oppression. The beats considered themselves oppressed and craved intimacy, and so made black culture the basis of their life-style. They favored the subdued, cerebral jazz played by artists like John Handy who conveyed the mood of depression so characteristic of their colony. They approved of and practiced miscegenation and assimilated ghetto slang into their vocabularies. And they used ghetto drugs. This led Norman Mailer to claim that "for all practical purposes, they could be considered white Negroes."

The Most Dangerous Toxic Chemical Ever Known

Although opiates, barbiturates and other compounds indigenous to the ghetto were available to the bohemians, their favorite toxic chemical in 1963 was probably ethyl alcohol. This drug, which results from the fermentation by yeast of a sugar, was known to Paleolithic man and has been employed as an intoxicant by almost every culture in human history. It has also been used therapeutically as an antiseptic, a sedative, an analgesic, an anesthetic, and a stimulant, although it has no stimulative properties.

Alcohol is still employed as a short-acting sedative, an antiseptic and an intoxicant today. It is classified pharmacologically as a nonselective central nervous system depressant because it can depress all excitable areas of the nervous system. Dr. Frederick Meyers further notes that alcohol should be considered a sedative-hypnotic-general anesthetic because graded doses of the compound produce four discernable stages of central nervous system depression. These include sedation and the relief of anxiety; disinhibition, possible excitation and hypnosis; general anesthesia; and complete respiratory and vasomotor depression.

When alcohol is taken orally, its most immediately noticeable peripheral effect is the stimulation of gastric acid secretion. This is followed by a slight increase in pulse rate and a dilation of surface and internal blood vessels that causes a flushed skin and a warm sensation. Small amounts of alcohol also produce an increase in the respiratory rate. These actions have led many to assume that the chemical has stimulative properties.

More pronounced are alcohol's central effects, which are initially experienced as a lessening of inhibitions and a characteristic feeling of euphoria and self-confidence. These are followed by increased sedation and an impairment of physical coordination. At a blood concentration of two-tenths of one percent, the equivalent of ten ounces of whisky, many drinkers become assaultive, stuporous and emotionally labile. When the alcohol in their blood reaches four-tenths of one percent, it makes most drinkers comatose. If the drug's concentration increases further, they may die of acute alcohol toxicity as their respiratory and cardiovascular functions are arrested.

This toxicity is often complicated by attendant shock, but it can be treated if the symptoms are diagnosed in time. Patients must receive respiratory and cardiovascular support and may require such postoperative stimulants as nikethamide (Coramine). If treatment proves successful, they gradually return to consciousness as the alcohol in their blood is metabolized. They are then administered supplementary vitamins and proteins to correct probable dietary deficiencies.

Acute alcohol toxicity is quite common in our society, and most urban medical facilities must deal with dozens, if not hundreds, of cases daily. Even more common is chronic alcohol toxicity or alcoholism, which ranks as one of America's most serious health problems. Alcohol is both psychologically habituating and physically addicting in high doses and can cause organic brain damage and personality change. It also has one of the highest abuse potentials known to man. Of the over eighty million people in the United States who use alcohol, at least seven million are estimated to be alcoholics. Robert S. DeRopp, in his book, *Drugs and the Mind,* states that there are almost one hundred thousand alcoholics in San Francisco, a city of seven hundred and fifty thousand.

The suffering of these and other alcoholics is severe. Alcohol is a protoplasmic poison which exerts a debilitating effect on the pancreas and other organs. It is also a fuel, and drinkers sometimes try to feed off of the calories it can produce. They receive enough energy to function by doing so but also incur vitamin, protein and mineral deficiencies. This often leads to two illnesses in addition to brain damage: cirrhosis of the liver, a degeneration and scarring of the liver tissue that is caused by protein deficiency; and peripheral neuritis, a disease characterized by sore and sensitive skin which is caused by a deficiency of vitamin B-1, or thiamine.

Thiamine is used in treating peripheral neuritis and is also employed in the treatment of three basic syndromes or psychoses often experienced by alcoholics. These include the Wernicke-Korsakoff syndrome or acute brain syndrome; delirium tremens, a withdrawal state which frequently follows addictive drinking binges; and chronic alcoholic deterioration, or chronic brain syndrome. Patients suffering this syndrome exhibit physical and psychological damage as a result of repeated attacks by alcohol on their nervous systems. They can be helped by medication and supplementary vitamins, but there is no way to undo the damage they have done themselves.

Nor is there an easy cure for alcoholism. Chronic alcohol toxicity is right-fully regarded as a behavioral disorder in our society and had been ex-plained by a number of theories which emphasize that alcoholics, like other drug abusers, are dependent people who have difficulty forming interper-sonal relationships and handling stress. Studies have also been made of alcoholics revealing that most of them have parents who themselves abuse alcohol. But no one has found a completely effective way to help alcoholics.

Psychotherapy is one method, but few alcoholics have the motivation necessary to undergo complete treatment. Alcoholics Anonymous, which bases its appeal on group confession and catharsis and attempts to replace the alcoholic's dependence on drink with a dependence on the organization, is only moderately successful with confirmed drinkers. So are other self-help groups in which alcoholics must surrender what little independence they have and usually operate psychologically at the level of a four- or five-year-old child.

Drugs are also employed to treat alcoholism, especially in Europe. Some doctors have administered hallucinogenic agents to alcoholics, hoping to give them intense spiritual experiences. Others have used calcium carbi-mide (Temposil) or tetraethylthiuram disulfide (Antabuse), two com-pounds that inhibit the complete metabolism of alcohol and thereby flood the body with its toxic by-product, acetaldehyde. These agents are likely to deter people from drinking when they are taken in conjunction with alco-hol, but their use is generally restricted to highly motivated spree drinkers. Unmotivated alcoholics rarely request drug or nondrug treatment. In fact, they may not admit to having personal problems and may want to see abus-ers of other chemicals jailed.

This results in part from the fact that alcohol is socially sanctioned and retailed in this country at an annual rate of over three hundred and fifty million gallons of hard liquor, in addition to several billion gallons of beer and wine. The companies responsible for this supply have never advertised the debilitating effects of their products, and few Americans even realize that alcohol is a drug. Fewer still are aware that alcohol is more harmful than heroin to the mind and body or that, as Dr. Joel Fort states, "in terms of individual suffering, crime and the total cost to society it is the most dangerous toxic chemical ever known."

Because of this public ignorance, most people take their first drink in a social setting under great pressure from their peer group to do so. Not all of them become alcoholics, and many derive more satisfaction from disinhibiting themselves, from relieving the tension of meeting others and from ritualistically sharing a nurturing substance than from its pharmacological properties. But millions who are more abuse prone proceed from periodic to habitual abuse of alcohol.

Although every pattern of alcohol use and abuse was found in the Haight-Ashbury during 1963, the bohemians there used the drug primarily as a social and medicinal agent, as most adult Americans do. Some drank beer and wine at their gatherings and rarely became intoxicated. Yet others began to abuse the compound by drinking to deaden their senses and to relieve anxiety. Many of these beats were aware of the price of chronic alcohol toxicity. They therefore tried to help themselves by transferring their dependence on alcohol into a dependence on marijuana.

"The Killer Weed"

Marijuana is derived from the resinous flowers and leaves of the female hemp plant, *Cannabis sativa,* which grows wild and is cultivated throughout the world. Cannabis was first described in Chinese literature around 2700 B.C. and has been employed as a euphoriant, a sedative and an analgesic by many cultures. It also has a long history of religious use in the Far East and among certain primitive African tribes.

The active ingredient in *Cannabis* is believed to be tetrahydrocannabinol or THC, a fusion product of a substituted resorcinol and a terpene ring. THC was first isolated from crude *Cannabis* by Dr. Roger Adams and his associates at the University of Illinois in 1942. It has since been synthesized by Dr. Alexander Shulgin and others as 1-hydroxy-3-n-amyl-6, 6, 9-trimethyl-1,7,8,9, 10-tetrahydro-6-dibenzopyran.

The strength of natural *Cannabis* is determined by the concentration of tetrahydrocannabinol in the plant, which itself varies with climate, cultivation techniques and soil conditions. It is strongest in Africa and Nepal, less strong in Central America and weakest in North America. The potency of the drug is also related to its preparation. In India, for example, *Cannabis* is legally obtainable in some states as bhang, a smoking mixture containing dried mature leaves with low resin content, and ganja, a specially cultivated grade used in making smoking mixtures, beverages and sweetmeats. Charas, the pure *Cannabis* resin, is also sold illegally. It corresponds to the hashish available in the Middle East and North Africa. American marijuana, or that grown in Mexico, is roughly equivalent to the Indian bhang and is called grass, pot, tea, or weed. It is usually smoked in this country, but some users also drink marijuana tea or eat marijuana brownies. Smoking the drug allows users to absorb it quickly into their bloodstreams through the lungs and thereby to regulate their consumption, as many people cannot or will not do while drinking alcohol.

Marijuana is considered a narcotic under federal and most state laws, but this classification is pharmacologically unwarranted. Yet scientists do not agree on the drug's proper categorization. Dr. William McGlothlin, for one, has described marijuana as a mild hallucinogen, indicating its similarity to drugs like mescaline and LSD. Dr. Leo Hollister says that marijuana lies halfway between alcohol and the hallucinogens, combining "the best of both worlds." Dr. Frederick Meyers feels that marijuana should be classified as a sedative-hypnotic-general anesthetic like alcohol and nitrous oxide, and cites research which shows that graded doses of the drug cause the same four levels of central nervous system depression as does alcohol. And Dr. Joel Fort believes that it should be called a mixed stimulant-depressant or listed in a separate category.

This difficulty in classification is compounded by the fact that marijuana is unique in the reaction it produces, although its peripheral effects have been likened to those of the sympathomimetic group of drugs and its central effects to those of alcohol. These peripheral actions begin shortly after the drug enters the bloodstream, when the eyes redden with conjunctivities, the tongue becomes tremulous, the mouth feels dry, and the skin feels cool. Cardiovascular changes consist of a slight increase in pulse rate. In addition, the extremities may become sensitive to pressure and pain.

Marijuana's central effects generally occur at the same time and are manifested by a high somewhat comparable to that of alcohol. This state may include a euphoric sensation of lightness in the head and heaviness in the limbs, with feelings of elation, satisfaction and well-being, as well as a possible increase in appetite and a release of inhibitions. At the same time, marijuana begins to alter perception, making time and distance intervals appear elastic, and distorting or amplifying sensory stimuli. As a result, users of marijuana often claim to be extremely sensitized while high, although these claims are inconsistent with the compound's depressant action. They rarely hallucinate, but the drug does alter their perception of sights, shapes and sounds.

The severity of these perceptual alterations appears to mount with the concentration of marijuana in the blood and is paralleled in many people by increased distortions in thinking, by memory lapses and by a decreased ability to recognize anger in others, according to Dr. Reese Jones of the Langley-Porter Neuropsychiatric Institute. The sedating effects of the drug also become so strong that although some users grow active and talkative, most prefer to become absorbed in internal or extrenal stimuli and to sink into a dreamy lassitude. They may then sleep and are likely to wake with some grogginess but without the racking hangover associated with heavy use of alcohol.

Most people who smoke marijuana do not consume enough of the chemical to cause extreme respiratory and vasomotor depression. But such self-regulation is an acquired process, and incidents of acute marijuana toxicity and overdosage, although rare, are not unknown. Overdosage can lead to nausea, dizziness and extremely impaired coordination. Marijuana can also trigger acute psychoses and induce anxiety in people who suddenly experience the compound's peripheral actions, as studies conducted in association with the Haight-Ashbury Free Medical Clinic have shown.

Such acutely toxic states and the infrequent cases of psychosis precipitated by the drug seem to be related more to the marijuana users' psychological condition and to the environment in which the drug is taken than to its pharmacological effects. Panic reactions are seen more often in older individuals with extremely negative expectations about marijuana, while some younger people with very positive expectations can actually become high from smoking placebos, as the studies of Dr. Reese Jones and a former Clinic volunteer, Dr. Andrew Weil, reveal.

Expectations and environmental and psychological factors also contribute heavily to chronic marijuana toxicity. The well-defined syndromes associated with alcoholism do not exist with marijuana in this country because the potency of the available drug is so low and because its users eat at least sweets regularly. Yet chronic marijuana toxicity is reputed to be as serious a health problem in the Middle East as alcoholism is in this country. The drug can irritate the mucosal lining of the lungs and bronchial passages and may therefore aggravate and/or cause such respiratory illnesses as bronchitis. It has also proven to be psychologically habituating, although the body does not develop a physical dependence on the drug as it does on alcohol.

Some habitual marijuana abusers resemble alcoholics in that they intoxicate themselves daily, become extremely anxious when deprived of the drug, and manifest what Dr. David Smith has called an amotivational syndrome in which they have no desire to work, to compete, or to participate socially. No one has determined to what extent this syndrome stems from marijuana's pharmacological effects or from the personalities of its users. But its existence has led physicians at the Clinic to compare dependence on marijuana to dependence on alcohol.

Such dependence has been traditionally limited in the United States to Spanish-speaking and Negro Americans who employ the drug as a euphoriant because it is so much cheaper to produce than alcohol. Marijuana use was also popular during the depression with low-income whites and was available for prescription in most states until the 1940's, when it was withdrawn from the market because of the restrictions of the Federal Marijuana Tax Act.

At that time the Federal Bureau of Narcotics persuaded most state legislatures to classify the drug incorrectly as a narcotic and to impose severe penalties for its possession and sale. The bureau mounted a propaganda campaign and convinced many people that marijuana served as a stepping-stone to heroin addiction. The media then accepted this unproven theory and helped propagate the myth that marijuana was a "killer weed" capable of triggering crimes of violence, acts of sexual excess, and insanity in anyone.

This and other absurdities were widely accepted by Americans during the 1940's and 1950's, but neither scare tactics nor strict law enforcement curtailed consumption of the drug. In fact, these efforts only seemed to have three undesirable results. They hampered scientific research on the chemical; they increased its price on the black market; and they prompted those who identified with minorities to begin using marijuana themselves.

Among them were bohemians who lived in areas like the Haight-Ashbury, where the drug was easily obtainable from Negro dealers and considered a natural part of the low-income life-style. Like millions of people today, the beats viewed the prohibition against marijuana as an inappropriate social sanction which conflicted with their own eupsychic ethic. Many were induced by peer-group pressure to try the drug, and their willingness to do so was increased by its illegality. In addition, the deceitful manner in which the Federal Bureau of Narcotics attacked marijuana only intensified their estrangement from society.

But marijuana use and abuse were too widespread in the Haight to be passed off as manifestations of conformity, alienation or rebellion. Indeed, most of the bohemians employed the drug as a cheap substitute for alcohol. Some used marijuana to induce sleep, for example, or as a tranquilizer. Others smoked the drug to disinhibit themselves or to relieve anxiety. Most, as many still do, believed it created a sensation of intimacy at their gatherings. This was ironic, for although they said that marijuana brought them closer together, they usually drifted apart and became less communicative while stoned.

For whatever purpose they employed marijuana, the beats seemed to get from it what they desired. The wide range of their expectations therefore led to many different patterns of use and abuse within their colony. Many of the bohemians consumed marijuana experimentally or periodically but a few became confirmed pot heads and smoked from ten to fifteen marijuana cigarettes, or joints, daily. Many of these habitual abusers were probably potential alcoholics who considered their health improved by marijuana and were therefore likely to look on the drug as a form of therapy.

Such therapeutic usage increased in the Haight-Ashbury in 1963, until marijuana all but replaced alcohol as the social and medicinal agent of choice in the colony. A few of the more disturbed beats even touted the chemical as a panacea for all personal problems, but most were sophisticated enough to realize that it offered only temporary relief. Because of this, they never invested marijuana with the same significance that their younger successors in the Haight and elsewhere were to do. The only drugs which they did exaggerate in importance were the hallucinogens.

The Unity of All Things

The hallucinogens are a number of compounds from different pharmacological classes that are able to disorganize nerve and ego functions and thereby induce a toxic psychosis or acute brain syndrome. The word hallucinogenic is most commonly used to describe their effects, but the terms "psychotomimetic" and "psychedelic" have also been employed. The drugs' toxic state is characterized by pseudohallucinative perceptual alterations which may culminate in real hallucinations and paranoid behavior.

Although a wide range of natural alkaloids and synthetic agents can produce such toxicity, Dr. Meyers divides the hallucinogens into several main categories. One of these contains four groups of sympathomimetic stimulants. The first two groups of stimulants include the amphetamines, which produce hallucinations in high doses but are more frequently abused for their euphoriant effects, and the hallucinogenic amphetamine congeners or psychotomimetic amphetamines, such as STP (DOM) and MDA. These latter compounds combine the mood-elevating action of amphetamines with the perception-altering effects of LSD.

Another group of sypathomimetic stimulants includes the phenylethylamine derivatives, of which mescaline is an example. This compound, which is known chemically as trimethoxyphenylethylamine, is an alkaloid derived from the peyote cactus, *Lophophora williamsii,* that grows wild in southwestern United States and Mexico. Peyote has been employed by Indians of these regions as a religious agent for centuries. It has also been worn as an amulet and has been administered by shamen to people suffering from alcoholism.

Mescaline was synthesized in 1918, but its use was limited to the peyote-using Indians' Native American Church until 1955, when Aldous Huxley took four hundred milligrams of the drug in the garden of his southern

California home. Huxley then published a report of his experience, *The Doors of Perception,* in which he argued for eupsychic education in the "nonverbal humanities" as well as book learning, and urged others "to take an occasional trip through some chemical Door in the Wall into the world of transcendental experience."

The fourth and final group of sympathomimetic stimulants used to obtain such experience are the tryptamine derivatives. The best known of these is psilocybin, or 4-hydroxydimethyltryptamine, an alkaloid of the mushroom *Psilocybe mexicana.* Two synthetic tryptamine derivatives, DMT (dimethyltryptamine) and DET (diethyltryptamine) have also gained popularity because they can induce a businessman's trip; that is, an intense and short-acting intoxication.

The second major class of hallucinogens includes the parasympatholytic agents. These include the belladonna alkaloids atropine and scopolamine, both of which cause a toxic psychosis that is distinguished by delirium and amnesia in addition to perceptual alterations. These compounds are available in such nonprescriptive medications as Sominex, Sleepeze and Compoz. They are employed occasionally for their hallucinogenic properties, although such use is deterred by their unpleasant peripheral effects.

Also employed are a third class of chemicals, the sedative-hypnotic-general anesthetics. These drugs are not true hallucinogens, but people have been known to take alcohol, marijuana and such dangerous agents as phencyclidine, or Sernyl, for the dreamlike state they can produce. Others have inhaled nitrous oxide, or laughing gas, the dental anesthetic praised by William James in *The Varieties of Religious Experience.* Still others have eaten nutmeg or inhaled the volatile hydrocarbons in model airplane cement, gasoline and cleaning fluids.

The fourth class of hallucinogens designated by Dr. Meyers is a miscellaneous category that includes narcotic antagonists and such medications as amantadine and methysergide. Although these drugs are available, they, the sedative-hypnotic-general anesthetics and the parasympatholytic agents are generally employed only in the absence of a fifth and final class of hallucinogens. This includes the lysergic acid derivatives, of which the most famous is LSD.

Lysergic acid diethylamide occurs naturally in plants and is common to the ergot alkaloids, a number of substances obtained from the fungus ergot, which grows on rye. Ergot gives rise to several compounds, including ergotamine and ergonovine, which are used in the treatment of migraine headaches and to contract the uterus after childbirth. LSD was first synthesized in 1938 by Dr. Albert Hofmann at the Sandoz Pharmaceutical Company in Switzerland as an intermediate leading to ergonovine. Seven years later, he accidentally ingested the compound, underwent a toxic psychosis, and discovered its effects for the first time.

As a sympathomimetic agent, LSD causes an increase in blood pressure, a dilation of the pupils, a relaxation of the bronchial muscles and other peripheral actions that are similar to, but less than, those generated by other stimulants. The drug is also unusual in that as little as one hundred micrograms can produce stimulative and hallucinogenic central effects which are three hundred times more powerful than those resulting from a much larger dose of mescaline. These effects last as long as twelve hours and serve as the prototype of the hallucinogenic or psychedelic experience.

The most spectacular phase of this intoxication includes a kaleidoscopic play of visual and auditory illusions. Perceptual distortions are so pronounced that users usually perceive objects and thoughts in a totally unfamiliar way. Memories and fantasies may rush before their eyes; colors may seem brighter and more beautiful; sounds may appear to be distorted and/or amplified. Hallucinogenic drug users may also experience synesthesia, a perceptual change in which one type of sensory input is translated into another, so that they "hear" colors and "see" sounds.

LSD and the hallucinogens also produce an emotional lability which is characterized not necessarily by euphoria but more often by marked changes in mood. All feelings may be magnified during the drug's intoxicating phase, and their users may go through highs and lows in which they become extremely sensitive to internal and external stimuli. They may become happy when they recall a pleasant moment, for example, and then grow increasingly sad when they remember or observe a painful scene.

Concurrent with this lability is an increased sensitiveness to interpersonal relations. Persons using hallucinogenic agents may become frightened by unfamiliar people and often develop an enhanced relationship with the guides who may — and should — lead them through their intoxication. Since the users are in a dependent state, they may relate to these guides as parents and grow increasingly suggestible to their instructions.

Users rarely lose consciousness, and can often recollect the entire content of their experience. But their thinking, capacity for making judgments and coordination are likely to be impaired. Thoughts appear to move much faster during the hallucinogenic intoxication than they do under normal consciousness, and they neither think in a logical nor in a causal way. Phenomena which are usually perceived as being opposite can therefore suddenly coexist; good and bad may appear equal, and people may feel light and heavy at the same moment. Most important, space and time orientation are frequently distorted much more than they are with marijuana, allowing past and future to merge with the present. People using the drugs seem to desire this state of timelessness more than any other effect and prefer to avoid anything that detracts from its intensity.

According to Dr. Dernburg, this intensity results from the fact that the hallucinogens can cause a dynamic psychological regression and temporarily suspend ego boundaries, thereby blurring the border between inner and outer worlds. Because these boundaries are absent at birth, the very young child cannot differentiate between itself and its environment and may actually consider its mother's breast an extension of its own body. The infant lives beyond time and space in a state of psychological symbiosis with the external world which is comparable to the physical symbiosis it enjoyed in its mother's womb.

From this original state, which the psychologist Jean Piaget has called "protoplasmic consciousness," the development of ego boundaries, ego functions and personal autonomy is a slow and often incomplete process. Sigmund Freud explained in *Civilization and its Discontents* that "originally the ego includes everything, although later it detaches from itself the external world. The ego feeling we are aware of now is thus only a shrunken vestige of a far more extensive feeling — a feeling which embraced the universe and expressed an inseparable connection of the ego with the external world."

Freud believed that artists and mystics strove to recapture this feeling through their creative and contemplative efforts. He also thought that it could be known to other people at the height of sexual intimacy. But subsequent investigation has revealed that the "oceanic oneness" of which he wrote can be artificially induced by hallucinogenic agents. As a case in point, the authors and many other individuals who take or have taken the drugs feel that they experience a form of protoplasmic consciousness which is so pronounced they seem to lose their personal identities and become parts of a larger whole.

This allows them to feel uniquely close to all living things. It also makes them think they have transcended so-called ordinary existence, as well as the shackles of time and space, and have understood the world. Central to this perception is the sensation that behind the apparent multiplicity of objects that are fragmented by ego consciousness lies a single, infinite reality. Some LSD users believe they have visited this reality. Others claim that the drug enables them to jettison their egos and join what has been called "the unity of all things."

This feeling of ego abandonment is sometimes accompanied by an extreme dissolution of the personality in which ego boundaries are severely disturbed. The dissolution leads people to lose their sense of self and can cause a terrifying feeling of unreality with messianic delusions. It can also result in depression and periodic flashbacks or perceptual distortions months after the hallucinogenic experience. In certain cases, people can be so panicked by these adverse reactions that they renounced the drug. In others, the toxic hallucinogenic psychoses seem to trigger more permanent disturbances.

Although many people interviewed at the Clinic enjoy becoming toxically psychotic, their condition bears a strong resemblance to that suffered by chronic schizophrenics. Because of this, the first scientists who worked with LSD believed that it induced a so-called model psychosis which might either provide a biochemical clue to the understanding of mental illness or lead to the discovery of an antidote that might prove effective in combating schizophrenia. This line of thought showed great promise fifteen years ago, but it was ultimately refuted by other scientists. It was learned, for example, that the toxic hallucinogenic psychosis only approximates that of schizophrenia, for schizophrenics have no insight into their mental states and experience many more hallucinations, including severe auditory recriminations, than do people using LSD. The model psychosis theory was therefore discredited, and biochemical research conducted on the drug also proved fruitless. But the medical profession was not willing to abandon LSD entirely. Further research was therefore initiated to determine whether the drug might be valuable as a therapeutic agent in itself or as an adjunct to psychotherapy.

The first investigators who worked therapeutically with LSD were enthusiastic. But while their glowing reports were coming in, scientists in the Bay Area and elsewhere were growing increasingly skeptical about the drug's promise. One was Dr. Jerome Oremland, a psychoanalyst who was treating patients who were concomitantly having carefully supervised LSD sessions at the Mental Research Institute in Palo Alto. These patients generally were moderately severe compulsive and obsessive neurotics. Many were engineers educated to the doctoral level who described symptoms similar to those seen in the Haight-Ashbury bohemians. The patients felt cut off from their own feelings and from other people. They complained of emptiness and meaningless in life and hoped that LSD would reduce their defensiveness and help them achieve spontaneity.

Dr. Oremland was initially impressed when his patients said that they felt improved by the hallucinogenic experience and could suddenly love, feel, and appreciate music for the first time. However, he ultimately concluded that LSD created only an illusion of improvement. The positive personality changes his patients reported seemed to be due either to messianic identifications or to the drug's toxic effects. Since many people spoke of their experience as an achievement, Dr. Oremland likened it to a test, a fearsome challenge which, once lived through, increased not a person's self-awareness but his self-esteem. This feeling of enhanced worth was a part of the hypomanic period that often follows the hallucinogenic experience with its characteristically wild flight of ideas.

Because the messianic state lingered in certain cases, Dr. Oremland realized that LSD could precipitate psychoses and permanent ego boundary disturbances. When this occurred, users often saw themselves as peace-loving spiritual leaders who were called upon to baptize others into the LSD fold. One striking example was a highly trained research worker who became an ardent proselytizer for peace, love and acid as his family life, professional standing and thinking disintegrated. Other experiences led Dr. Oremland to realize that psychotics were occasionally using the drug and its effects to disguise their own mental dysfunctioning and hide their psychoses under a chronic LSD state. He feared that they might attempt to introduce others to hallucinogens to disturb their functioning. This would allow them to avoid recognizing how disturbed they themselves actually were.

The possibility of such massive psychological disturbance, the lack of objectivity in LSD research, and the realization of the drug's probable chemical dangers, led in 1963 to LSD being discounted as an adjunct to or as primary agent in psychotherapy by the San Francisco Psychological Association, which anticipated Dr. Oremland's and other's findings. But neither that organization nor similar groups across the country could dampen public interest in the compounds. They had entered their popular era by this point, and thousands who should have known better were enraptured by LSD.

Among them were bohemians in the Haight-Ashbury and elsewhere who were tired of book learning and eager to take the "occasional trip" Aldous Huxley recommended. They believed that LSD could heighten their esthetic and philosophic acumen. They looked upon the hallucinogens as therapeutic agents which could give them instant satori and help them feel.

The beats viewed their guides as peyote shamen and established a ritual around the hallucinogens in the Haight and elsewhere. At the same time, they became interested in the American Indian, whom they saw as a noble savage mistreated by the white man. Some bohemians endowed the Indian with their own alienation and were attracted by his naturalistic religion, his tribal culture and, most important, his supposed psychological primitivism.

They had once looked to black culture for similar reasons, but the Negro had little use for the inner trip enjoyed by his white companions. Black Power was also forcing the races apart at this point, and the failure of the civil rights movement and the emergence of Vietnam as a more consuming white issue tended to lessen the beats' involvement with the Negro. Although many still thought of themselves as "white Negroes," some began to follow American Indian–oriented messiahs who were creating a new, psychedelic life-style.

New Heroes to Join the Old

Drs. Richard Alpert and Timothy Leary were two such messiahs. They began taking psilocybin and other hallucinogens in the early 1960's and subsequently administered them to students at Harvard. This led to their dismissal from the university in 1963, but they continued to proselytize for LSD in a drug manual they wrote, *The Psychedelic Experience*. Drs. Alpert and Leary then became involved in the Esalen Institute at Big Sur, an organization inspired by Aldous Huxley's call for the "nonverbal humanities," established a League for Spiritual Discovery in upstate New York, and assembled a road show to deliver the now famous gospel of "turn on, tune in, drop out" to the world.

Their California counterpart was Ken Kesey, whom Tom Wolfe has recreated in *The Electric Kool-Aid Acid Test*. Kesey was studying writing at Stanford and researching a book on North Beach in 1959, when he participated in a series of drug experiments at a hospital in Menlo Park. The experiments were soon concluded, but he continued taking hallucinogens and writing down his fantasies. The result was *One Flew Over the Cuckoo's Nest*, a novel narrated by a schizophrenic Indian named Chief Broom. It became a best seller in 1962, while its author emerged as a folk, as well as a literary, hero.

Kesey's next novel was also well received, but he had moved from art to chemicals by this time and was acting out his fantasies instead of turning them into literature. To facilitate this, he rented a house in the hills behind Stanford and began activities which made the League for Spiritual Discovery seem like a finishing school by comparison. Kesey called himself the Chief after Chief Broom and surrounded himself with admirers whom he dubbed the Merry Pranksters. Then, anticipating Marshall McLuhan, he invested his royalties in sound and film equipment and began holding parties at which Allen Ginsberg, Neil Cassady and other bohemians could sample hallucinogens.

The parties continued until 1964, when Kesey and crew bought an ancient school bus and painted its body in fluorescent, Day-Glo colors. They then loaded the bus with sleeping bags, DMT, DET, mescaline, LSD and other drugs and set off across the country. The Pranksters took nicknames and started calling themselves acid heads en route. When they finally re-

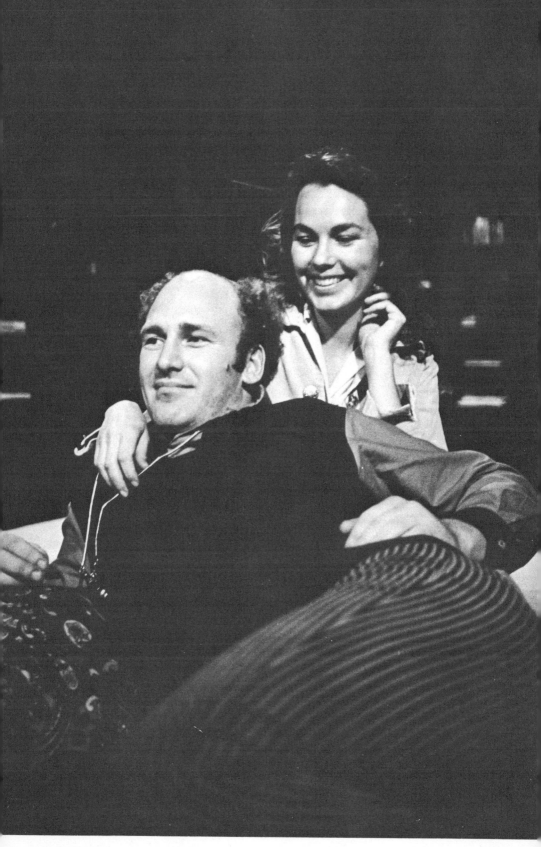

La Honda: Ken Kesey and his wife Faye.
(Jim Marshall)

turned to La Honda, they had institutionalized nomadism as an integral facet of their new life-style.

The close living arrangement on the bus had also given them a feeling of group protoplasmic consciousness which apparently appealed to the Chief. So did a book entitled *Stranger in a Strange Land*. This science fiction novel by Robert Heinlein concerns a character named Valentine Michael Smith, a human who is raised from infancy by Martians and in the process acquires hypnotic and magical powers. He returns to earth and is tutored in and shielded from temporal reality by a lawyer named Jubal. He then sets out, in a panoply of disguises, to save mankind from itself by propagating children who possess his abilities and by "discorporating," or casting into another dimension, those who stand in his way.

One of Valentine Smith's first acts is to establish a "nest," or extended family, with some twenty members, most of them women, who follow him in worshiping children for their so-called innocence, lack of socialization and intrinsic virtue. Smith sexually initiates the female members into the family. They eat, sleep and "share water" (possibly a hallucinogenic substance) together, while existing in a state of undifferentiated consciousness in which they "grok," or telepathically understand one another. From this womblike nest, Smith emerges as a Christ figure who ultimately saves the world.

Kesey apparently assumed that *Stranger in a Strange Land* had been inspired by his odyssey. He had already rendered the beats' gripe sessions obsolete with his La Honda parties and therefore set out to initiate others with LSD. In August of 1965, he introduced the Hell's Angels to hallucinogens after explaining that "you bust people's bodies — I break their minds." He then came up with new entertainments to win younger, straight people (who were once called squares) to his side.

These were the acid tests, all night carnival-cum-revival meetings at which costumed celebrants could prove their ability to survive hours of psychedelic art and superamplified music after drinking a sacramental punch — Electric Kool-Aid in Tom Wolfe's idiom — laced with LSD. The sacrament for these soirées came from Augustus Owsley Stanley III, the first person to amass a fortune from the manufacture of nonpharmaceutical hallucinogens. The art consisted of body painting and a rudimentary light show. The music, later identified as acid rock, was furnished by the Grateful Dead, a group which tried to produce a sensory bombardment that duplicated and enhanced the hallucinogenic experience.

While the Dead was playing at acid tests through the Bay Area, other long-haired musicians in the Haight-Ashbury were also spreading word about LSD. Most of these musicians had been folk performers who traced their origins through Bob Dylan and the Beatles to Negro blues. The musicians formed small groups and went by such names as the Charlatans, Quicksilver Messenger Service, Big Brother and the Holding Company and Jefferson Airplane. They and the Grateful Dead were initially responsible for what Ralph Gleason of the *Chronicle* has called the San Francisco Sound.

Also essential to the Sound were two promotors. One was Chet Helms, a dropout from a Baptist college who belonged to a communal organization called the Family Dog that eventually sponsored weekend acid tests, now called dance concerts, at the Avalon Ballroom in San Francisco. The other was Bill Graham, an intense Jewish war orphan, former office manager for Allis-Chalmers, and producer of the radical San Francisco Mime Troupe, who rented the Fillmore Auditorium, a dilapidated dance hall once used by Negro entertainers at the northern mouth of the Fillmore ghetto, and gave dance concerts of his own.

The final ingredient for the dance concerts was their audience. The beats had originally popularized the acid tests, but these events were now being attended by younger people as well. Some were merely curious onlookers. Others were students and dropouts in their early twenties from San Francisco State, the University of California and other local colleges. Many of the young people were passive members of the New Left who saw Kesey's eupsychic life-style as a peaceful and productive alternative to Vietnam and President Johnson's Great Society. Most lived in the Haight-Ashbury, where they were accepted by the old community. Few knew their numerical strength, but they would soon.

The person responsible was Ken Kesey, who held a huge coming-out party for his followers with Bill Graham and a Prankster named Stewart Brand in January of 1966 at the San Francisco Longshoremen's Hall. Over ten thousand participants attended this three-day orgy of sight and sound, and although the Chief left the city a few days later to escape prosecution for possession of marijuana, the press was alerted to the existence of the psychedelic movement he and Drs. Leary and Alpert helped establish in the Bay Area. A reporter from the *San Francisco Examiner* then studied the rapidly swelling colony in the Haight-Ashbury. In February of 1966, the media term "hippie," a derivation of Norman Mailer's Hipster, was born.

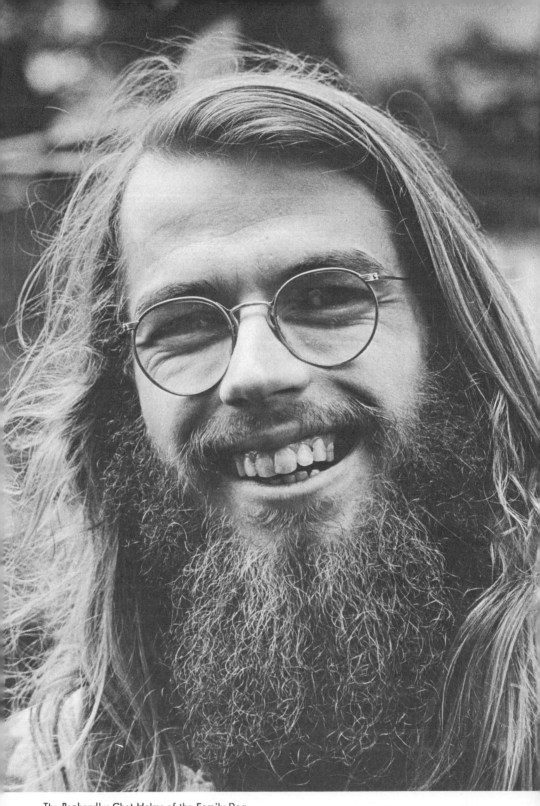

The Panhandle: Chet Helms of the Family Dog.
(Jim Marshall)

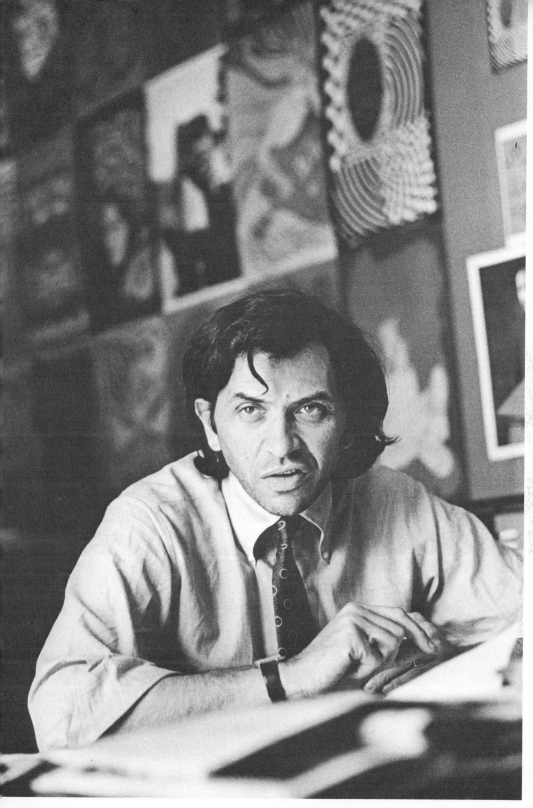

The Fillmore Auditorium: Bill Graham — "The P. T. Barnum of rock and roll."
(Jim Marshall)

From Bohemian
Colony to New
Community: The
Birth of Hip

The Birth of Hip was recognized by the hippies two months earlier when Ron and Jay Thelin, two San Francisco State students who took LSD on Dr. Alpert's advice, opened the Psychedelic Shop on Haight Street. Theirs was the first headquarters in America where acid heads and pot heads could meet. The Thelins stocked a small supply of books and pamphlets, including *Stranger in a Strange Land,* J.R.R. Tolkien's fantasy, *The Lord of the Rings, The Psychedelic Experience, The Doors of Perception* and the works of Marshall McLuhan. They also sold papers for rolling marijuana cigarettes. Their store did very well.

Other long-haired merchants soon followed the Thelins onto Haight Street. A former airline stewardess opened Mnasidika's, one of the first boutiques in the country to stock Carnaby Street clothes and American Indian costumes. Two men from Berkeley started the Print Mint, America's first psychedelic emporium, which featured the work of Alton Kelly, Rick Griffin and other poster artists and offered space to Allen Cohen's *Haight-Ashbury Oracle,* an underground paper livened by psychedelic art and utopian prose. In addition, a group of local hippies leased and began refurbishing the old Haight Theatre.

While these and others were transforming Haight Street, a similar facelifting was underway in the Flatlands, which were being mentioned in the Bay Area's oldest underground paper, the *Berkeley Barb.* Hundreds of young people were flocking to the area, but instead of living as couples in pads, they rented larger flats and entire houses that they turned into urban communes. Like the Grateful Dead, they decorated their residences with posters and LSD inspired art and spread mattresses on the floors. Over their doorways they hung God's eyes, peyote symbols made of twigs and yarn. The total effect was something never seen in San Francisco — or anywhere else — before.

The same could be said of the residents. These hirsute young people wore leather and paisley and looked like circus performers when compared with the colorless bohemians of years past. A few were older beats like Allen Ginsberg, who had adopted an Indian identity and the new psychedelic life-style. But most were self-acknowledged "gypsies" who never fully enjoyed the bohemian living arrangements. Most of these hippies saw themselves as cowboys or as "white Indians" who belonged to tribes.

The communes they occupied were loosely structured organizations which were based on an ideal of participatory democracy. Some were inhabited by several couples who engaged in little or no mate-swapping and

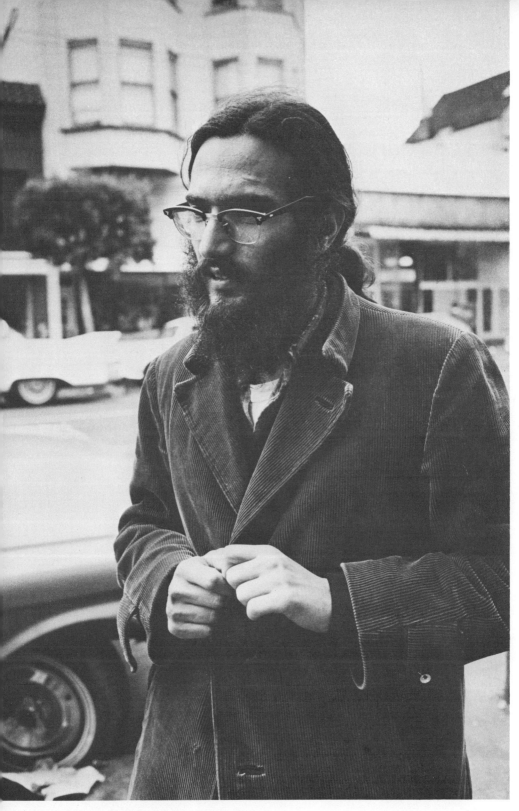

Haight Street: Allen Cohen of the Haight-Ashbury Oracle.
(Jim Marshall)

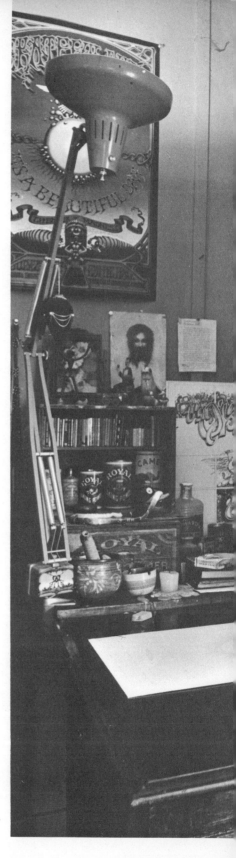

In his studio: Rick Griffin — "Zap."
(Elaine Mayes)

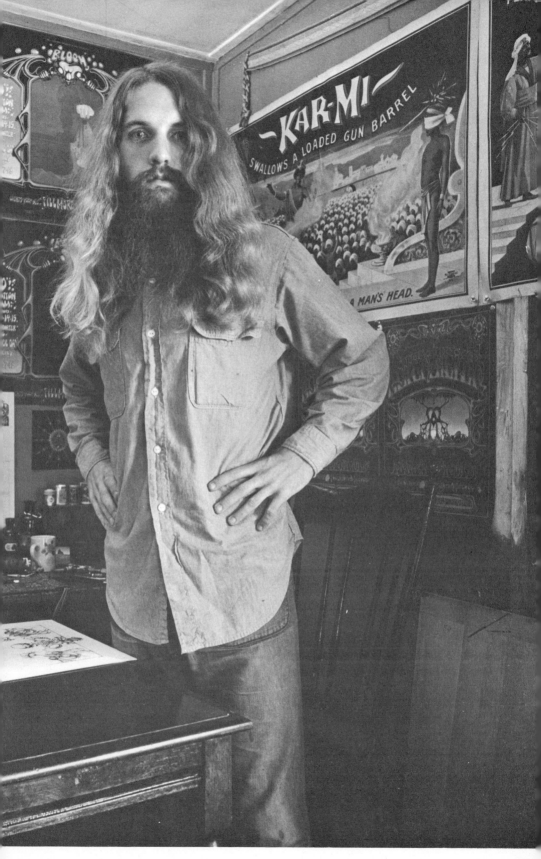

lived as one family. Others were group marriage communes similar to that described in *Stranger in a Strange Land* which were based around one young man or woman and the children they held in common. Most of these parent surrogates were experienced LSD gurus or maternal earth mothers who provided economical and/or emotional support for their extended families.

The young people who belonged to these families were only occasionally employed. Some worked at the post office or in the shops on Haight Street. Others ran errands for the rock groups, received allowances and tuition money from their parents, peddled underground papers, or sold the marijuana and hallucinogens that they more frequently gave away. The hippies often contributed their earnings to their families and tried to achieve a domestic tranquillity while exercising a eupsychic ethic of individual freedom based on Norman Mailer's sanction of psychopathy. This ethic was described by Ron Thelin as "the inalienable right of each person to act upon his impulses, to work out his creativity, to pursue his trip so long as he doesn't lay it on another man. It's called doing your thing."

Such philosophic anarchy often ran counter to the esprit de tribe, but the young people made every effort to maintain their precarious solidarity. They also extended their personal ethic into a political philosophy. Believing as Mailer did that man would prove to be more creative than destructive without social restraints, they wanted to tear down America's jails and provide unlimited freedom to all people, including the Hell's Angels. Their utopian model was an antiauthoritarian state with no regulations; as Mailer had suggested, the Hipster had no need for rules at all. The hippies viewed the Haight as a functional aggregation of tribes which belonged to a larger, Neo-American Church comparable to that of the peyote-using Indians. Theirs was a loose structure applicable to all society, they said. It was the basis of a brand-new kind of community.

This new community was characterized by four words its members used. The word nature conveyed their spiritual aspirations and identity with the Indian. The word peace meant a conclusion to the war in Vietnam and an end to hassles at home. The word free meant the same emotional spontaneity and permissiveness towards drug abuse, sexual experimentation and psychological problems that it had to the beats. But it also referred to a profitless and egalitarian distribution of the educational, medical, housing and nutritional resources of society.

Advocates of such freedom were the Diggers, young people who drew their name and thinking from a band of seventeenth-century English farmers who practiced utopian communism and considered private property the root of all social ills. The Diggers were alleged to have no leaders, but their

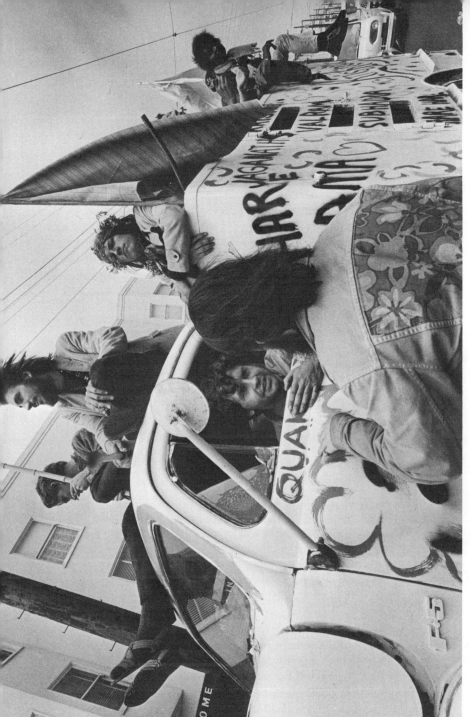

Haight Street: a Digger express, Arthur Lisch at the wheel.
(Elaine Mayes)

most avid spokesmen were Emmett Grogan, a former mental patient, and Arthur Lisch, a Quaker street worker who conceived of the new community as a national spawning ground not for drug abuse but for alternative social institutions. Lisch and other Diggers used the Hell's Angels as their police force. They set up a free soup kitchen in the Panhandle with food which they stole and scavenged, opened free stores where clothes were distributed to needy hippies, and supervised a number of large communes.

Although the Diggers were overtly hostile people, they used a fourth word common to the new community: love. The hippies invested love with a great many meanings, but it signified less an intimacy and mutual respect between two people than an all-embracing feeling for man and nature. This feeling was probably an extension of the oceanic oneness associated with LSD and the toxic afterglow of hallucinogenic experience — a toxicity so strong that the young people sought to dispense with ego boundaries and see themselves as part of a psychologically undifferentiated organism, a group mind.

The hippies wanted to include others in their collective organism. They knew that they had a better chance than the bohemians did before them. The beats had their therapies, but they could offer new converts only alcohol, marijuana, gripe sessions and philosophy and had little more than a small and rather limited colony to supplant the status quo. The hippies and the bohemians who identified with them had unlimited quantities of acid and saw their community as an open and accepting therapeutic alternative to middle-class white society. They therefore did everything in their power to help the new community grow.

But they soon encountered opposition. The first came in October of 1966, when a new law went into effect in California banning the possession of LSD. This statute did little to curtail consumption of the drug, and although the Sandoz Pharmaceutical Company removed its product from the market, Owsley and his imitators continued to make acid by the case, if not the carload. Yet the police from Park Station were encouraged by the state's action to begin raiding the local communes.

A second blow fell a few weeks later, when Ken Kesey returned to San Francisco, was apprehended by the FBI, and was denied another Trips Festival by Bill Graham, who feared the Chief might become the Elmer Gantry of the psychedelic movement. The hippies then ran afoul of merchants and homeowners, who asked the police not to allow them to lease property on Haight Street. The long-haired merchants countered by forming an independent association, H.I.P. — Haight Independent Proprietors — and securing representation in the Neighborhood Council. But tension continued to mount between the new community and the old.

It finally came to a head in December, when Richard Alpert and the Thelin brothers decided to hold a huge assembly in Kesey's absence at which they could collect their collective and show its strength to the world. A list of celebrities was drawn up, the Hell's Angels were signed on for protection and posters were passed out announcing "A Gathering of the Tribes for a Human Be-In — Saturday, January 14, 1967 — on the Polo Fields of Golden Gate Park — a Pow-Wow and Peace Dance to be Celebrated with Leaders, Guides and Heroes of our Generation."

It was hot and clear in San Francisco on January fourteenth, and more than twenty thousand people showed up on the Polo Fields in costumes as brief as the weather permitted. The Thelins were there, in light-colored robes, as thousands of LSD tablets were distributed among the multitudes. Allen Ginsberg, forty years old but dressed in the white coat of a hospital intern, smiled ecstatically as he delivered a short Buddhist prayer and introduced the master of the San Francisco Zen Center to start the event rolling. The Angels screamed up on their Harley-Davidsons shortly thereafter and guarded the sound truck on which the Grateful Dead and Jefferson Airplane were playing. Dr. Timothy Leary made his speech. A young man floated down from the sky on a paisley parachute, prompting groundless speculation that even the Chief had arrived.

The day continued peacefully, marred only by a prophetic scuffle between two innocent blacks and a few dozen Angels. Then, after the Quicksilver Messenger Service finished its performance, Ginsberg led the new community in a Hindu mantra. The sun sank slowly into the Pacific, as the bearded guru blew on a conch shell to herald the end of a perfect afternoon — and the beginning of a new age.

The Hippie Modality

Allen Ginsberg was not alone in thinking that the be-in had ushered in a new era. The hippies' spirit was infectious, and their gathering in Golden Gate Park sent emotional shock waves across the country. In fact, Bishop James Pike and several other prominent clergymen compared the young people to early Christians and interpreted their emergence as the first step in a long-awaited religious revival.

Equally impressed were those media which had hitherto dismissed the new community as an insignificant social phenomenon. More reporters were dispatched to the Haight-Ashbury after the be-in, some sporting beards and bohemian costumes, to infiltrate the tribes and document their occupants' supposed ecstasy. Lurid stories about "Life With the Love Gen-

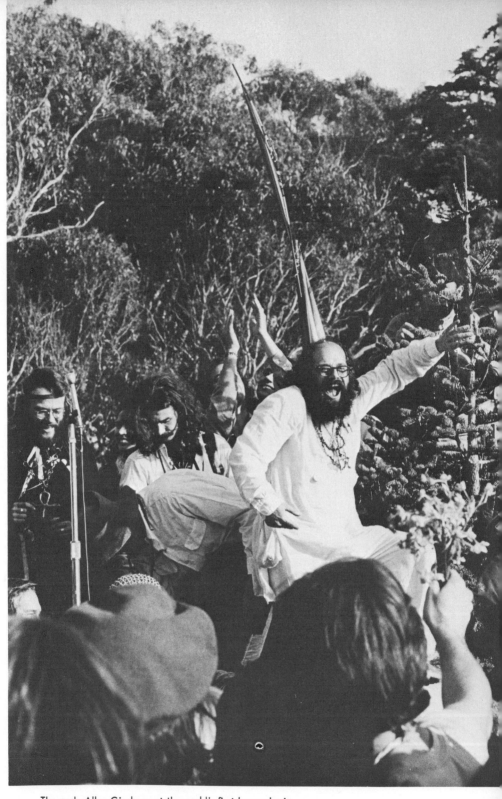

The park: Allen Ginsberg at the world's first human be-in.
(Jim Marshall)

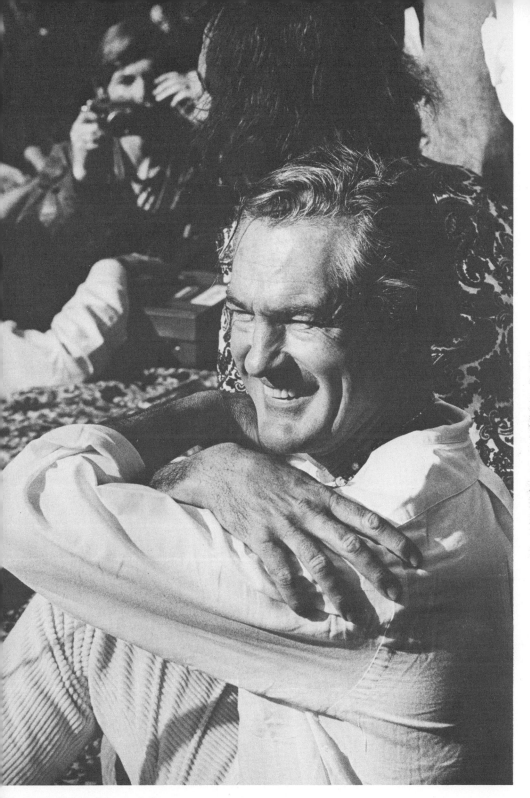

he park: Dr. Timothy Leary at the be-in.
(Jim Marshall)

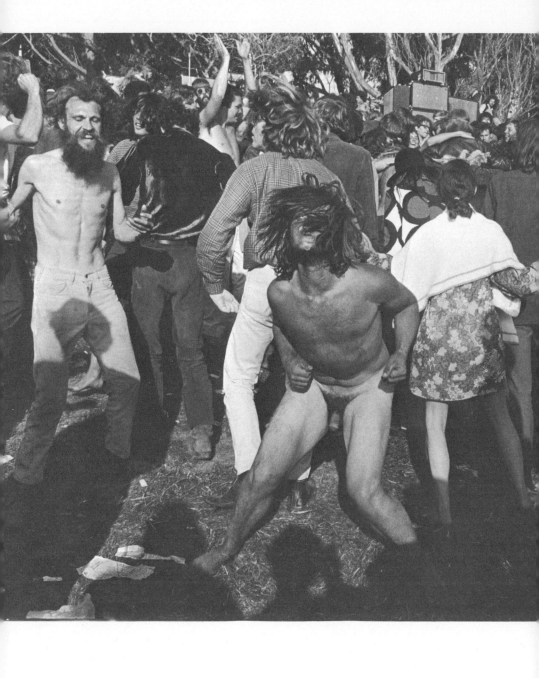

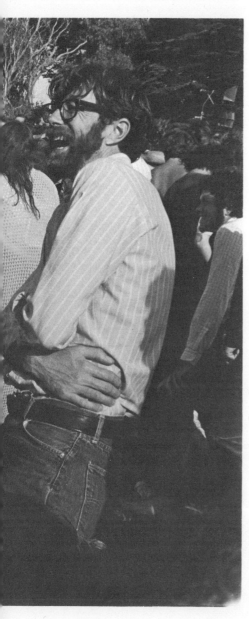

The park: a gathering of the tribes.
(Michael Alexander)

The park: backstage at the be-in.
(Jim Marshall)

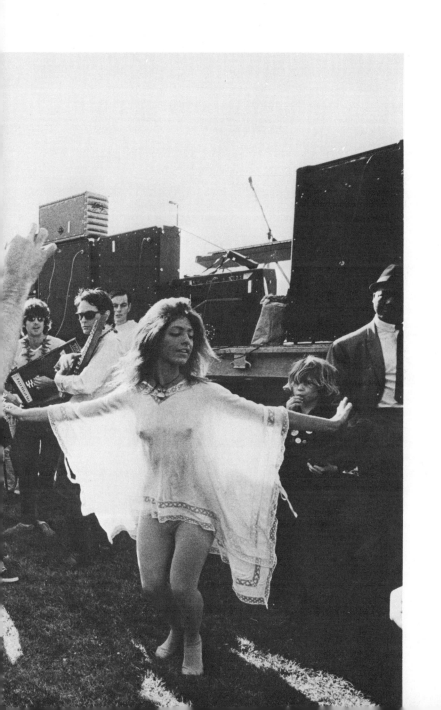

eration" started appearing in the straight press as a result, alongside glowing accounts in the *Oracle* and the *Barb*. By February of 1967, television crews were already bumping into one another on Haight Street and preparing the footage which would soon send the so-called flower children into living rooms around the world.

The media also helped create several "experts" on LSD in the process. One such authority, Marshall McLuhan, came to San Francisco, singled out the Haight's residents as a uniquely turned-on species, and then told the public not to be alarmed by their chemical consumption. These young people are on an exciting inner trip, he said; hallucinogenic drugs duplicate for them the tactile sensory experience others obtain from watching TV. Television is retribalizing the young, teaching them to absorb life through all their senses. The life-style of the Electronic Age is turning today's adolescents into evolutionally superior human beings.

McLuhan and others who claimed to speak for youth may have intended their remarks to ease pressure in the Haight-Ashbury. Yet they and the media only increased it by reinforcing the self-consciousness of the hippies. As the intellectual and religious worlds paid them homage, the young people began to see their new community as the national center of a counterculture, not a subculture, that was morally and spiritually superior to American society. This thought intensified the hippies' sense of independence. It prompted the Diggers and other leaders to increase their proselytizing. And it helped attract hundreds of people to the area.

Some were society matrons shopping in the H.I.P. boutiques or record company scouts bidding for their slice of the San Francisco Sound. Others were undercover narcotics agents and disturbed persons who hoped to hide their pathology in the all-accepting hip scene. But most were hippies who used marijuana and the hallucinogens exclusively, followed the eupsychic ethic of their spiritual forefathers, and continued to bring the Haight international fame.

They also brought it a host of new problems. The young people began gobbling up much of the available acid after they reached the district in their campers and school buses and prompted several second-rate Owsleys to start manufacturing LSD. They also squeezed into the crowded communes, thereby creating a housing shortage, a lack of sanitation and a rash of adverse hallucinogenic drug reactions the likes of which the Haight had never seen.

The housing shortage led in turn to the creation of crash pads, former communes that were turned into more transient quarters and often degenerated into flophouses because of their open occupancy. The Diggers established several crash pads in the property they rented, while the Thelin brothers converted the back of their Psychedelic Shop into a calm center for young people freaking out on LSD. An organization called the Hare Krishna Movement then opened the Krishna Consciousness Temple, a storefront shrine on Frederick Street, and offered refuge and free meals.

At the same time, Allen Ginsberg and other older beats and hippies apparently became upset by the confusion and alarmed by the prospect of even more overcrowding. They had helped establish and publicize the psychedelic movement, but they took no responsibility for their homeless followers. Instead, they left the district, swearing that whatever plans once existed for a therapeutic alternative had perished January fourteenth on the Polo Fields.

While this was occurring, a physician who would play an important role in the Haight-Ashbury Free Medical Clinic was coming to a similar medical appraisal of the new community. He was Dr. Ernest Dernburg, who was then serving as chief of outpatient psychiatric services at Letterman General Hospital in the San Francisco Presidio, training psychiatric residents at Mt. Zion Hospital near the Haight-Ashbury, and treating a number of hippies from the district in his private practice as well.

Dr. Dernburg initially felt that these young people resembled the older bohemians he had known in several ways, including their introversion, their spiritual searching, their alienation and the attention and self-protection they achieved through their costumes. But he soon realized that the two groups differed in other respects. In the first place, the hippies were much more anxious, depressed and passive than his earlier patients. And while the beats had wanted but could not obtain psychological primitivism, the hippies seemed to be so primitive in their mental functioning that they could not be considered bohemians.

Because of this, the young people could not be called eccentrics or schizoid characters. They could not be called psychopaths, either, for they generally exhibited a strong, if not harsh and punitive, sense of conscience. And not all of them could be labeled psychotic, although some seemed to be seriously disturbed. Because the hippies did not fit at first glance into the traditional psychiatric categories, Dr. Dernburg was reluctant to describe them diagnostically. Instead, he tried to understand them in terms of the psychological deficiencies and the impoverishment which appeared to distinguish them not only from the beats but also from others their age.

This impoverishment was perhaps most obvious in their poor symbol formation. When most people think or dream, they make up linear "movies" or "talk" to themselves. But many of the hippies apparently lacked this ability. Instead of dreaming or thinking sequentially, some of them experienced and focused on only immediate sensations of light, color and sound, a

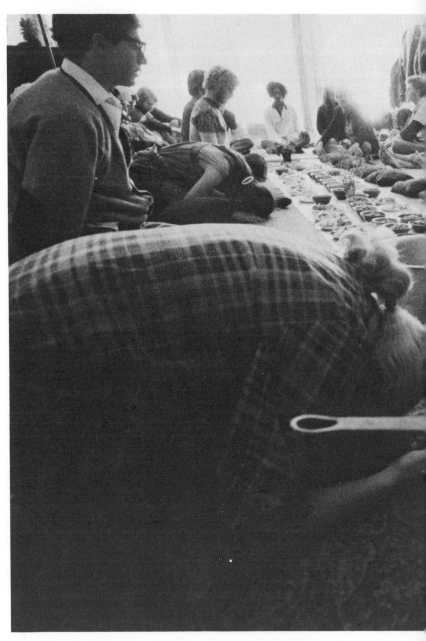

Frederick Street: a free meal at the Krishna Consciousness Temple.
(Elaine Mayes)

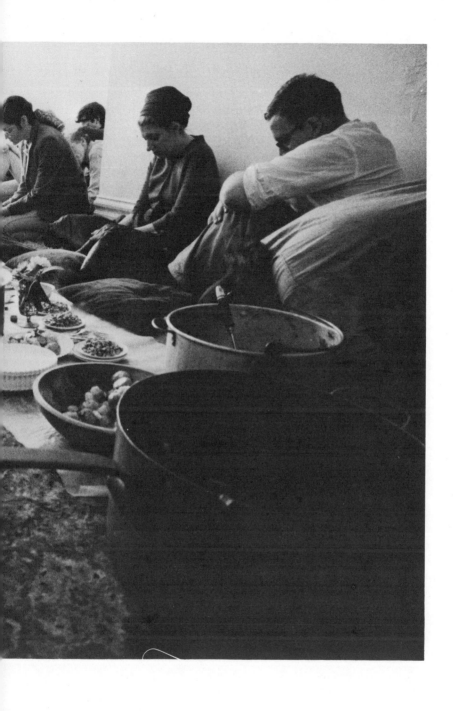

state which one patient compared to "having a screwed-up circus in my mind." Others exhibited more inner life, but their circuses were more chaotic and their feelings more confused.

This condition may have seemed promising to McLuhan and others who considered it an inner trip, but for most of Dr. Dernburg's patients the circuses never seemed to end. They either had such a limited fantasy life or such a tangle of painful emotions that they had nothing to make trips out of. In fact, they appeared to be stuck on a sensory level of psychological functioning and had great difficulty in using verbal and symbolic modalities.

Because of this, they could not make much sense out of the random impressions they received. And they could not create, for they had nothing cohesive enough to channel into artistic production. If creativity represents a "regression in the service of the ego," as Freud believed, it necessarily requires a reasonably intact ego to begin with. The bohemians seemed to possess this intactness, but their successors did not. Most said they wanted to be artistic and thought drugs would help them do their thing. Yet although some managed to join rock groups, shaking tambourines was all that others could do.

Furthermore, very few of the hippies could or would express themselves with words not included in their own special jargon. While the beats employed ghetto slang occasionally, the young people who followed them into the Haight-Ashbury took no pleasure in verbal gymnastics and apparently had to rely on the hip idiom all the time. Many described their reaction to every experience with such global terms as "groovy," "heavy," "wow," "far out" and "too much" and called everybody, including women, "man." McLuhan and others may have assumed that this jargon was simply part of a secret tribal language. Yet its vagueness and constant usage suggested to Dr. Dernburg that some hippies could not particularize their thoughts and feelings, that they assumed everyone saw the world as they did, and that they had neither the ability to communicate nor the desire.

Concomitant with this deficiency in the use of symbols was their lack of general knowledge. Most of Dr. Dernburg's patients had received some college education, but the information at their command was comparable to that seen in seventh- and eighth-grade students. They seemed to be totally ignorant about elementary mechanics, cooking, health and diet matters, first aid and personal hygiene, for example. Since the hippies were not unintelligent, their paucity of information seemed to indicate either that they had repressed previous knowledge or that experience had poured through them like water through a sieve.

Although this situation could have changed after they reached the new community, few of the young people appeared eager to learn. Some beats stopped reading to stress the liberation they allegedly achieved from taking drugs, but they generally did so only after years of serious study. Yet many of the hippies could not concentrate enough to read. The only books Dr. Dernburg's patients enjoyed were fantasies and science-fiction stories like *Stranger in a Strange Land* and *Lord of the Rings,* which were so concrete they were not called upon to fill in the chinks with their own imagination. Other material they found too taxing and not immediately gratifying. So, apparently as a corollary to their deficiency in the formation and use of symbols and their inability to delay gratification, they sought a constant and direct bombardment of the senses, particularly when they could regulate their sensory input with marijuana and the hallucinogens.

Here again, they differed significantly from the early bohemians. Both groups employed marijuana primarily as a social and medicinal agent, but only a few beats abused marijuana enough to be considered pot heads. Many hippies, on the other hand, exhibited the amotivational syndrome associated with chronic marijuana abuse to a marked degree. This suggested that some of them were so overwhelmed by anguish that they had to continually anesthetize themselves with marijuana. It also suggested that they employed the drug as a source of nurturance far more than the bohemians did. One patient indicated this when he said that "smoking pot is like plugging a breast into your brain."

Furthermore, while many of the young people insisted that they used LSD as a religious and therapeutic agent, they actually seemed less interested in acquiring philosophic insight then in taking chemically induced trips night and day. Some of them established elaborate and compulsive drug rituals as the beats did; they would meet at a prearranged hour, for example, select popular records to listen to, drop acid at the same moment, and repeat prayers as they became intoxicated. But others appeared to be so eager for the hallucinogenic experience that they would smoke or swallow almost anything said to be psychedelic in unsupportive settings to get high.

This suggested that some hippies had to subject themselves to potentially fatal acid tests to prove their mastery of the drugs and of their psychological processes. It also suggested that the more messianic and overtly disturbed were confusing themselves with the hallucinogens to disguise the fact that they were already quite confused, as Dr. Jerome Oremland observed several years earlier. And the quantities of chemicals they consumed seemed to indicate that those hippies who suffered from inner emptiness had to fill themselves up in every possible way.

This emptiness was so pronounced in certain cases that the young people appeared to be starved not only for strong emotions, but also for some tangible evidence that they were really alive. By upsetting their mental functioning with LSD, those with a limited fantasy life could turn the external world into a circus similar to their own mental states and thereby gain a feeling of vitality that masked their internal deadness. The more disturbed young people could create comparable circuses that masked their internal confusion. And by submitting themselves to their disordered environment, both types could obtain a sense of mastery over the chaos which had probably beset them since their early lives.

Both types also seemed to acquire some relief from their chronic depression and to convince themselves and others that they were turned on by obtaining a stimulation and a lingering hypomania with the drugs. This procedure may have led McLuhan and others to think that the hippies were ecstatic. But they appeared to be almost totally turned off to Dr. Dernburg. Why else, he wondered, would they continuously need to stimulate themselves?

Such selective self-stimulation showed up in many areas of their behavior. Dr. Dernburg's patients did not enjoy reading or engaging in intellectual pursuits, but they did spend hours drinking in bright colors, staring at sunsets and watching television. They also loved to taste exotic flavors, to wear textured fabrics, to inhale incense and to drench their bodies with patchouli and other scented oils. As McLuhan observed, they did soak up life through their senses, if not through their pores.

Yet they never seemed able to engage it. The beats who first popularized dance concerts would snake their way through the Fillmore Auditorium and the Avalon Ballroom, but many hippies merely sprawled before the bandstand, stoned on drugs. A few rose to dance, to shake their bodies, or to stick their heads into speakers that blasted out music so loud it could literally move their inner organs. Yet the rest stayed rooted to the floor. Most of them said they were excited in such situations. But with their dull and vacant faces, they looked as though they were watching TV.

This comparison was further suggested by the nature of the dance concert form. Because the auditory and visual stimuli were omnipresent in Bill Graham's and the Family Dog's environments, the young people could follow them with a minimum of mental effort and tune in and tune out of the sensory barrage at will, as they could while observing television. They could also stimulate themselves impersonally with color and music, instead of by interacting with their companions. Thus, they seemed to employ dance concerts, as they did drugs, to avoid close personal contact and to substitute for it the sensory richness and/or distraction they seemed to require. Such avoidance may have been necessary in many cases, for they appeared to relate better to electronic media than to other human beings.

This impoverishment in their relationships was not initially obvious to Dr. Dernburg, for his patients and the hippies he was observing talked about love and spent much more time with one another than the beats did. Yet although most of them lived, ate, and slept together, many told him that they still felt alone. The young people seemed to gain genital gratification from members of the opposite sex, but their relationships were usually of an anaclitic, or leaning-on, variety. Instead of maintaining individuality, they would cling together for support, feed one another, and smother their companions with a nurturance which seemed to be unconsciously intended for themselves.

Many hippies had pets, not the vicious Doberman pinschers and German shepherds later seen in the Haight-Ashbury, but meeker cats and stray dogs to which they would also allot their nurturant feelings and their food. Some of the young women also had children whom they treated like strays and orphans, a fact which probably revealed how they thought about themselves. Other females appeared anxious to have babies on whom they could bestow a similarly self-directed tenderness. Men and women alike related to their contractual or common-law spouses as pseudoparents and called them "my old lady" or "my old man."

The young people invested little intimacy in these relationships; instead of communicating and growing together, they appeared to engage in impersonal and rather monotonous sex, especially in those communes whose population changed from day to day. Although McLuhan apparently found these living arrangements fulfilling, they may actually have been an escape from involvement, for by surrounding themselves with people, the hippies could partially relieve their loneliness and still keep from encountering one person at a time. The shallow and transient quality of their relationships suggested to Dr. Dernburg that they were both unable to differentiate one person from another and unwilling to become involved.

Underlying this unwillingness, he believed, was a third area of impoverishment: their difficulty in handling sexual and aggressive drives. According to psychoanalytic theory, these drives are genetically determined psychic constituents that act like biological live forces and can be separated in infancy into erotic and aggressive components. They fuse during late adolescence and early adulthood to a certain extent, finding their ultimate expression in sexual intercourse between partners of the opposite sex who are not excessively attached to their parents and can therefore display tender and loving, as well as sexual and aggressive feelings. But if the Oedipal relationship is not resolved in growing up, people may experience a "failure of fusion" which manifests itself in so-called perversions, in excessive passivity or aggressiveness, in erotic preoccupations, in promiscuity and in other extremes.

It was these extremes that Dr. Dernburg noticed in the hippies. Although few of his patients and the young people he was observing in the Haight were overtly homosexual, they did pal around with members of the same sex to a marked degree. Many of the males also seemed much more passive and the females much more aggressive than others their age. Some of them shied away from any and all sex, even though it was often thrust upon them. Others apparently could not sublimate their sexual impulses and had to ball several times daily. Most could not show tenderness and aggressiveness concurrently, seemed to enjoy sex only for its impersonality, and valued others not for who they were but for whatever need they could satisfy.

These facts, coupled with their avoidance of involvement, suggested to Dr. Dernburg that leaving home was a precipitously employed defense for his patients, particularly those confused ones who tried to screen out all intrusive stimuli. He decided that many of them had not resolved their Oedipal attachments before coming to the Haight-Ashbury. They had probably been overstimulated by their parents and were therefore unable to deal with the seductiveness of others or with their own sexual drives.

While he was coming to this conclusion, Dr. Dernburg was seeing a similar difficulty in the hippies' handling of aggressive impulses. Instead of channeling their aggressiveness into physical competition as many do or into the intellectual and esthetic competition preferred by the bohemians, many of these young people professed no desire to compete. The Diggers could be combative, but their companions often associated aggressiveness with violence, dismissed the assertion necessary for success as an ego trip, and projected an attitude of the utmost submissiveness and humility.

The hippies' anger did manifest itself in their provocative attitude toward policemen, in the assaultive lyrics of their music and in their desire to blow other people's minds. Yet they insisted that they had "stopped feeling angry" after they started taking LSD. In addition, many indicated that they dropped acid when they were becoming annoyed by their companions and said that they sustained a better chance of having bad trips when others riled them.

Because of this, Dr. Dernburg suspected that the only way the young people could fight off their hostile feelings was to distract themselves with music, to direct the emotions against themselves and thereby intensify their depressions, or to depersonalize their feelings by losing themselves in the hallucinogenic experience. They also seemed to reinforce the peaceful aspects of their behavior by becoming involved in a nonviolent community which also enhanced their self-esteem. The early bohemians had used their colony for a similar purpose, but they also had psychologically sophisticated defense mechanisms to deal with unwanted feelings. Apparently the only defenses at some of the hippies' disposal were a repression, projection and/ or denial of all aggressive impulses, the isolation from potential anger-producing stituations they achieved in the new community, and the emotional defusing they gained from LSD.

This fact, coupled with their drug consumption, suggested that the dynamic regression characteristic of the hallucinogenic experience meant much more to the young people than it did to the beats before them. Many of the hippies seemed to require not only a defense against impulses and an amplification and regulation of sensory stimuli but also a continual feeling of protoplasmic consciousness through which they could reconstitute an earlier mother-child relationship and thereby obtain a sensation of nurturance and security.

Although the regressive pull that motivated them was not so powerful in the young people as it was in the habitual and multiple drug abusers who were then coming into the Haight, it was much stronger than that seen in the earlier bohemians. In fact, while the beats appeared to use hallucinogens primarily to achieve a feeling of rebirth and emotional liberation, the hippies apparently wanted to remain at or return to a primitive level of psychological functioning akin to becoming children again.

This was further indicated in a fourth area of impoverishment: the infantile and superstitious nature of their thinking. Whereas the bohemians dabbled in Zen, yoga and other disciplines, the young people who followed them into the Haight were fanatical about so-called therapies. Some of them jumped from one faith to another as often as they changed communes. Others seemed to settle on astrology or Krishna Consciousness at least temporarily and then attempted to understand the entire world through the narrow shutter of their new-found philosophy. In some cases, this behavior emphasized the extreme suggestibility of the young people and their need to have decisions made for them. In others, it indicated that they were either trying to impose an external order on their internal confusion or were groping for a belief to hang on to.

Ignorance of hygiene and physical reality also permeated their life-style. Some of Dr. Dernburg's patients stayed up on drugs for days, denying their need for rest and depriving themselves of REM sleep in the process. Others slept more often, but they did so in crowded and unsanitary crash pads or communes. Few of the hippies brushed their teeth, bathed regularly, or used their own sheets and towels. They went without shoes, allowed the lacerations they sustained to go untreated, and burned their skin by sitting in the sun.

In addition to this general neglect, the young people showed little sense in their diets. Some would shop at straight supermarkets, but others followed the nutritionally deficient vegetarian and/or macrobiotic regimens and would eat only organically grown cereals and grains they found at the Krishna Consciousness Temple or at health-food stores. And although these people ate religiously, if not regularly, many of their companions fasted at one time or another, went on exotic food trips, or tried to exist on brown rice alone.

Yet they insisted that these habits were therapeutic. They also professed a primitive faith in magic, believed that gurus and witch doctors could heal them, chanted such words as "Om" and "Hare Krishna" to get their heads together, and tried to cure psychological problems and physical sickness with incantations and spells. Their health code was far more at variance with reality than the Christian Science–like belief of the beats. Like their mystical aspirations, it was predicated on the infantile assumption that wishing can make things so.

The strength of this assumption suggested to Dr. Dernburg that the thought processes of some hippies were generally prelogical and similar to those observed in psychotic patients. Thus, whereas the early bohemians he treated had their share of illusions but still maintained a link with reality, many of the young people who followed them into the Haight had far-ranging and poorly organized delusions and were deficient in their reality-testing to a marked degree.

Such a deficiency undoubtedly contributed to a fifth area of impoverishment: their poor self-images and sense of identity. Although the beats also experienced complex identity problems and felt different from other people, the hippies considered themselves freaks, showed a singular lack of self-respect, and carried their differentness to a ridiculous extreme. Most did not attempt to make sickness a virtue as the speed freaks would. But they were so confused and/or hungry for stimulation that they had great difficulty taking care of themselves.

This inability, coupled with their other impoverishments, led Dr. Dernburg to conclude that many of his patients and some of the young people he was observing in the Haight-Ashbury were either overtly psychotic or borderline psychotics who probably externalized their confusion as the Hell's Angels did and thereby created a chaotic and self-destructive living pattern.

Both types of hippies had somehow regressed and/or plateaued in their psychological development, he decided. Both were trying to disguise their dysfunctioning and to deal with their problems by abusing drugs and by wearing the protective mantle of the psychedelic scene.

The young people were also using the Haight to sustain the illusion of evolutionary superiority to which Marshall McLuhan apparently subscribed. But superiority in biological terms is a measure of adaptability to stress and change. The hippies apparently lacked this adaptability. They seemed to be limited to an environment and a life-style that reflected and reinforced their psychological primitivism. Their community was not the independent counterculture they might have wished. It was actually a subculture which mirrored the straight world in its shortcomings, allowed its members to continue in their regression and/or plateauing, and depended on society.

Dr. Dernburg realized that the subculture contained many young people who differed from his patients. He was also aware that the hippies as a group were not totally representative of modern youth. Yet he felt that the personality traits of his patients and the hippies he was observing were common to a certain extent in many young Americans. Dr. Dernburg saw the members of the new community as an extreme of the social spectrum, an extreme which would grow and influence the entire spectrum in the future. Anticipating the clinical implications of this growth, and aware of the danger of clinical overgeneralization, he collectively identified their psychological dynamics as the hippie modality.

After reaching this rough diagnosis, Dr. Dernburg then addressed himself to the question of how the hippie modality arose. Other than social factors, one possibility was that his patients had become disturbed by hallucinogens and were exhibiting a chemically induced confusion. Another was that LSD had biochemically produced a permanent regression. A third possibility was that they had been born with ego defects which impaired later development. A fourth was that they had been psychologically damaged by their parents in their early lives.

Dr. Dernburg leaned toward the last possibility. He felt that the hippies' homes were similar to but significantly more harmful than those of the bohemians. The hippies whose thinking was extremely disorganized seemed to have been overstimulated in infancy by emotionally inconsistent mothers whose ego boundaries were severely disturbed. Others who were starved for sensation and protoplasmic consciousness appeared to have been deprived of nurturance by their parents. Although Dr. Dernburg supported the ideals of the hippies he felt that many had come to the Haight-Ashbury primarily to find families. Some of them reminded him of hospitalized infants who are not mothered sufficiently and therefore develop anaclitic depressions and become both psychologically moribund and inordinately susceptible to physical disease.

I Don't Feel So Dead Inside

One patient who prompted this thought was a thin, pale and anemic-looking young man named Alan. He was raised in southern California by strict Catholic parents who had little time or use for him. His father was brusque, distant, and greatly involved with his job as a minor executive in an electronics firm. His mother was preoccupied with achieving status in suburban society. Instead of caring for Alan and his younger sister, she treated the children like pieces of furniture to be shown off in front of friends. Instead of giving them her own limited warmth or even the maternal support of a babysitter, she left them in front of the TV.

Because Alan was never read to by his parents or encouraged to read by himself, he never gained an interest in literature. And because he rarely played with other children, he recalled few companions from his childhood other than his sister and the characters he saw on television. His parents fought frequently, and when they did, the TV room, which was located on the children's wing of their large ranch-style home, promised sanctuary. Television also provided a means through which Alan could obtain stimulation and sedation selectively.

By doing so, he never learned how to deal with other people. Alan developed asthma during grammar school and was kept from roughhousing with his peers. He took no pleasure in dating, sports or school work during high school but he did try to attract his parents' attention by earning good grades. When he was fourteen, his mother became seductive toward him, apparently to blackmail her husband into spending more time at home. Alan apparently started drinking to screen out his mother. Two years later he entered the University of California at Berkeley, where he hoped to escape her and find friends.

Alan initially enjoyed Berkeley and participated in campus political activities. But such issues as civil rights and the war in Vietnam soon began to worry him. Although his asthma made him draft-exempt, he sympathized strongly with those students who feared they would be forced into military service. And although he adopted an antiwar stance, he seemed to be upset by the anger sparked in him at protest rallies.

In 1966, halfway through his sophomore year, Alan gave up politics, grew his hair long and started hanging out at the coffeehouses on Telegraph Avenue. Yet he could not hold his own in conversations with the older bohemians. Unable to cope with the confusion on Telegraph Avenue, he soon turned to marijuana to relieve his anxiety. He went to southern California for the summer and was finally noticed by his father, who told him either to cut his hair or leave home. He left without an argument, returned to Berkeley, began wearing beads and buckskin and taking LSD. He then dropped out of school and joined a coeducational commune in the Haight-Ashbury.

Alan identified completely with the new community, channeled most of his energy into drugs, and became an authority on astrology. Although he was not old enough to be a guru, he gave free horoscope readings for the members of his commune. He also threw himself into rock music, went to the Fillmore on weekends, and tried to sign on as an equipment manager for one of the bands. This naturally increased the opportunity of having sex with the female groupies who also followed the musicians. But although Alan did have sexual intercourse on several occasions, he never permanently shacked up with an old lady and found that balling frequently brought him down. He therefore gave up women. By the time of the be-in, he was "spending more time in my head," and looked like a cross between Jesus Christ and Robinson Crusoe.

This martyr role did not make Alan unique in the Haight, but he took the Jesus trip very seriously. He was a firm believer in universal brotherhood and extended his acceptance to everyone. When he was stared at by straight people, he would smile gently as if forgiving them. When tempers threatened to flare up in his extended family, he would soothe his companions, often with LSD. He did all he could to maintain his faith in peace and love.

Alan's faith was fragile, however, and he suffered continual attacks on his self-esteem whenever he left the new community. This happened twice during January of 1967, when he visited downtown San Francisco to sell the *Oracle*. On his first afternoon there, Alan was berated by two intoxicated stockbrokers. On the second, he was harassed by a policeman and told to peddle his papers elsewhere.

A few days later, Alan was taking acid when one of the more aggressive females in his commune attempted to seduce him. He panicked; the girl turned to another man. This incident stirred his feelings, for he soon began to see hideous monsters — creations of his own projected anger — which threatened to engulf and devour him. The anxiety caused by these hallucinations then precipitated an acute asthma attack which was complicated by the bronchial-constricting effects of LSD and by the dust-filled atmosphere in which he was taking the drug. His panic mounted to the point where he thought he was going to die.

Alan survived this acute episode by smoking marijuana and by taking a massive dose of antipsychotic medication. But three days after his first adverse hallucinogenic reaction he began to experience uncontrollable flashbacks in which he recounted several unpleasant childhood memories. He was so frightened by the emotions generated during the flashbacks that he sought psychiatric help at Mt. Zion Hospital, where he was eventually seen by Dr. Dernburg, to whom he explained his feelings about drug consumption.

I just don't know what's happening. I got so paranoid I thought everyone was after me — Like I've dropped acid maybe fifty times in the last couple months and nothing like that — I don't — it just never happened before. I mean I dig acid. I never take anything else excepting grass and I never will. Acid is the key, man, like Kesey says. It gets you beyond games. I never — like we've all got this potential for joy, for being our true selves and really living every minute. It makes life possible, see what I mean?

Can you feature what would happen if everyone dug that? My father — he's so hung up, into his work and the office game but he doesn't have time to just sit still and groove. And my mother, always moving chairs around — It's like those two guys on Montgomery hassling me, two sad guys with no life left in them, all sucked dry. I don't hate those cats, man, I just feel sorry for them. So many good things to do and they're caught up in that shirt-and-tie crap. I've seen more beauty in the Haight than in all downtown San Francisco. Some kids who you'd probably call freaks but they feel nothing but love.

Like we have such a good thing. In school, all they do is fill you with facts and history instead of helping you live Here and Now. They call it education, teaching people to be machines. What about living? What about stars and flowers and just being alive? Life is beautiful, man . . .

So I'm teaching myself now. My parents, they wouldn't understand it but I'm happy here. I'm learning more than I ever did in school. Wow, you walk down the street, you see eyes blazing, full of love. My brothers and sisters — I feel close, you know? Oh, I guess you think we're all terrible freaks: we smoke dope and take acid and don't cut our hair. But we have a good thing. Where does it go? — I don't know — you just let it happen, follow your karma and don't try to explain it, right? What's going to happen is going to happen and there's nothing you can do about it. It just is. The kids are hip to that, they know it's going to work out. Over half the population is under twenty-five now, you dig? That's a lot of energy . . .

I've found my way, I know it. Don't try to analyze it or put it in words. I can't really explain it. What good are words anyway? Saying something doesn't make it more true. I know what's happening to me, without having to put labels on it. It just is. Lao-tse knew that, Buddha did, Christ did. You remember the lilies of the field?

So I just do my thing. I've given away my clothes, I share my food but there's always more. If your head's in the right place, good things just happen to you. No sense getting hung up on material things — I'm as much a man as my father without clothes. I can go into the park. I don't need anything. Did you know you can get high off the right foods? And by drinking macrobiotic tea? Far out — they've even got this place, the Krishna Consciousness Temple, where you get stoned on brown rice and like by chanting these things. I'm a Leo — I don't need acid — I can get high just listening to the Airplane or the Dead — in the Panhandle, people just come up and lay things on you, no hassle, nobody cares what you look like or whether you cut your hair.

But that's what we need, none of the politics or the games. You just don't need games. It's like hate, people say you've got to hate, they give it to you in school, how there were always wars and there always will be but that's just not true. Hate is just your ego talking because you're scared. You can get beyond that — hate never did anything. If people only knew — everybody's God, we're all God if only we knew.

That's what I want to do, to show people that they can love, that they're all part of the same universe, they're all the same thing. Acid showed me that. Sometimes, I walk around this city and want to cry. You see some cop, probably a nice guy but he's so into his role he forgets he's a human being. The same thing all over, people in a hurry to do what? If we could only slow it all down, bring it all to a stop people might look around and say, "hey, that's cool!" What if we brought the Dead downtown, could you see that? Take a bunch of crazy long-hair freaks down to the Bank of America and set up right there on a sound truck. Would that ever blow their minds!

So maybe that's all LSD is for, just to open you up, to clear out the crap they've been feeding you all your life. I know for me acid was the best thing that ever happened. Before I was just hanging on, trying to find some place to plug myself in. Well, I've got a place now. I had one bummer, but most of my trips have been good, man. Before I turned on, life was just a blah. It didn't make sense — I was just doing the same thing over and over again but never getting up, never feeling alive. I really bloomed on acid, like I was a flower. You can pick me apart all you want, but I tell you, man, I'm not going to stop taking drugs. For the first time in my life, I don't feel so dead inside.

Dr. Dernburg felt that Alan's deadness could be alleviated through psychotherapy. But he was less optimistic about those young people who never saw their possible need for treatment because they stayed in the circus atmosphere of the new community. He also feared that few of them were amenable to the gradual process of psychotherapy because they were unable to delay gratification and because they externalized their internal confusion as Alan did and therefore saw the source of all their problems in society.

Yet Dr. Dernburg knew that the hippies needed help. The Haight-Ashbury was filling up, and they were exposing themselves to more infection, confusion and irritation every day. If the confusion continued to escalate, it might prove psychologically fatal to those overtly psychotic persons who were already working overtime to control their own confusion. And if the irritation also increased, it might have equally grave consequences for the borderline cases like Alan who seemed to have achieved a shaky stability by avoiding anger, by maintaining interpersonal distance and by regulating their sensory input with LSD.

Given this possibility, Dr. Dernburg decided that special health measures would have to be taken in the Haight. He hoped that a center could be established in the district that would be geared to treating bad trips, physical illness and long-term psychological problems. He was not optimistic that such a facility could reach all the young people because of the reality-denying nature of their subculture. But Dr. Dernburg wanted to help the young people. And he knew they would have to be approached on their own terms.

Stimulus

While Dr. Dernburg was coming to these conclusions, a thirty-one-year-old bohemian and hallucinogenic drug user named Robert Conrich was independently envisioning the center he desired. Conrich was the son of a San Francisco architect and was also a frustrated doctor. He worked as a private investigator until 1966, when he took acid and dropped out of business to help form the new community. His paternal feelings towards young people then led him to wonder about creating a medical institution in the Haight-Ashbury.

Conrich conceived the center as a privately financed facility, administrated by himself, for the treatment of adverse hallucinogenic drug reactions. He felt that the beats and hippies would serve as volunteers and seek help in the center if it accepted their differentness and was designed with their tastes in mind. And he knew a local physician who might take a leading role.

This was Dr. David Smith, a twenty-seven-year-old toxicologist whom Conrich had seen often since the be-in. Dr. Smith was living across from a Digger free store on Frederick Street in January of 1967 and spending much of his time at the University of California Medical Center on Parnassus. There he was conducting experiments on the hallucinogens and amphetamines and also participating in the Psychopharmacology Study

Group, a research and educational organization supervised by Dr. Frederick Meyers.

In addition to these activities, Dr. Smith was serving as chief of the Alcohol and Drug Abuse Screening Unit, a division of the Center for Special Problems run by Dr. Fort. The center, which was located across the city, offered counseling and several types of psychotherapy in a warm and accepting setting where patients were approached nonpunitively. The screening unit was a referral agency that was housed on the psychiatric wing of San Francisco General Hospital. It was a prime location from which to observe and treat the difficulties which beset the new community.

Before 1967, Dr. Smith had worked primarily with older alcoholics, heroin addicts from the Fillmore and Mission districts and amphetamine abusers from the Tenderloin. But after the be-in, he began to see more and more hippies from the Haight-Ashbury who were suffering adverse hallucinogenic drug reactions. Some of these young people had been picked up by the police from Park Station. Others were brought in by the Thelin brothers and by Emmett Grogan, Arthur Lisch and the Diggers, who apparently found their intervention ineffective in dealing with intoxicated people who wanted to walk on water or to fly.

Most of the hippies who came to the screening unit were experiencing acute anxiety, not the psychoses and chronic problems seen by Dr. Dernburg, whom Dr. Smith did not yet know. Many of these patients had been turned on without their knowledge or consent or had dropped acid at dance concerts or in crowded communes. As a result, they had become terrified by other people, by the police, by perceptual distortions, by paranoid projections, or by a sudden rush of painful memories and feelings. All were desperate for a guide to help them down.

Dr. Smith's first concern with these patients was to provide detoxification in a supportive atmosphere. He did all he could to make them comfortable in his cramped office and urged them to concentrate on a fixed object, such as a candle flame, to help them get their heads together as Conrich and the Diggers recommended. Then he tried to assure them that their perceptual distortions would eventually subside. If their panic increased, or if the young people were seriously disturbed, he administered a sedative or, if necessary, a more potent antipsychotic drug like Thorazine. If their anxiety persisted, he provided additional sedatives and talked with the hippies until they were composed enough to go on their way.

Most of the patients left the screening unit and were not heard from again. But many returned later to request additional medication and to discuss their recurrent symptoms. Some of them were still experiencing panic and flashbacks long after their trips had ended. Others suffered severe anxiety. By February of 1967, Dr. Smith knew that acute psychological crises were prevalent in the new community.

At the same time, he also realized that the Public Health Department was actually complicating the hippies' problems. The institutional trappings and the risk of arrest at San Francisco General were preventing some potential patients from seeking help there and exacerbating the anxiety of those who had the courage to ask for treatment. Furthermore, because the screening unit was open only from eight to five on weekdays, young people who came to the hospital complex for detoxification at other times were sent to Mission Emergency Hospital across the street, where they were usually denied treatment, thrown in with alcoholics and accident victims, or locked in padded isolation cells.

Even worse was the situation at Park Emergency Hospital, where the Public Health Department physicians appeared to be harassing the hippies incessantly. When young people arrived at Park Emergency, they either had to go through a long registration process or were snubbed completely by the staff. Then, since there were no available facilities for treating adverse drug reactions, they had to be taken by ambulance to San Francisco General. Their acute symptoms were so often intensified by this inhumane and drawn-out procedure that what began as mildly bad trips for them frequently turned into horrifying nightmares.

The extent of this damage was seen in the case of a nineteen-year-old girl who was crossing the Panhandle one afternoon with her boyfriend when she saw something move in the shadow of a eucalyptus tree and became convinced that the police were after her. The girl was carrying eight LSD tablets at the time, which she immediately swallowed to avoid detection. As the drugs took effect, she started hallucinating wildly and threatened to kill herself. Her boyfriend rushed her to Park Emergency.

The girl saw one of the uniformed attendants there, assumed he was a policeman, and became hysterical. She was then removed to an examining room, while her friend was ordered to remain outside. The girl became even more hysterical in his absence and had to be subdued by three attendants. Four of her ribs were broken as she was forcibly given a sedative by injection. After waiting for twenty minutes in a straitjacket, she was taken to San Francisco General in an ambulance by an attendant who called her a dope fiend. She was then sent to the psychiatric wards, where she spent three days experiencing flashbacks and perceptual distortions. When Dr. Smith finally saw the patient, her anxiety attack had blossomed into a full-blown psychosis. Most of her suffering, he felt, had been precipitated by the treatment the Public Health Department had provided her.

This particular patient was quite unwilling to seek assistance from the city again. But even more important was the fact that experiences like hers were making it increasingly difficult to reach the new community. Word about such incidents spread quickly through the Haight, and Dr. Smith could see that more and more hippies were becoming hesitant about asking for medical attention. This was potentially tragic, for in addition to adverse drug reactions and psychological difficulties, they also suffered a host of physical health problems as a result of their crowded living conditions, their drug abuse and their debilitating life-style.

Dr. Smith had been able to handle some of the acute medical needs of his patients by sending them to such city agencies as the Venereal Disease Clinic at 33 Hunt Street, the Pediatrics, Hepatitis and Oral Surgery units at General Hospital, the Immediate Psychiatric Aid and Referral Service and the Center for Special Problems. He had also made some progress with those young people who refused to use the Public Health Department by referring them to Planned Parenthood and to the University of California Medical Center, where they were treated by Charles Fischer at the Dental Clinic and by Dr. Meyers.

Nevertheless, Dr. Smith knew that he was only scratching the surface of the new community and not even touching the hippies who did not know their way around town. Bob Conrich believed those hippies required an on-the-spot facility in the Haight-Ashbury, open twenty-four hours a day and seven days a week, where they could be detoxified, counseled, treated for acute symptoms, referred elsewhere for extensive treatment and educated about drugs, nutrition, preventive medicine and proper hygiene.

If such a center were not established, the district might experience a rash of psychological and health problems. VD and infectious hepatitis were increasing dramatically in the Haight; fifty-two rapes, three hundred robberies, two hundred and twenty assaults and sixteen hundred cases of burglary were reported during 1966 in the district, and the crime rate was still on the rise. Park Emergency and Park Police Station seemed unable to stem these mounting statistics, but a more youth-oriented facility might heal sickness and exert a positive moral influence in the area, thereby keeping the crime rate down.

It might also be able to prevent other devastating infections from developing. The new community was growing daily and bearing more and more resemblance to a gypsy encampment. It was thus becoming a breeding ground for measles, mumps, influenza, dysentery, typhoid fever, mononucleosis, meningitis, tuberculosis, plague and other infectious diseases. If these contagions appeared, they might sweep through the Haight-Ashbury and then spill over into other sections of San Francisco as well.

Although preventing these problems was his primary objective, Dr.

Smith had other reasons for desiring a regional health facility in the Haight. Prior to the be-in he had dated Florence Martin, a black nurse who worked in the Medical Center and who informed him about a facility created to meet the needs of poverty-stricken patients in Watts after the riots there in 1965. The Watts Clinic was highly effective in providing care for black patients who previously had to travel several miles to receive medical attention. It also served as a neighborhood center with political influence that gave its patients and volunteer paramedical staff members a stake in the system they despised.

Dr. Smith realized that a similar center could be an important addition to the new community. He had treated hundreds of beats and hippies by this point and had begun to look on them as members of a minority group who were estranged from the dominant American culture by their beliefs, language and life-style. He had experimented with several of their drugs. He had also come to support their opposition to the Vietnam war and to respect their search for alternatives to the status quo.

Indeed, Dr. Smith identified with the young people. He shared their frustration and disillusionment with society and their Rousseauian faith in the virtue of natural, presocial man. He subscribed to the eupsychic belief that man could achieve a greater spiritual dimension through the release of repressed or suppressed instincts. He felt that progress could be accomplished if people did their thing — and he wanted to do his thing too.

This desire probably stemmed from his background. Dr. Smith was born and raised in Bakersfield, California, where his grandparents had settled as farm workers after the depression drove them from the Oklahoma dust bowl. His father was a railroad clerk; his mother, a nurse, developed cancer when Dr. Smith was three years old. Both had encouraged his medical ambitions and had guided him towards a straight life. Both had died before he graduated from college; his mother a week before his seventeenth birthday, his father when he was nineteen.

Dr. Smith respected his parents' wishes and remained achievement-oriented. But although he once accepted the conservatism of medicine and the inevitability of middle-class existence, he began to have second thoughts after he worked with two father figures following medical school. One was Dr. Frederick Meyers, who testified before the Kefauver Crime Commission about the unethical practices of the American pharmaceutical industry and argued for a nonrepressive approach to drug-abuse problems. The other was Dr. Joel Fort, who helped bring Dr. Smith out of the research laboratory.

Dr. Smith was also influenced by Bob Conrich and the other bohemians he had met in the Haight-Ashbury. He enjoyed existential literature, identified with minorities, and was envious of their supposed sexual freedom — and that of the beats. He wanted to become bohemian, to free himself of inhibitions. Although his clothes and profession were conventional, his desire for freedom and the feeling of lack of contact which probably prompted it made him more bohemian than he ever realized.

Dr. Smith was also unaware of his parental attitude towards young people. This attitude stemmed in part from their life-style — they were living out his own fantasy of the free life. But his primary motivation was probably nurturance by proxy. Dr. Smith, who had no family, felt protective towards homeless adolescents in the Haight. He related to them like a parent and thereby protected himself too.

Although Dr. Smith followed Conrich in helping the new community, he disagreed with him in several ways. Like its other members, Conrich saw the new community as a counterculture capable of caring for itself. But Dr. Smith felt that the community was a subculture that had failed to provide itself with adequate institutions. He was not entirely aware of the psychological dynamics and possible psychopathology of the beats and hippies, in part because he knew few hippies well, because he assumed that drugs were the sole cause of their dysfunctioning and because he had been treating only acute problems. Yet he still regarded his patients as members of a minority group who needed help from the straight world.

Conrich and Dr. Smith also disagreed on the scope of the proposed center. Dr. Smith conceived of it as a halfway house which should attempt to alter and improve its patients' life-style. But Conrich, who valued their psychedelic living pattern, opposed such intervention. He wanted the crisis center to be a permissive and accepting facility. Conrich ultimately had his way.

A final area of disagreement related to the issue of sponsorship. Conrich planned a private facility but Dr. Smith thought the responsibility for treating the new community rested with the Public Health Department. He saw it as a logical extension of the Center for Special Problems and the Alcohol and Drug Abuse Screening Unit. The proposed center reflected his and Dr. Fort's ideals of community medicine.

But these ideals had little official support in San Francisco. Mayor John Shelley had a limited medical knowledge and seemed apathetic towards the hippies and other minorities. Chief Administrative Officer Thomas Mellon, a former businessman who supervised the Health Department and had permanent tenure because of the city's antiquated charter system, was opposed to treating people within their communities. Public Health Director Ellis

Sox resisted the community model because it jeopardized his authority. He apparently wanted to isolate the Haight-Ashbury and let its young residents die.

Dr. Smith detested this approach but believed that the Health Department could be reformed and induced to create a health center for the new community. He wanted to stay in the Establishment and keep a foot in both the hip and straight camps. Uncertain about his own identity, he saw the proposed center as a way of demonstrating that the straight world had room for the hippies and the beats. He wanted to nurture the love philosophy of the young people. And he hoped to show the hip world that its philosophy required responsible care.

Thus, the center that Conrich and Dr. Smith were discussing was to be a symbol encompassing the best of two worlds. It might make the Health Department become more responsive to minorities. It might educate the beats and hippies. It might serve as a model in the treatment of drug abuse. It might emerge as an inspiration for communities everywhere.

The desire for such a symbol was shared by several members of the Psychopharmacology Study Group. Included were a dental student named Charles Fischer, who knew the needs for his specialty in the Haight, and Dr. Meyers, who had treated dozens of longhaired patients since the be-in and was convinced that new chemicals hallucinogenic and otherwise, would soon appear in the district. Dr. Meyers believed that a regional health center would be an ideal place to collect and identify those drugs and to work out new treatment procedures which might be useful to other doctors. Although he hoped that the city would establish the facility, he had little faith in the Public Health Department. For this reason, he agreed to the idea of establishing a medical center with or without San Francisco's official support and offered to serve as its research director if the city did not respond.

Dr. Smith talked the matter over with Dr. Fort before he considered any independent action. Dr. Fort recognized the need for a center and felt that San Francisco should and would come up with the necessary funds. He also saw the facility as a logical extension of his activities and offered to approach the Health Department. Primarily because of this, Dr. Smith decided to stay within the system until the city took a position on the Haight-Ashbury.

Response

He did not have to wait long, for conditions worsened considerably in the Haight during the spring. The Thelin brothers' calm center was filled to overflowing by this time, and Arthur Lisch and the Diggers were also out of space in their communes and crash pads. They had managed to recruit several interns from Kaiser Hospital and an ex-mental patient named Doc, who served as a witch doctor to the Hell's Angels, to treat people at their free stores, but they were faced with an impossible patient overload and had few medical supplies.

Yet the Diggers would not admit defeat. In the middle of March, they reported that the Haight-Ashbury had filled up beyond their expectations and predicted that one hundred thousand young people dropping acid in Des Moines and Sioux Falls would flock to the district after school was out for a Summer of Love. They then demanded that the city give them the food, shelter and medical services necessary to care for the coming invasion.

But San Francisco was unwilling to accept any summer influx unless it brought tourist dollars. Two days after the Diggers made their demands, the chief of police ordered more men to Park Station and promised that law and order, if not health, would prevail in the Haight. Mayor John Shelley asked the Board of Supervisors to pass a resolution warning hippies away from the city. Thomas Mellon suggested erecting "Hippies Not Welcome Here" signs on the bridge approaches into San Francisco. The Municipal Railway Company sought the board's permission to reroute its buses around Haight Street, while a local sightseeing company was seeking sanction to bring its buses in. And the Recreation and Park Commission declared Golden Gate Park off limits to young people with sleeping bags.

At the same time, Dr. Ellis Sox closed several Digger establishments for so-called health reasons and ordered a sanitation- and housing-code crackdown in the Haight-Ashbury. His sanitation sweep was a surprising failure; the inspectors who visited six hundred and ninety dwellings in the district found only thirty-nine code violations, most of which were in buildings occupied by black families. Several supervisors questioned Dr. Sox's motivation, and Dr. Fort told the press that the Haight needed help, not harassment. Dr. Sox replied that the city could not afford to broaden its health program and said that if he extended "special services" to the Haight-Ashbury he would also have to open medical centers in districts like the Mission and the Fillmore, where the poverty was not voluntary. Dr. Fort said that this was a splendid idea. A few days later, he was fired.

Dr. Fort's dismissal was interpreted as a declaration of war in the new community. It also prompted the young people to make another show of strength. In early April, the Diggers, H.I.P., a recently formed free school and other self-help agencies formed an organization for mutual protection. They then announced that a Council for the Summer of Love had been created to coordinate a Summer Solstice Festival in the park, where the one hundred thousand people coming West could congregate on their arrival in town.

The thought of such an assemblage led several people in turn to help the hippies help themselves. The first was Al Rinker, a former marine who leased a flat on Fell Street across the Panhandle and set up the Haight-Ashbury Switchboard as an answering, housing and referral service. The next was Father Leon Harris of All Saint's Episcopal Church on Waller Street, who created a Community Affairs Office in his basement, invited the Diggers to use the space, and established an emergency housing program with members of the Neighborhood Council. He was followed by Howard Rochford, a Catholic layman who founded a coffeehouse and counseling center in Hamilton Methodist Church, and Reverend Larry Beggs of the United Church of Christ, who launched Huckleberry's for Runaways in a brown Victorian on Broderick Street to counsel young people, help them contact their parents, and provide a neutral setting wherein both parties could thrash out their grievances in family therapy.

Therapy was also the goal of Dr. Harry Wilmer, a psychoanalyst from the Langley-Porter Neuropsychiatric Institute, who was so convinced that the beats and hippies had failed to found a therapeutic community that he created one of his own. Dr. Wilmer believed that the young people were dependent on television but also felt that their dependence could be positively utilized if TV were employed as a therapeutic tool. For this reason, he conceived of an experimental electronic environment called the Youth Drug Unit in which approximately twenty patients could act out psychodramas before closed-circuit television and use group methods before going on to more intensive psychotherapy.

Another therapeutic effort was underway at the Mendocino State Hospital, two hours north of the city, where a social worker named Wayne Wilson was developing the Mendocino Drug Abuse Program and Family as an extension of the Center for Special Problems. In keeping with his philosophic debt to Dr. Fort, Wilson stressed voluntary admissions and maximum participation from his patients. He also offered detoxification on the wards of the hospital, along with various encounter-group methods used by Synanon and Esalen Institute to bring the patients into a communal family.

A seventh attempt to aid the new community was made by Stuart Loomis and Leonard Wolf, a professor of English at San Francisco State College. Professor Wolf lived near the University of California Medical Center and had been impressed by Allen Cohen of the *Oracle* with the need for a youth-oriented educational program in the Haight. In April, he and Professor Loomis raised a small grant for rent money from a local church foundation, recruited a number of their colleagues, and set out to establish somewhere in the Haight-Ashbury an educational project called Happening House.

The leaders of the new community lacked only medical services now that Happening House was underway. They therefore approached Dr. Smith and Bob Conrich, who had concluded that the Public Health Department would not act in the district after the firing of Dr. Fort. Conrich saw his dismissal as proof that change could not be accomplished within the system and interpreted it as an act of war. He convinced Dr. Smith that they had to attempt an alternative with the help of the Psychopharmacology Study Group and the beats and the hippies. Dr. Smith therefore decided to start a private and nonrepressive crisis center in the Haight-Ashbury.

Love Needs Care

After making this decision, he and Conrich met in Dr. Meyers's pharmacological laboratory to implement their plans. Their most pressing problems at this point were staffing and financing, but they felt that they could count on liberal physicians and students at the Medical Center, in addition to young people from the Haight, and also secure donated supplies. This would allow them to offer free treatment in keeping with the tenets of the new community.

Dr. Smith and Conrich named their center the Haight-Ashbury Free Medical Clinic to further this point and picked themselves as its medical director and administrator respectively. They also chose for their logo and letterhead a design of a white dove of peace on a blue cross created by

Conrich's girlfriend, Janie Lucas. And they decided on a slogan for their facility, one which would also be used by the city's VD clinic: "Love Needs Care."

The concept of Love Needs Care was first made public by Dr. Smith at the Haight-Ashbury Roundtable, an invitational conference held at the Medical Center on the thirteenth of May. Dr. Smith was encouraged by the number of students and doctors who offered to help the Clinic at this meeting, although he was unable to recruit Florence Martin, Dr. Price Cobbs and other black nurses and physicians who were working with the health problems of the black ghetto. He was also surprised when Dr. Ellis Sox pulled him aside after the Roundtable and told him to save his patient records because the Public Health Department might want to contract retroactively with the Clinic for services rendered during the Summer of Love.

Equally surprised was John Luce, who was covering Dr. Smith for *Look* magazine. Luce was twenty-five years old the day of the Roundtable. He had worked as an editor and free-lance writer since the fall of 1966, when Ronald Reagan's election preempted his position as a campaign press secretary to California's former governor, Pat Brown. Luce first visited the Haight with his younger sister, who lived in the Western Addition but considered herself part of the new community. He then wrote a *Look* piece on the Jefferson Airplane. Now he was seeing the Haight-Ashbury through Dr. Smith's eyes.

His interest in Dr. Smith was prompted by several factors. First was the similarity of their backgrounds: Luce's parents divorced early; his father, a retired military officer, was in a rest home; his mother, an interior decorator, had died from cancer when he was fourteen. Luce was also interested in medicine and drugs. And while Dr. Smith was fighting the medical Establishment, Luce was trying to resist political conservatism in California.

Because of this, Luce saw the symbolic value of Dr. Smith's mission. Although he considered the doctor naïve, he had given up on organized politics and believed that private initiative was the best answer to public problems. Luce did not think that San Francisco would ever aid the Haight-Ashbury Free Medical Clinic. But he offered to publicize Dr. Smith's efforts and to help the Clinic as time went on.

Dr. Smith welcomed this participation after the Roundtable. He then spoke with Professor Leonard Wolf, who had chosen the conference as a place to announce his plans for Happening House. Professor Wolf had not found a classroom for his project yet, so he suggested that Happening House and the Clinic combine their operations under one roof. A joint arrangement was reached, and Bob Conrich set out to find space for the

Haight-Ashbury Free Medical Clinic and Happening House in the new community.

Conrich first looked for a house but met with little success because many merchants and homeowners were opposed to the project. He was then helped by Robert Laws of the Neighborhood Council, who volunteered to serve as legal counsel to the Clinic and offered to establish a referral program with the Neighborhood Legal Assistance Foundation whereby patients could gain free advice and secure admission to Mendocino and the Youth Drug Unit. After being turned down by several dozen landlords, they found an abandoned dentist's office on the second floor of a pale yellow building at 558 Clayton Street.

This small office was divided into two seven-room suites, the first of which contained two bathrooms and five small cubicles packed with dust and painted a bilious green. Two of the cubicles could be used as examining rooms; the third could house Conrich's office; the fourth could be turned into a receiving and waiting area and an impromptu classroom; the fifth could serve as the calm center. Conrich obtained a one-year lease on the sorry space at one hundred and fifty dollars a month from Professor Wolf's budget. He was also given an option for an additional one hundred and fifty dollars on the second seven-room suite in the rear.

The Clinic had a home now, but it still had another obstacle to overcome. For when Dr. Smith checked with the city, he found that local zoning and building ordinances made the charity operation he and the organizers envisioned impossible. Their plans ground to a halt until he and Laws talked with Jack Morrison, a supervisor and antiwar mayoralty candidate who lived in the Haight, and hit upon a legally acceptable idea. The facility could function as the private office of Dr. Smith, doing business as the medical director of the Haight-Ashbury Free Medical Clinic. He could then see patients as he wished, while his malpractice insurance could cover volunteers.

With this procedure established, the organizers started to equip their office. First, they scavenged furniture and secured wastebaskets, chests, mattresses and chairs, including several donated by Roger Smith, whom Dr. Smith had met while lecturing at a drug symposium. Dr. Conrich talked with a janitorial supply house that promised free toilet tissue and towels. He then visited private hospitals in the city, from which he received an odd assortment of medical equipment, including scales, stethoscopes, cabinets and such pieces as an 1890 pneumothorax machine that qualified more as pop art than as medical supplies.

Following this, the organizers obtained free medication from several detail men, or salesmen, representing the major pharmaceutical companies.

They also wrote pharmaceutical houses for samples, collected what they could from sympathetic physicians, and utilized the Medical Center Pharmacology Department. They then raised a few hundred dollars from friendly doctors and purchased analgesics, antibiotics, antibacterial detergents and, most important, sedatives and antipsychotic tranquilizers. The perishable items were kept in a donated refrigerator. All other drugs were stored in a broom closet under lock and key.

The organizers then held a meeting on June third at 558 Clayton Street to size up their staff. Several Neighborhood Council members were present, along with Doc and the Kaiser Hospital interns who had been helping the Diggers and a number of hippies who were perched on packing crates or huddled together with their animals on the floor. Dr. Smith began the meeting with a pep talk but was interrupted by a boy in a paisley poncho who lit a marijuana cigarette and passed it among his companions. This inspired Conrich to write down the Clinic's first house rule. It read: "No Holding, No Dealing, No Using Dope, No Pets. Any of These Can Close the Clinic. We Love You."

The organizers discussed their immediate goals after the joint was extinguished. They emphasized the importance of the calm center and signed up Doc and several local gurus to act as guides under the supervision of legitimate physicians. They told their potential volunteers that the facility's future success would depend on its acceptance within the new community. They assigned certain volunteers to act as liaisons with the other hip and straight service organizations in the district.

Dr. Smith then noticed a girl in a fishnet sarong who was seated on the floor in a lotus position, humming softly to herself. He assumed that she would continue tripping quietly, so he concluded the meeting with a discussion of the psychiatric program he hoped to offer. At this, the girl suddenly stopped humming and stood up. "Psychiatrists?" she asked of no one in particular. "What the hell good are psychiatrists going to do? Man, this whole place is fucked."

Dr. Smith could hardly disagree. He had counted on help from the new community, but most of the hippies who showed up at the meeting looked more like potential patients than volunteers. Nevertheless, he and Conrich invited everyone present to return on June seventh, when the Clinic would open. They then met with several people who arrived late at the meeting and subsequently became the nucleus of their staff.

The first was Peggy Sankot, a nurse who had just quit her job as an intensive-care specialist for heart surgery patients at San Francisco General Hospital. Miss Sankot came to the city in 1963 after graduating from Mercy School of Nursing in Cedar Rapids, Iowa and was close to dropping out of her profession by June of 1967. Although she visited the Clinic on June third almost by accident, she immediately saw the need for her services and offered to assist for free. She started wearing beads over her white uniform and would soon be recognized by the press as "the Florence Nightingale of the Haight-Ashbury."

The second staff member present that evening was Peter Schubart, a chemistry student from the University of California at Santa Cruz. Schubart was a stable young man with only a slight hippie identification. He became a political activist during college and was arrested with folk singer Joan Baez at an Oakland protest rally. He looked on the Clinic as a place to put his principles of social involvement to the test, and was named its assistant administrator.

After Schubart came Alan Rose, a twenty-one-year-old former student from Shaker Heights, Ohio. Rose had intended to become a rabbi until psychological difficulties cut short his stay at Ohio State and Tioga Community College. After dropping out of school in 1966, he worked in a Shaker Heights delicatessen until he moved to the Haight in response to a television show. Rose was a lonely person with a limited sense of self-esteem and personal accomplishments. He hoped to find friends and involvement at the Clinic and asked to work with the calm-center volunteers.

The fourth new staff member was Dr. Robert Morris, a thirty-one-year-old pathology resident from Children's Hospital. Dr. Morris was the son of a prominent general practitioner in the city and hoped to become the drug expert of the San Francisco Medical Society. Because he saw 558 Clayton Street as a way station to other facilities, he was most interested in establishing referral procedures. Shortly after the organizational meeting, he began negotiations with the Board of Directors at Children's to arrange for patients to be treated there.

Dr. Morris was also instrumental in formulating the Clinic's operating procedures and floor plan. Under these procedures, all patients would be required to fill out personal histories when they arrived, and to see a doctor before they could receive medication. All drugs were to be carefully controlled and could be issued only by a pharmacist or by the head nurse, when and if the Clinic could obtain one. Physicians volunteering at the facility would have to show their medical licenses and could not go to work until they had done so. Paramedical staff members could assist in the calm center, take patients' histories, file charts, answer questions over the telephone and supervise the volunteers.

One procedural problem the Clinic faced related to its patients' ages. The California laws which existed in 1967 classified individuals between the ages of eighteen and twenty-one as minors, and those eighteen and under as juveniles. Legally, only people twenty-one and over could authorize medical treatment without some form of parental or court consent, a limitation that caused considerable difficulty with young people living away from home who contracted communicable disease.

Because of this limitation, many physicians in San Francisco illegally treated patients over eighteen as if they were adults. Dr. Morris felt that this practice could be followed at 558 Clayton Street. He was supported in his belief by Father Larry Beggs, who was encountering similar difficulties with the legal age classifications at Huckleberry's, and by the San Francisco Medical Society, with which he was working to amend the state laws. After discussing the situation, the organizers decided that they should treat patients over eighteen for acute medical problems if they had established residence away from home or could not contact their parents. People under eighteen should be given referrals, although they might secure treatment by lying about their age.

The organizers next decorated the former dentist's office to suit their prospective patients' tastes. Bob Conrich painted the doorways of the Clinic and brought some color to its drab interior. The chairs, mattresses and tables were placed in the waiting room, along with a radio, a coffee maker and a large can for donations. An artist present at the organizational meeting created a collage of dance-concert posters for the wall of the waiting room. The sign prohibiting dealing and using drugs was posted at the top of the stairs.

Posters spelling out other house rules ("No Smoking Except Tobacco" was one) were also put up, as were lists of the available housing and employment opportunities and information about Huckleberry's, the Switchboard, Father Harris's and Howard Rochford's services, the Mendocino Drug Abuse Program and Family and the Youth Drug Unit. More graffiti and posters followed, including a masterpiece from the Print Mint. It showed a nude girl crouched in a rocky cave in the fetal position. Below her was a single word: "Return."

All that remained now to be recruited for the Clinic were its patients. The organizers were still not convinced that young people would use their facility, so they spent several days soliciting moral support from leaders like the Thelins and talking with beats and hippies on the street. Leaflets were passed through the new community. Posters were put up in Mnasidika's and at other H.I.P. shops. The *Barb* and *Oracle* were asked to inform their readers. Two volunteers painted poster boards announcing the Clinic opening and paraded with them on Haight Street.

Finally, a sign reading "David E. Smith, M.D. and Associates: Haight-Ashbury Free Medical Clinic and Happening House" was posted on the weathered door at 558 Clayton Street on the morning of June seventh.

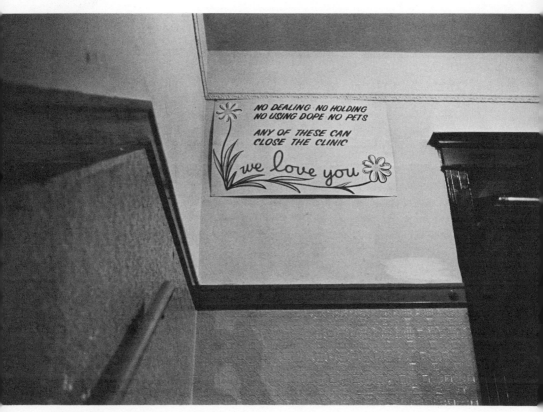

Clayton Street: house rules.
(Jim Marshall)

Underneath it was painted the Clinic logo. Underneath this was written the slogan Love Needs Care.

That afternoon, when the front door was opened, hundreds of patients pushed their way inside. Love did need care.

Part III

Summer
of
Love

Love consists of this, that two solitudes
protect and touch and greet each other.

Rainer Maria Rilke, **Letters to a Young Poet**

She's leaving home after living alone
for so many years.

John Lennon and Paul McCartney, "She's Leaving Home"

Extreme remedies are very appropriate
for extreme diseases.

Hippocrates, **Aphorisms**

The First Wave

The opening of the Haight-Ashbury Free Medical Clinic and Happening House coincided with the beginning of perhaps the most serious medical emergency to hit San Francisco since the 1906 earthquake and fire. The earthquake was a natural disaster which resulted from unexpected shifts in the earth's crust along the San Andreas Fault. The Summer of Love was man-made. It might have been prevented if the city had heeded the Diggers' warnings about an invasion of young people to San Francisco that summer. And the fissures which appeared in the Haight in subsequent months were surface manifestations of deep cracks in the social core.

The two cataclysms invite further comparison. The 1906 earthquake and fire devastated much of San Francisco but left the Haight-Ashbury intact. Yet in 1967 the Haight had been so isolated by the city and so identified by the media that it bore the entire brunt of the summer onslaught. The earthquake resulted primarily in property damage. But the Summer of Love was characterized both by the destruction of a district and by the suffering of thousands of people who turned its circus atmosphere into a horror show.

Although young people sustained most of the suffering, many of the spectators were adults. Included were the tourists, journalists and social scientists who had first revealed their presence at the be-in. There were also well-meaning nuns and wildly erratic street preachers who hoped to convert the hippies and few remaining beats. There were postcard salesmen and bead-bearing merchants who opened headquarters on Haight Street. There were hustlers and hardened criminals who moved over from the Tenderloin district. And there were white, Negro and American Indian alcoholics who wandered up from Skid Row.

These people expected to see, save, study and/or exploit the one hundred thousand young people in the Haight-Ashbury that summer. They were not disappointed, for an even larger number passed through the area over the summer months. Yet most of the new arrivals were not true bohemians or hippies. Ken Kesey was in jail at this point, and the new community's

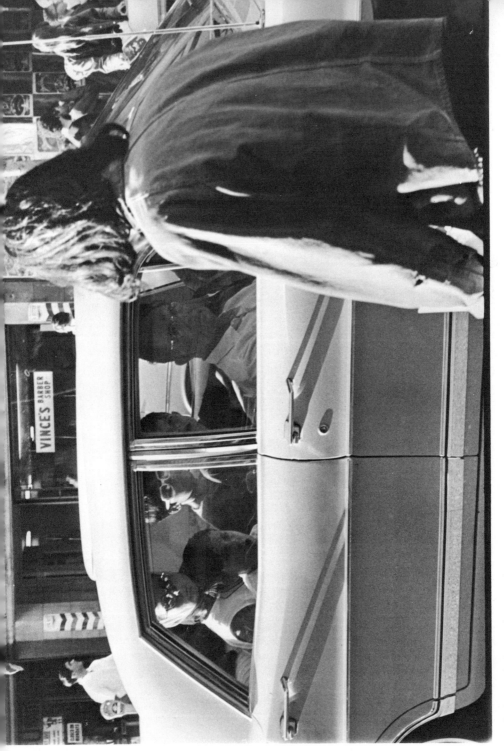

Haight Street: don't stop the carnival.
(Michael Alexander)

membership was already depleted in early June when the first wave of summer visitors washed over Haight Street.

Some of the young people had left the Haight-Ashbury to join satellite communities around the Bay Area or the new subcultural enclaves which were springing up in most major American cities. And while they were spreading the psychedelic movement into urban centers, others were taking it back to the land. The Haight was still a spiritual home for these hippies, but they had become depressed by drug-taking, by the city's harassment during the spring and by the impending invasion that summer. They had therefore decided to sit out the next few months at such nearby rural communes as the Morningstar Ranch, one hour north of San Francisco, where they planned to turn on to nature, take their trips in private, and practice their exotic therapies.

Thousands stayed in the Haight-Ashbury, but they too went through their changes as the summer progressed. Many hippies had become depressed through their involvement with LSD by this point and were bothered by flashbacks and perceptual distortions and by the overpublicized possibility of chromosomal damage and birth defects. Some were therefore switching to other hallucinogens like mescaline or were looking for new compounds to bring themselves up. Others were becoming interested in offshoots of the psychedelic movement that promised instant intimacy, spontaneity, heightened functioning and protoplasmic consciousness without drugs.

One was the Human Potential Movement of the Esalen Institute, which now sponsored allegedly therapeutic encounter groups and gestalt therapy sessions in addition to seminars devoted to the hallucinogens. Another was the Meher Baba Movement, made up of people trying to get their heads together through yoga and meditation. A third was the Transcendental Meditation Movement of Maharishi M. Yogi, the smiling swami who was credited with weaning the Beatles away from LSD. A fourth was the Hare Krishna Movement that had operated since January out of the Krishna Consciousness Temple on Frederick Street.

This storefront shrine was once known mainly for its free meals, but it had become a haven for young people preoccupying themselves with chants, prayers and the ever-popular Eastern spiritualist trip. Among them was Alan, Dr. Dernburg's patient, who had donned a peach-colored robe, shaved his head, and changed his identity once more to that of a wandering monk. Alan was optimistic about his new mission, so much so that he swore off acid temporarily and distributed free incense at the corner of Haight and Clayton for two weeks. Yet his anxiety and depression lingered, and his ability to tolerate intrusions remained at a painfully low ebb.

Part of Alan's problem related to the new population which was gradually taking over the street. In it were servicemen, Hell's Angels and other bikers, blacks from the Fillmore, habitual abusers like Randy, and hoodies. Many grew their hair long, dropped LSD, and talked about love. But the word was not a natural part of their vocabularies. If the true hippies stood for peace and acid, the psychopathic hoodies represented the opposite: violence and speed.

Somewhere in the middle were several thousand impressionable white adolescents whom Dr. Dernburg described as active or summer hippies to distinguish them psychologically and historically from the other types of people on Haight Street. These young people, who were also often called teeny-boppers, weekenders or plastic hippies, came from middle-class homes in every urban, suburban and rural area in America. Most of them looked like hippies, emulated their eupsychic ethic, and partook of the hippie modality to a certain extent. Their great numbers and wide geographical distribution stressed how common, if not yet universal, the modality had become.

But there were differences between the two groups. The summer hippies were generally younger, more psychologically malleable and less committed to hallucinogenic chemicals than their mystically oriented elders. They were neither as isolated, primitive and passive as the young people who proceeded them in the district nor as disturbed, uneducated and antisocial as those who would soon rule it. By and large, these adolescents came from intact, if not "ideal" families, according to Dr. Dernburg. They may have appeared unusual because of their costumes, yet they were rather typical teen-agers underneath.

Typical or not, the summer hippies had their share of hang-ups. In particular, many experienced the same conflicts regarding unresolved dependence that the beats and early hippies did. Some were runaways who were attempting to force concessions from their parents by bcoming psychedelicized for the summer. Others had been encouraged to leave home and either erected defenses against familial rejection or used toxic agents to deal with their anger and resentment. A few either found their feelings intolerable or suffered from inner emptiness.

But most were merely lost and lonely youngsters who hoped to conceal their problems, create a group identity, and thereby find themselves in the Haight. They had apparently been influenced by the hip heroes, by the media and by McLuhanistic pronouncements to look on the new community as a playground, and hoped to squeeze all the stimulation from it they could. The summer hippies spoke about the Summer of Love as the time for a temporary regression in which they might explore freedom, obtain sex, and experience Now-ness. In earlier years, they might have flocked to well-publicized locations like Fort Lauderdale to achieve these purposes. But the Haight-Ashbury was the place to do your thing in 1967. And doing your thing in 1967 meant taking drugs.

Few of the adolescents actually began their chemical consumption in San Francisco. Indeed, most of them acted as if they had always considered mind and mood alteration a normal part of growing up. Although they came from every corner of the country, many reported that they had been influenced by high school and college companions, by local beats and hippies, by television advertisements and/or by the plethora of psychoactive compounds in their parents' medicine cabinets to try different kinds of chemicals. Many began with marijuana instead of, or in addition to, alcohol. Most had tried acid by the summer or were now eager to sample it.

Some of the summer hippies followed their spiritual elders in regarding the hallucinogens as therapeutic agents for self-discovery and psychic release. Others employed the compounds as the hippies did to regulate stimuli and to disguise their dysfunctioning. Many felt that they would mature more quickly in a drug-based subculture where they would face more constant and demanding tests. Yet there were limits to their self-imposed challenges, for these adolescents were neither quasi-ritualistic abusers like Alan nor multiple and habitual abusers like Randy and his ilk. Experience was their primary objective in consuming chemicals. They could therefore be described as experimental drug users, at least when they first reached the Haight.

But few of them remained for long in this experimental category. Thousands of the summer hippies came West on the words of a popular song that recommended wearing flowers to San Francisco and arrived in the Haight-Ashbury with little else. Although they hoped to play with fellow flower children, they usually had to cope with hoodies and street spades who wanted to rob them, rape them or beat them up. Although they planned to be met by psychedelic welcome wagons, they were often either rolled on arrival or picked up by the police.

Those who survived this negative screening found themselves in an environment for which they were pathetically ill-equipped. The summer hippies were not trained in alley smartness and had to make their living by shoplifting, panhandling, selling underground papers or peddling drugs. Yet even this was difficult, for although there was slightly more money on Haight Street in 1967 than a year later, the competition was much more intense. Because of this, many of the summer visitors soon realized that they needed help.

Some left at this point, preferring the hassle at home to the agony of the

Haight. Others were taken in by the remaining beats and hippies, found temporary brothers and sisters with whom they could rent communes, secured space through Father Harris and the Neighborhood Council, crashed in places like the Psychedelic Shop and the Print Mint or slept in the Panhandle and on the street. Few of the adolescents became prostitutes, for love was still free in the Haight-Ashbury. But many did sell their autonomy either to homosexuals, tourists and servicemen who operated on a pay-as-you-lay basis; to the bikers, who turned them into errand boys or mamas who serviced the gangs; or to older psychopaths, who taught them street wisdom and organized them into drug-dealing packs.

Because of their exposure to such people, many active hippies learned criminal skills as part of their summer schooling. They were also introduced to chemicals far more powerful than those to which they were accustomed, for almost every toxic substance known to science was now available in the Haight. Several clandestine laboratories were supplying the district with speed and acid by June of 1967; blacks and whites were bringing even more amphetamines, barbiturates and opiates into the area; and the adolescents themselves often arrived with contraband drugs. Few could refuse all the compounds offered them. And since they were subject to several kinds of peer-group pressure, they had to swallow some chemicals to demonstrate their love to the hippies and shoot others to convince the hoodies that they could handle life.

Yet these young people were not as durable as they pretended. In fact, they were prone to adverse reactions both because they were experimental users and because they were taking adulterated drugs in such a confusing and congested place. Their bad trips and acute health problems often diminished the longer they stayed in the district, but their anxiety, depression and physical symptoms invariably increased. Many of the active hippies were already sick by June seventh. Some had turned to black-market medications. But others who knew about the new Clinic were waiting alongside the beats, hippies, hoodies, bikers, alcoholics and other patients pouring into 558 Clayton Street.

A Field Hospital in a Combat Zone

Two things distinguished the line leading into the Clinic that afternoon and evening — its diversity and its length. Most of the prospective patients strung around the corner of Haight and Clayton were beats and older hippies, wearing beads and buckskin, who had not seen physicians in months. Some came with their commune-mates, made music together, and passed out flowers. Others stood quietly, cradling their infants to their breasts. Standing with them were Arthur Lisch and other tribal elders eager to inspect the new facility. And off to the side slouched new arrivals carrying bedrolls and clad in lightweight clothing that offered little protection against the San Francisco fog.

Around them swirled the sights, sounds and smells which would permeate the Haight-Ashbury for many months. Tourists were present, paying Alan to pose for photographs and purchasing postcards for the home folks. The Angels were also visible, as were winos sprawling against the unboarded storefronts and sailors searching for fresh meat. The air hung with incense, patchouli, marijuana and body odor. It rang with the tinkle of camel bells, the rattle of tambourines and the eerie whistle of wooden flutes. Haight Street looked like Rio during Carnival; like New Orleans at the height of Mardi Gras. But while some of its healthier celebrants danced and frolicked, others who were already hung over from the permanent party crowded onto the Clinic's front steps.

The cacophony they created was barely tolerable, but the pandemonium inside never ceased. Peter Schubart and several persons from the organizational meeting had stationed themselves behind the front door when it was opened, where they tried to keep the line in order and urged the more suspicious adolescents in off the street. Other volunteers were positioned at the top of the stairs, underneath the sign that prohibited dealing, holding dope and pets. They smiled at the patients who climbed the stairway and then gestured them into the receiving and waiting room.

There the young people were met by Peggy Sankot and a half-dozen nurses. Miss Sankot and her co-workers were wearing street clothes; some also went barefoot. They were calm and reassuring as they asked the patients for their names, ages, addresses and chief complaints. The nurses allowed the more frightened patients to use false names on the forms they were filling out but urged them to remember their aliases so that their case histories could be retrieved if they ever returned to 558 Clayton Street. They also let the young people lie about their ages, although many were not even adolescents yet. The nurses often touched the patients. They were tolerant when they inquired about their problems and drug abuse.

After giving the necessary information, the young people tried to find space in the waiting room. This was difficult, for the area was even more crowded after the Clinic first opened than Father Grosjean's Episcopal Peace Center would be over a year later at 409 Clayton Street. Yet the patients were willing to crush together on the chairs and mattresses and on the single couch. Some of them chatted with each other. Others talked with Stuart Loomis and with Leonard Wolf.

But talking was so difficult in the waiting room that only those who found furniture to sit on could really converse. Because of this, most of the young people turned within themselves, tripped out on the wall decorations, or listened to Grace Slick and the Jefferson Airplane on the house radio. They also drank coffee, dropped their change into the donation can, leafed through the health pamphlets and housing information which the organizers provided, or read comic books.

While this was occurring, several dozen patients were spilling into the hallway, lining up outside the single toilet or drinking water from the bathroom sink. Arthur Lisch and three other older leaders were crowded into Bob Conrich's cubicle, where they were trying to determine if the facility was turning out to be satisfactorily hip. Conrich was digging through a card file to find transportation for patients to nearby hospitals and could not really spare the time to talk. Yet he responded to their questions. "Look, this is a cool place — you know we're here to treat people, not to bust them," he said. "It doesn't matter if some of the doctors have short hair now. You wait — how could anyone work in these conditions and stay straight?"

Lisch and his allies could have verified this assertion by stepping into the two examining rooms a few doors away. In one of these small spaces, Dr. Meyers was working alongside his wife, a physician at the student health service at San Francisco State College. She was treating a young girl for a skin problem, while he was explaining the value of personal hygiene to a boy with slashed feet. Dr. Meyers was in his shirt-sleeves, his hands and arms well scrubbed. He looked clean, even spotless, when compared to the two patients. Yet concern and sympathy showed on his face.

The same emotions could be seen in the second examining room, where the Kaiser interns were treating young people whom they had formerly attended at the Diggers' free stores. A half-dozen doctors and students from the Medical Center who had been introduced to Love Needs Care at the Haight-Ashbury Roundtable were also on hand to make diagnoses, dispense medication, and write referrals. One peered out of the front window around ten o'clock that evening and nearly fainted. He had already helped twenty patients since the Clinic opened, but for every one he treated there were two dozen others waiting outside on the street.

The Clinic administered care to over two hundred and fifty people during its first twenty-four hours of operation. On at least thirty occasions carloads of summer visitors and tribes of older veterans of the district trouped up the front steps with problems ranging from severe vitamin deficiencies to cold sores. Two young men stumbled in with second-degree burns which they sustained by touching their legs to hot motorcycle exhaust manifolds. Twelve patients were seen for infectious hepatitis, three of them jaundiced. Alan and fifty other hippies complained of bronchitis. Another thirty had colds and other infections of the upper respiratory tract.

Although most of these young people were well aware of the severity of their symptoms, some were too stoned to notice. An example was one twenty-three-year-old woman who wandered up to the registration desk at midnight wearing little more than a pink bed sheet. After Peggy Sankot spent fifteen minutes coaxing her into talking, the patient said that she had a severe cough and chills generated by a nagging cold. She then asked for medication, but Miss Sankot explained that she would have to see a doctor before she could receive any drugs.

The patient pondered this restriction and finally agreed to visit a physician. He in turn found that her problem was due not to a cold but to lower-lobe pneumonia. The Clinic was low on penicillin at this point, but Bob Conrich secured three ampules from a doctor with samples in his medical case. Peggy Sankot then urged the patient to go to the hospital. The young woman insisted that she had to hitchhike to Big Sur the following morning. Miss Sankot pleaded for reason. Conrich intervened and almost literally dragged the patient to San Francisco General. He learned en route that she had been up on acid for ten straight days.

This particular crisis passed, but the case load continued to mount. More than three hundred patients arrived at 558 Clayton Street on June eighth, many of them severely malnourished and weak with disease. Sixty-seven of the young people suffered from sprains, fractures and/or infected lacerations. Eighty-five had eczema, athlete's foot, ringworm and other skin infections. Six sustained attacks of asthma which they aggravated with LSD.

Fourteen were treated for nausea and diarrhea after they dropped acid and then consumed a week-old communal stew containing rancid vegetables and bone marrow scavenged from the San Francisco Produce Mart.

Twenty-three females were sent to Planned Parenthood during the same period for birth-control pills or pregnancy tests. Fifteen patients were taken to the Hepatitis Section at General Hospital. Twenty were treated for trichomoniasis, nonspecific urethritis and vaginitis or for other infestations of the genitourinary tract. Forty were chauffeured in private automobiles to the 33 Hunt Street Clinic for VD.

While all this was occurring, several volunteers were talking over the telephone with members of the new community who thought that the Clinic was too good to be true. Older people were also calling with medical questions; parents were inquiring after lost children; the police had questions about runaways and drugs. Middle-aged members of the Neighborhood Council who had come to 558 Clayton Street were finding housing for adolescents through Al Rinker of the Switchboard, Father Beggs of Huckleberry's, Howard Rochford, and Father Leon Harris of All Saints' Episcopal Church. Other volunteers were in touch with Robert Laws, who was trying to place patients in the Mendocino Drug Abuse Program and in the Youth Drug Unit.

At the same time, Peter Schubart and his co-workers had abandoned their position in the doorway and taken to the street. Some were restationing themselves in front of the liquor store at the corner of Haight and Clayton. Others were picking up prospective patients in the Panhandle. Still others were talking up the Clinic at Mnasidika's, the Straight Theatre and the Psychedelic Shop. And Schubart was distributing pamphlets and literature to poster buyers in the Print Mint.

Meanwhile, several of the other organizers were still trying to make arrangements with the local facilities which had agreed to take the young people whom Schubart and crew rounded up. Dr. Smith spent much of the evening of June eighth on the phone with Dr. Arthur Carfagni of the Immediate Psychiatric Aid and Referral Service. Dr. Meyers was engaged with the Pediatrics Department at the University of California, while Dr. Robert Morris was concluding his negotiations with Children's Hospital. The organizers' efforts were successful. But although they initiated a round-the-clock shuttle service, the waiting room remained stuffed with patients queuing up to see the doctors, marking time before their admission to local facilities, or merely coming in from the cold.

Even more crowded was the calm center, where Alan Rose, Doc, several other gurus and witch doctors and a handful of physicians were seeing better than fifteen adverse hallucinogenic drug reactions an hour, in addition to a few cases of acute alcohol and amphetamine toxicity. The small storeroom in which they labored was so congested that some patients who came to be detoxified had to comfort their companions before they could be assisted themselves. Sixteen people were talked down while standing up in the calm center. Many others were helped by young doctors who had never before treated a bad trip.

At least twenty patients who could not be given immediate treatment were urged to concentrate on candles. Dozens more were allowed to crash on the calm center floor. Four packing crates which had been left in the storeroom were converted into temporary sleeping pallets. One young man passed out in a mummy bag and was wakened by two patients trying to snuggle in with him. Four patients came down from hallucinogens simultaneously on a well-worn psychiatrist's couch. Two were treated together for adverse reactions in a collapsible lawn chair that often collapsed.

Such forced intimacy was seldom disastrous, but it did trigger an inevitable number of bad trips. On the evening of June ninth, for example, Al Rose returned from an emergency ride to Mission Emergency to find that an eighteen-year-old girl had freaked out on acid and was trying to throw herself through the calm center wall. After quieting this patient, Rose turned to talk down another who was prancing nude through the waiting room. He then attempted to detoxify a third hallucinating hippie, only to discover that 558 Clayton was out of medication.

"I never dreamed a crisis like that could happen," Rose recalled later. "The Haight-Ashbury I saw on television was a quiet place, a place with no violence, far away from Vietnam. But we were waging our own kind of war in the calm center: it was like working in a field hospital in a combat zone. There was noise and sweat and freaky things happening every minute. And all we had to work with after the tranquilizers ran out were candles — and love."

Yet candles and love could not keep the Clinic going. All of its penicillin and most of the antibiotics as well as the tranquilizers were depleted by June ninth, and many of the medical supplies the organizers collected had been stolen by the patients to use as souvenirs. The donated icebox had broken down and blown the fuses on three occasions. The facility needed bandages and disinfectant. Even the towels and toilet paper were running out.

558 Clayton was low on manpower as well. Drs. Smith and Morris and most of the other physicians had regular jobs and could only come to the Clinic before and after their other responsibilities. Dr. Meyers and his wife were worn out after working at the facility until four A.M. the previous two evenings. Dr. Charles Fischer, who had somehow found the time to take his final exams and receive his dental school diploma, had treated many young

people sent to the University of California Dental Clinic. Bob Conrich, Peter Schubart and Peggy Sankot were close to collapse after staying up for seventy-two hours.

Stuart Loomis and Leonard Wolf were also exhausted. Professor Loomis had counseled dozens of patients and decided that his services would be called for at 558 Clayton Street throughout the summer. But Professor Wolf, who was still intent on teaching, had concluded that the Clinic would never be quiet or roomy enough to house his Happening House. He therefore told the organizers that he would move his operation to the relative sanctity of All Saints'.

"There was simply no other alternative," he insisted. "After three nights in the waiting room I realized that not even Allen Ginsberg could hold classes there. We knew the Haight needed help in the spring. But no one ever suspected until the front door was opened that the kids were so sick."

And this was only the beginning. The organizers had once feared that their facility would not be welcomed by the new community. Now, they knew that it had been accepted — perhaps too much. If anything, the Clinic should have been expanded after its initial opening. It was only three days old at that point, and already it looked to John Luce as if it would have to close.

Reinforcements

The closing seemed imminent, but help was on the way. On the night of June tenth, just as Bob Conrich was preparing to drive yet another infected adolescent to General Hospital, David Perlman, science editor of the *San Francisco Chronicle*, walked into 558 Clayton Street and was almost floored by what he saw. Perlman put down his notebook, pitched in to take patient histories, and served as a volunteer for three hours before he could buttonhole Dr. Smith long enough to conduct an interview. He then returned to the *Chronicle*, where his impressions of "A Medical Mission in the Haight-Ashbury" were turned into a front-page story.

Perlman's article proved to be one of the most accurate ever done on the Clinic. It also set off a public response to the health emergency which made up for the city's inaction in the Haight. Less than an hour after the *Chronicle* hit the streets, the facility was besieged by phone calls from physicians and visits from friendly journalists. Herb Caen, Art Hoppe, Charles McCabe, Ralph Gleason and other *Chronicle* columnists then began to publicize the activities at 558 Clayton Street.

When their columns appeared in the *Chronicle*, checks for five, ten, twenty and even one hundred dollars started coming in through the mail. Some people walked in off the street to donate their services. Others arrived with furniture, food and medication in their cars. A doctor donated his Peugeot station wagon to be used as an ambulance. At least two dozen attorneys volunteered to assist Robert Laws in his legal aid program. Kathy Grant, the wife of Bing Crosby, drove up from her home in Hillsborough to work as a nurse on three successive evenings. Hume Cronyn and Jessica Tandy dropped by after their performances at a downtown theater one night to consult with Dr. Smith and talk with lonely adolescents in the waiting room.

At the same time, the Clinic was favored by several older bohemians who became members of its fledgling staff. One of the first to arrive was Kurt Feibusch, a forty-one-year-old actor and amateur therapist with Esalen experience who offered to supervise in the calm center and set up gestalt therapy sessions and encounter groups. He was followed by Lowell Pickett, a hard-drinking underground film maker who asked to assist in fund raising and subsequently became the first business manager.

Alan and over one hundred other hippies also responded to news of the facility and became important additions to its paramedical and clerical staff. Few could tolerate the tempo at 558 Clayton indefinitely, and many tended to turn the Clinic into the same sort of circus they had created earlier in the district. Yet, in spite of their lack of staying power and stability, the young people gave generously of their time and energy and were invaluable in writing up histories, passing out literature, taking temperatures, and talking patients down.

Equally important, they lent a spirit of acceptance to the former dentist's office and continued to win its approval on the street. Their backgrounds and motivations varied: some came to the Clinic for sex and stimulation, while others hoped to help their brothers and sisters or save themselves. Most seemed to profit from their experiences. The Clinic may have been a shaky structure, but it was a comparatively stable rock in the Haight-Ashbury storm.

One person who grew though her involvement was Laurel Rowland. She had been a college student in the East Bay before the be-in, when she left school to join the new community. But Miss Rowland was depressed by months of taking acid until she began volunteering seven days a week at 558 Clayton Street and was appointed night manager. "The Clinic gave me something other than drugs to believe in," she said. "It was the only bridge in the city between hip and straight worlds."

Although few hippies used this bridge to reenter square society, well over a hundred and fifty health professionals did employ it to come the other

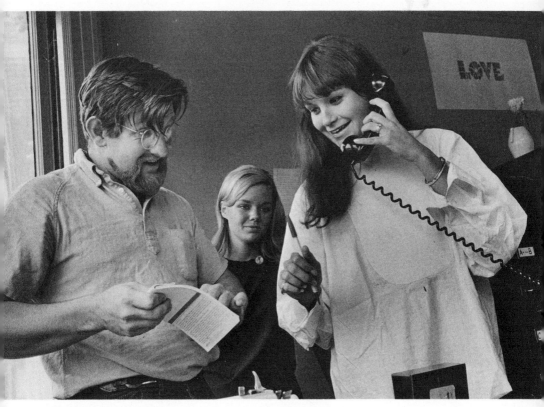

558 Clayton Street: Lowell Pickett, a volunteer, Laurel Rowland.
(Elaine Mayes)

way. Many of these medical volunteers were students, nurses, interns, residents and young physicians from the University of California and other local and out-of-town hospitals. Some belonged to the Medical Committee for Human Rights, an organization devoted to securing equal treatment for patients regardless of race, income or philosophy. Others identified with the psychedelic movement and shared a commitment to community medicine and a dissatisfaction with both the conservative stance of the American Medical Association and the bureaucratic rigidity which characterizes so many public health departments.

Some of these activists admittedly were interested in action for its own sake. Others saw the Clinic as a viable alternative to existing institutions and as a symbol of shifts to come in medical treatment practices. Most used the facility as a vehicle to bring health services to poverty-stricken patients on their own level and learned a great deal of emergency medicine in the process.

The volunteers often said that public and private medical organizations required them to spend more time arguing over fees than treating patients. They recalled having to turn away people who could not pay for treatment after being advised to offer less comprehensive care to so-called second-class citizens. 558 Clayton Street gave the volunteers a chance to practice their skills without worrying about discrimination or administrative inflexibility. It thereby afforded them one of the few opportunities in medicine to do their thing.

One physician who used the facility for these and other purposes was Dr. Eugene Schoenfeld. He was a twenty-nine-year-old general practitioner who had assisted at the Albert Schweitzer Hospital and Leprosarium in West Africa while a medical student. Dr. Schoenfeld became interested in the hallucinogens in Africa and participated in several drug experiments with Dr. Smith, Dr. Charles Hine and Charles Fischer at the Medical Center in 1967. After working at the Center for Special Problems in the winter and spring and in the Haight that summer, he became famous as the author of "Dear Dr. Hip Pocrates," a syndicated health column that first appeared in the *Berkeley Barb*.

Although most of the medical volunteers were young and of Dr. Schoenfeld's persuasion, over fifty older doctors also came to the Clinic. Among them were Dr. Richard Gleason, a general practitioner from Oakland who commuted to the Haight-Ashbury twice weekly with his nurse; Dr. Norman Sissman, chief of pediatric cardiology at Stanford University and his wife Hallie, a social anthropologist; Dr. David Breithaupt, a San Jose internist; Dr. Bertram Meyer, a forty-six-year-old internist and friend of Florence Martin; and Dr. Alan Matzger, a local surgeon who was having difficulty establishing himself in private practice. Dr. Matzger became interested in community medicine and realized that "in terms of adolescent drug and health problems, 558 Clayton Street stood on the medical frontier."

Like Dr. Matzger, some of the older professionals came to the Haight to help young patients and to acquire an understanding of them. Others had high school or college-age children and were prompted primarily by guilt or parental anxiety. Still others were military physicians who enjoyed working in a nominally structured situation. Many considered themselves overspecialized and looked on the Clinic as a place where they might broaden their medical experience. Most were so disappointed by the city's unresponsiveness to the Haight-Ashbury that they donated large amounts of time, money and medicine to 558 Clayton Street, always at the risk of censure or ostracism from their peers.

Another risk they ran was more serious, for in spite of house rules to the contrary, illegal drugs were often possessed and/or dealt by patients at the Clinic. Park Station was apparently aware of this, as were the San Francisco Narcotics Detail and the State Narcotics Bureau, all of which sent men through the facility on occasion. Yet Matthew O'Connor of the state bureau offered sound advice to Dr. Smith, and although the local police approved neither of the drug abusers nor of the doctors at 558 Clayton, they never tried to bust the Clinic. "The beat patrolmen came in periodically, usually looking for runaways," Dr. Bertram Meyer remembered. "They never really liked us, I guess, but they always let us get our work done."

Dr. Meyer was a regular volunteer at 558 Clayton Street during the summer of 1967. He was therefore well qualified to speak of the potential hazards he and the other physicians faced. He also resembled the other volunteers in his liberal attitude towards young people, his belief in nonviolence, his opposition to the Vietnam war and his commitment to the Haight. He could give, therefore, several reasons for his involvement with the Clinic.

I have a teen-age son. But equally important was the fact that the Clinic provided me with an outlet for my idealism. What excited me most was that we were trying to evolve a new and badly needed approach to community health problems, providing services to one disposessed minority which should be afforded to all. The approach was never finalized, because we were in a constant state of flux and had to respond to new crises every day. But our adaptability was intentional. We wanted to answer the needs of our patients as they, their problems and their abuse patterns changed.

This was something nobody else was doing, something that ran counter to standard operating procedures at the time. Instead of selecting patients on the basis of their finances or supposed moral suitability, we went out to find them in their own environment. Ours was a revolutionary concept — a real experiment — but it proved its worth. And though the facility always had problems, it also had the potential for becoming what every neighborhood health center should be.

Several organizational changes were in order before this potential could be actualized. The first was initiated by Dr. Dernburg, who arrived at 558 Clayton Street five hours after reading about it in the *Chronicle* and worked there the next twenty-six nights in a row. Although long-term psychological problems were his primary objective, Dr. Dernburg was so struck by the physical sickness and acute drug difficulties he saw at the Clinic that he gave them top priority. As a result, he spent most of his nights examining patients, treating their cuts and bruises, and helping with bad trips. He also trained volunteers for the calm center, counseled some persons about draft problems, took others into his private practice, and made house calls.

These various activities kept Dr. Dernburg busy, if not satisfied, for several weeks. But he began to scale down his medical involvement to establish a psychiatric service as the summer progressed. After obtaining the approval of the chief of psychiatry, he recruited a number of psychiatric residents and older volunteers from Mt. Zion Hospital. He also arranged to have psychiatric patients hospitalized at Mt. Zion and at St. Mary's Hospital. Then, aided by Stuart Loomis and two dozen psychiatrists and social workers who had independently come to 558 Clayton, he instituted group and individual therapy sessions when conditions permitted. These services were gradually expanded, and Dr. Dernburg became psychiatric director.

The next alteration in its structure was accomplished by Donald Reddick, the thirty-four-year-old president of Medical Logistics. Reddick was the son of a doctor. He was born and raised in the Haight-Ashbury, attended Temple University in Philadelphia, and served as a corpsman with the army in Korea before returning to San Francisco. Reddick thought of himself as a bohemian and felt protective towards the hippies. When he came to 558 Clayton Street, it reminded him also of a field hospital in a combat zone.

Reddick was eager to aid in the war the Clinic was waging. He offered to obtain cases of drug samples from the detail men who did business with Medical Logistics and donated stethoscopes, storage chests, examining tables and other equipment from his own company. He and his business partners then established a more efficient bookkeeping system at the facility and streamlined the procedures for writing up histories and regulating the pa-

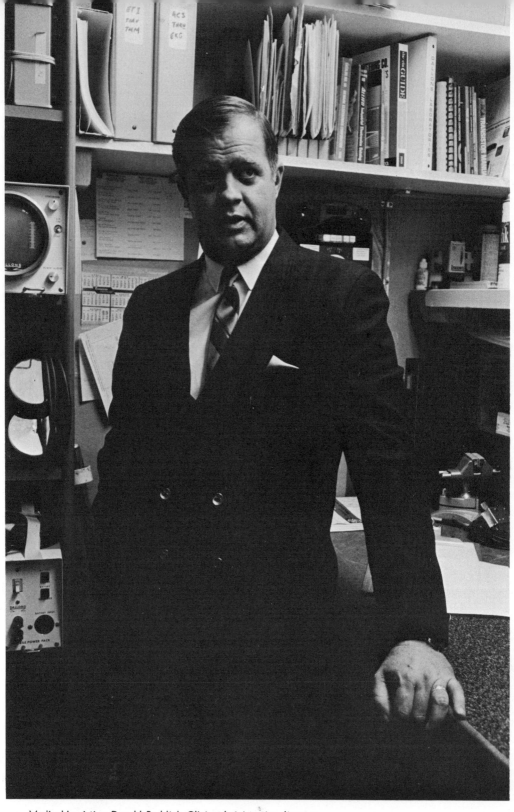

Medical Logistics: Donald Reddick, Clinic administrative director.
(Elaine Mayes)

tient flow. Reddick came to the Clinic almost every night after work that summer. He was named administrative director, in charge of all clerical and paramedical personnel.

While this was occurring, a third organizational step was taken by Dr. William Nesbitt, a general practitioner from the town of Fairfield, an hour and a half east of San Francisco. In 1966, he and four others founded a nonprofit corporation called Youth Projects to design a treatment program for emotionally disturbed adolescents. Although they had little money, they read the *Chronicle* article and sensed that the Clinic was the realization of their plans.

Dr. Nesbitt inspected the facility a few days later and learned that the organizers were having some difficulty in securing donations because they had not been able to obtain a nonprofit status through which gifts could be declared tax deductible. He then invited them to join Youth Projects and use its tax shelter as their own. The organizers agreed enthusiastically. The Haight-Ashbury Free Medical Clinic and its as-yet-inoperative Happening House thus became a field project of Youth Projects, and Dr. Nesbitt began driving regularly from Fairfield to volunteer.

Because of these several developments, the Clinic was better organized and outfitted at this point in its brief history than ever before. And although its operating budget was a mere three thousand dollars a month, the facility was treating more than five times as many patients as Park Emergency Hospital at less than one-fifth the cost. Chaos continued at 558 Clayton, but the Clinic's unqualified success in reaching alienated young people was making a profound impact throughout San Francisco.

It was also becoming somewhat of an embarrassment to the Public Health Department, which was under attack by the *Chronicle* for its failure to act in the Haight-Ashbury. The department's response to the attack was suggested on June twentieth, when Dr. Ellis Sox announced that the city planned to allocate two hundred thousand dollars to open a more "proper" health center in the district before the end of July. And it was confirmed a few days later, when Mayor John Shelley told the press that the free facility already operating in the area was supported by public funds.

Whether misinformed or intentionally malicious, the mayor dealt a near fatal blow to 558 Clayton Street. In fact, the Clinic soon received over fifty phone calls from people who felt they had been duped into becoming its friends. As word spread of Dr. Sox's supposed center, other potential donors decided that the Haight no longer needed their support. Mail contributions slackened, and the organizers were forced to start a second desperate drive for financial aid.

Their efforts were fruitful, but barely in time. Although they obtained enough private pledges to keep going until August, when they assumed the Public Health Department would open its own center and perhaps reimburse them for the patients they were treating, many of the organizers doubted that the Haight-Ashbury would last that long. School was out across the country by this time; the Monterey International Pop Festival had been held, attracting over thirty thousand people to San Francisco and its rock groups, the Summer Solstice Festival was approaching, and the presence of thousands of young people was bringing significant changes in the drug traffic on the street.

Chemical Shift

One factor which underlay the shift in chemical consumption was the weakened position of the new community. The beats and hippies still set the ethical tone of the district, but their specious community solidarity and love philosophy had less and less influence over the hoodies and habitual abusers as the summer progressed. The summer hippies also had little spiritual hold over the new population because they were too caught up in their own survival to care for the welfare of other people streaming into the Haight.

Another reason related to the scarcity of good LSD in the area. Owsley and several of his imitators were still turning out pharmacologically respectable hallucinogens, yet they could not begin to supply the entire Haight-Ashbury with unadulterated drugs. Indeed, Haight Street was already resembling the smorgasbord that Matthew O'Connor would call it in 1968. Commercialism and mass consumption had been added to the new community's chemical search for a better life.

A third factor was the recent change in public tastes. Some hippies had developed psychological problems through LSD and were now amenable to more intense central stimulation for medicinal purposes. The summer hippies also had problems and were attracted to amphetamines because of their natural curiosity and their need for instant courage. And although Randy and others like him abused LSD when it was available, they were temperamentally more suited for speed.

These facts, coupled with the comparative cheapness and the ease of production of counterfeit amphetamines, all served to influence the laws of supply and demand which operated in the Haight. This in turn led several local cooks and large-scale manufacturers to start mixing speed and acid together to maximize the hallucinogenic and stimulative properties of their products while minimizing the possibility of bad trips.

Needless to say, these new chemicals did nothing of the sort. In fact, they actually increased the occurrence of panic reactions seen at the Clinic, because the tachycardia, muscle tremors and anxiety induced by the amphetamine components were magnified in minds sensitized by LSD. Yet thousands of young people in the Haight-Ashbury continued to swallow adulterated drugs. Some summer visitors treated at 558 Clayton Street were so ingenuous that they assumed protoplasmic consciousness could be had from all toxic substances, including alcohol. Others preferred the speed-acid mixtures. Many were so confused that they neither knew what they were taking nor had any way of determining the percentage composition of the chemicals they took.

Furthermore, these compounds were identified not generically but by misleading brand names comparable to those used for legitimate pharmaceutical medications. Over two dozen preparations purported to be LSD were sold with Madison Avenue techniques for from fifty cents to four dollars per tablet during the summer with such esoteric labels as "white lightning," "yellow flats" and "blue dots." Few of these drugs remained on the street long enough for their quality to be determined. They were seldom manufactured in quantities sufficient to sustain prolonged sales campaigns, and once a particular product was accepted as righteous, or pharmacologically dependable, cheap copies were immediately introduced.

The blue dots were a case in point. They were Vitamin C tablets splashed with acid and food coloring which proved to be quite popular during June for their health-giving, as well as hallucinogenic effects. But soon after they won customer approval, similar tablets without LSD were distributed. The original product then had to be withdrawn from the market and another series of dots appeared on the street.

Such chemicals continued to proliferate over the summer, reinforcing the changes in drug-taking as they did. Thus, although most members of the new community stayed loyal to acid, some were either so discouraged by the scarcity of righteous acid or so eager for stimulation that they began swallowing or injecting speed, while others who tried to remain psychedelic began experimenting with certain prescription and underground products because of their supposedly hallucinogenic properties.

One of these substances was amantadine or Symmetrel, a compound which inhibits the penetration into cells of viruses like influenza A and is employed medically to prevent development of the flu. Another was methysergide or Sansert, an expensive ergot alkaloid similar to ergonovine that is used in the prevention of migraine headaches. Neither Sansert nor Symmetrel was ever widely popular, but the psychotomimetic amphetamines were.

The psychotomimetic amphetamines are called hallucinogenic amphetamine congeners by Dr. Meyers. They are a number of compounds that combine the central nervous system stimulation of amphetamines with the psychotomimetic, or mind-alerting qualities of mescaline and other true hallucinogenic drugs. They are distinguished by a molecular structure which tends to intensify and accelerate their action on the central nervous system while lessening their peripheral effects.

The psychotomimetic amphetamines were so named by Dr. Alexander Shulgin, a Bay Area chemist who synthesized dozens of the compounds during his association with Dow Chemical. Dr. Shulgin hoped that his creations might proved useful either as therapeutic agents or as adjuncts to psychotherapy, but his employers gave them to the army for its chemical warfare work. Their formulas were then reportedly released "for identification purposes" and found their way to the underground. Because the drugs are difficult to synthesize, their manufacture was restricted to the more chemically sophisticated individuals, like Owsley, who supplied the Haight.

The first two major psychotomimetic amphetamines created by Dr. Shulgin were MDA, which is known chemically as 2,3-methylenedioxyamphetamine, and MMDA, or 3-methoxy-4,5-methylenedioxyamphetamine. These two compounds are comparable to mescaline in several of their properties and produce a six-to-eight-hour hallucinogenic experience that is accompanied by a dilation of the pupils, an increase in heartbeat and other peripheral effects.

MDA and MMDA also induce a pronounced memory recall, a fact that interested certain physicians when Dr. Shulgin reported his findings in 1964. But the medical profession looked with disfavor on the compounds by 1967, when they were well thought of by certain more sophisticated members of the new community. Their use was limited to intimates of Owsley, and neither MDA nor MMDA ever appeared in bulk form on the street.

In fact, the only one of Dr. Shulgin's creations which was seen in substantial quantities during 1967 was DOM, or 2,5-dimethoxy-4-methylamphetamine. DOM contains several modifications not found in the two earlier compounds: it is almost eighty times as potent as mescaline in its hallucinogenic properties and may also cause extreme perceptual distortions and persistent flashbacks at a higher dosage level. When taken in ten- to twenty-milligram doses, the drug's central action may last as long as twenty-four hours, during which time the toxic psychosis often produced may be aggravated by attendant overstimulation and loss of sleep. Although now common knowledge, this information was not available at the start of the Summer of Love either to members of the new community or to the Clinic doctors, some of whom were familiar with Dr. Shulgin's work. This was because DOM was not sold as such in the Haight-Ashbury. Instead, it was marketed as STP.

According to hippie legend, Owsley named STP after Scientifically Treated Petroleum, the popular American oil additive, "because it makes your motor run smoother and lubricates your head." The chemical was given a slightly different connotation by the *Oracle* and *Barb,* which praised it in May of 1967 as a legal substitute for LSD that allegedly produced three days of Serenity, Tranquillity and Peace. STP was handed out to a few select customers during June, so that the Haight was soon prepared for the new panacea. But when it showed up at 558 Clayton Street, the drug caused nothing resembling serenity, tranquillity — or peace.

The first case of STP intoxication was seen at the Clinic on the frantic evening of June ninth, when a nineteen-year-old boy said that he had ingested the chemical two days earlier and had not managed to regain his senses. The facility was short of Thorazine at this point, so the attending physician gave the patient a mild sedative, which helped him go to sleep. Dr. Smith then obtained some STP and sent it to Dr. Meyers, who made preliminary judgments before forwarding the sample to the Food and Drug Administration for further inspection.

Dr. Smith saw several more STP cases at San Francisco General Hospital while he and Dr. Meyers were awaiting word from Washington. The first occurred on June sixteenth, when two nineteen-year-old boys were brought into Mission Emergency for detoxification. Although both were hallucinating wildly, only one patient was given a high dose of Thorazine; the other received no medication because his mother, a Christian Scientist, would not allow it.

This was actually beneficial to the second individual, for while he came down eventually, his companion became even more agitated after the medication was administered and had to be placed in an oxygen tent. Dr. Smith presented these findings to Dr. Meyers and they reasoned that STP was probably an atropinelike substance whose effects were intensified by antipsychotic agents. Knowing that many young people in the Haight kept their own supplies of Thorazine, they feared that an epidemic of STP reactions would be precipitated if the drug were ever distributed en masse.

These fears were realized at the Summer Solstice Festival on June twenty-first. This event had been billed by the Thelins and others during the spring as a climax of the summer migration to San Francisco which would be bigger and better than the be-in. But it proved to be a real bummer from the start. Although a huge sunrise service was planned prior to the day's festivities, most of the planners overslept. Only a few dozen young people attended the service, and no more than five thousand assembled later that morning on Speedway Meadows in Golden Gate Park.

The entertainment was also tardy, and when the Grateful Dead finally pulled up on a stake truck, the generator would not start. The group therefore had little influence over its audience, which had swelled and gathered by now around an impromptu barbecue and was wolfing down spoiled hamburgers and water-stained buns. Then, to top everything, five thousand STP tablets were passed through the crowd like after-dinner mints. After the Dead drifted away and the Clinic physicians were alerted, the festival casualties started stumbling into 558 Clayton Street.

First to arrive was a twenty-three-year-old earth mother who was convinced because of recurrent palpitations that she was having a heart attack. Next came two young men who said their pulses were racing and their "brains were on fire." They were followed during the evening by over twenty young people, many of whom suffered from hyperventilation, hallucinosis, food poisoning and fatigue. The Clinic doctors were cautioned against using antipsychotic agents with these patients. They therefore tried to calm them with antianxiety agents but were forced to send several patients to Mission Emergency Hospital.

The physicians eventually left much of the detoxification up to a familiar bearded witch doctor named Swami or Superguru, who sat five STP victims in a circle in the calm center, instructed them to stare into candles, and intoned at length about vibrations and love. He was still talking later that night when several more patients reached the facility and reported that they had been able to tolerate the first hours of the experience but were exhausted now and unable to turn themselves off.

This complaint was heard often over the next two days, until the STP taken at the Summer Solstice Festival finally ran its course. Almost every patient who sought help at 558 Clayton Street during that period said that the worst thing about this so-called miracle substance was his own inability to master it. Several adolescents also revealed that they had taken Thorazine at some point during their experience and had become even more anxious when they were still unable to control themselves. Most eventually left the Clinic in good condition. But all were somewhat embarrassed after flunking the STP test.

Although these young people sustained only severe blows to their egos, others suffered more devastating long-term effects. An example was one twenty-year-old boy who originally asked for treatment of a panic reaction and was seen two weeks later for a complete loss of body sensation. This patient said that he initially felt a tingling in the bottom of his feet which spread up his legs until he experienced a lack of feeling in his scrotum. Because he was also incoherent and paranoid, the doctor in charge concluded that his condition was due to a drug-induced psychosis. He then referred him to the Immediate Psychiatric Aid and Referral Service where the patient was encouraged without success to begin psychotherapy.

Dr. Carfagni and his staff saw a number of other psychotic patients over the next few weeks, many of whom were delivered by the police. One, a seventeen-year-old girl who was arrested for "aberrant behavior" and then manhandled by two officers at Mission Emergency, had to be held in the psychiatric ward for five days until she stopped hallucinating. Another patient, a twenty-year-old male who had taken one STP tablet orally and another intravenously, was found racing nude through the park. He was kept under sedation for several days and eventually reported that he had removed his clothes so that he might be arrested and taken to the hospital, where "the Mafia couldn't get at me." The patient was discharged shortly thereafter, claiming that he had enjoyed his drug experience in spite of his delusions and occasional flashbacks. One month later he was arrested after an abortive robbery. The diagnosis: psychosis probably precipitated by STP.

As such cases mounted, particularly those in which patients manifested tachycardia, flashbacks and paranoia, Drs. Smith and Meyers became more and more convinced that the chemical acted not like atropine but like a combination of acid and speed. Then, just as they set out to inform their patients of these findings, word arrived simultaneously from the Food and Drug Administration and from Dr. Shulgin that STP was in fact a psychotomimetic amphetamine. The physicians therefore increased their distribution of a poster outlining the dangers of self-medication. It read: "STP Users — Do Not Take Thorazine, Seconal or Other Downers for STP Bum Trips. Call the Free Medical Clinic If You Need Help."

Thanks largely to these efforts, STP all but disappeared from the Haight-Ashbury over the summer, only to return later as a component in other drugs. But although this particular problem passed, the emergence of the psychotomimetic amphetamines marked an important transition in chemical consumption on the street. Many young people had been exposed to intense central nervous system stimulation for the first time through these compounds and were also introduced to a new and much more demanding chemical challenge. Thus, although the hallucinogens remained the drugs of choice in the district for several months after the STP episode, their prominence was gradually undercut by such destructive substances as speed.

Heads and Freaks

At the same time, this transition in drug taking was paralleled by the evolution of two separate subcultures in the Haight. The first was made up of hard-core hippies like Alan and summer hippies who sampled amphetamines occasionally but still maintained their faith in peace, love and LSD and considered themselves members of the new community. These young people and the few beats who had adopted the psychedelic life-style seldom referred to themselves as hippies. Following Ken Kesey, they called themselves acid heads.

The second subculture consisted of elements of the new population that sanctioned violence and crime and contributed to what Roger Smith would eventually describe as the Marketplace of Speed. Because the members of this group looked like hippies, the public had trouble differentiating them from the other young people in the Haight-Ashbury. The media oversimplified the situation by calling everyone on Haight Street hip.

Both groups kept to themselves as much as possible during the summer, the hippies spending more time in their communes, the hoodies and habitual abusers shooting chemicals in their crystal palaces and roaming the street. Both groups also grew more defensive, the first chiding the second for being unconcerned about transcendence, the second ridiculing the spiritual aspirations of the first. And both groups competed for the attention of those uncommitted summer hippies whose psychological makeup determined their heroes and the patterns of their drug abuse.

Some cross-fertilization went on between the two subcultures, particularly because some speed freaks wanted to be psychedelic and because the new arrivals borrowed from both groups in creating their own life-style. But by and large, the subcultures became more self-contained, each manifesting its own kinds of psychological problems and physical illnesses as the summer progressed.

Although this distinction may have been lost on the media, it was all too apparent at 558 Clayton Street. Many amphetamine abusers were initially reluctant to use the facility because of its strong hippie identification, but some, like Randy, swallowed their suspicions when they became unduly sick. As a result, certain physicians began to gather patients because they were considered tolerant of, if not friendly toward, speed freaks. Dr. Morris, for one, regularly treated amphetamine abusers. Dr. Dernburg was also accepted by the second subculture. He was therefore afforded an early opportunity to investigate its magnitude when Randy escorted him to a hotel on Haight Street one evening to assist a patient who had overamped.

Randy had established a semipermanent residence at this crystal palace and was therefore able to get Dr. Dernburg past the heavily armed manager who sat at the front desk. Yet Dr. Dernburg was given a thorough going-over by three speed freaks as he climbed the first flight of steps. Gaunt and menacing faces peered out at him as he walked down the second-floor hallway, and he noticed corpselike figures stretched out on the floors and the furniture in several shuttered rooms.

When Dr. Dernburg reached the third-floor landing, Randy went ahead to give some sort of password to a handful of half-dressed young people who were standing in the hallway. This screening procedure lasted a full ten minutes, during which time Dr. Dernburg was prohibited from looking into the adjoining doorways. He was then confronted by Randy's companions, who ordered him to produce credentials verifying his association with the Clinic.

After this was accomplished, he was ushered toward a locked door behind which he could hear high-pitched screams. Randy and his other escorts shouted through the thin partition, and after a few seconds the door was opened to reveal a thin, deathly white female face. Dr. Dernburg entered a room that was strewn with needles, piles of white powder, bed sheets, sleeping bags, soft-drink cartons and cat dung. He was then directed toward a bed over which three people were leaning. Beneath them lay a six-foot AWOL serviceman who weighed less than ninety pounds.

He was lying in a foul pool of sweat. Beside him was a much-used needle with a broken, rusty tip. His jaundiced face glistened with perspiration and was sunken around the eye sockets. His heart raced. His arms, visible under the shreds of a long-sleeved uniform, were covered with fresh tracks or needle punctures and swollen with abscesses the size of baseballs. Running up to one shoulder was a darkened blood vessel, the sign of septicemia, or blood poisoning. He mumbled incoherently and writhed under Dr. Dernburg's touch. He screamed: "Let me die; don't bust me; I've had enough."

Dr. Dernburg sent Randy to 558 Clayton Street to get the house ambulance. He then turned to find that his first set of escorts had vacated the room. After picking up the patient, who was too weak to walk, he carried him to the landing. There he was assaulted by a psychotic young man in a grimy trench coat who apparently mistook him for an undercover narcotics agent. Dr. Dernburg calmed his assailant by providing proof of his identity as a doctor. Once again, he was allowed to pass.

More furtive glances followed his progress down the stairway and into the street. Randy and Bob Conrich had arrived by this time; they helped Dr. Dernburg deposit the serviceman in the Peugeot station wagon. A half-dozen Hell's Angels then appeared and demanded to know what was happening. One of them recognized Conrich; they then volunteered to run interference for the ambulance through the traffic on the street. The Clinic staff members lost their motorcycle vanguard near the Fillmore district. They arrived at San Francisco General twenty minutes later, where their patient was treated for septicemia, malnutrition, cellulitis and serum hepatitis, and was subsequently sent to the psychiatric ward.

This incident was the most bizarre in Dr. Dernburg's experience to date. Yet it was not an isolated example, for amphetamine abuse had become a fact of life in the Haight-Ashbury by the beginning of July. Over three hundred speed freaks came to 558 Clayton Street or were treated by physicians in their crystal palaces over the summer. Although few asked for long-term psychiatric intervention, Drs. Charles Fischer and David Smith were able to analyze their chief clinical complaints.

They found that eighty-eight percent of these patients overamped or experienced acute anxiety reactions at some point during the summer. Fifty-seven percent apparently had amphetamine-induced or precipitated psychoses of a paranoid-schizophrenic nature. Thirty-seven percent were completely exhausted. Only eight percent were either undergoing or willing to begin abstinence from drugs.

In terms of their physical symptoms, thirty-eight percent of the patients manifested malnutrition and general debility. Twenty-four percent were seen for serum hepatitis; twenty-four percent for abscesses and cellulitis; twenty percent for gastrointestinal disturbances; eight percent for muscle cramping and/or hyperventilation; seven percent for migraine and other forms of headache; five percent for extreme tachycardia; and forty-seven percent for traumatic injuries.

The speed freaks also suffered from upper respiratory tract infections and venereal diseases. But the drug-related problems that Drs. Smith and Fischer analyzed were so common that they constituted an independent health entity. Because of this, the Clinic physicians ultimately lumped the symptoms together as a medical syndrome associated with amphetamine abuse. They then used this syndrome to distinguish the speed-dominated subculture in the Haight.

At the same time, Dr. Smith postulated the existence of a psychedelic syndrome to describe the problems which stemmed from hallucinogenic drug abuse. He included in this category the bad trip or acute anxiety reaction, flashbacks and recurrent perceptual distortions, the messianic delusions characteristic of the toxic LSD psychosis, and the same psychological deficiencies, emotional impoverishments, defenses against feelings, inhibited aggression and superstitious beliefs that Dr. Dernburg linked with chronic hallucinogenic toxicity.

This syndrome encompassed the hippies' psychological difficulties, but it could not be so readily extended to their physical complaints. Since these young people seldom injected chemicals they spared themselves the abscesses, cellulitis and serum hepatitis so often seen in the speed freaks. They also avoided such symptoms as the excessive tachycardia and muscle cramping which were related pharmacologically to amphetamine consumption. Some did become nauseated or aggravated their asthma attacks with acid, but their physical problems were caused much more by their life-style than by their drugs. Because of this, the speed- and LSD-oriented subcultures differed in kind as well as degree.

This difference was illustrated in their eating and sleeping habits. While the amphetamine abusers went for weeks without nourishment or REM sleep, most of the hippies paid nominal attention to their health. Some ate either macrobiotic foods or followed esoteric diets. Others, especially the summer visitors, survived on Digger stew or on high-carbohydrate meals made up of hot dogs, bakery products and potato chips. Such practices were far from exemplary, but because the hallucinogenic abusers ate at least something and did not take sleep- and appetite-suppressant compounds, they were less advanced in their malnourishment and general debility than the speed freaks. The former were deficient in their vitamin intake, while the latter were also deprived of proteins.

The vitamins the hippies were often deficient in included B-1, or thiamine, which is used for carbohydrate metabolism and is usually lacking in many alcoholics and in people with beriberi; vitamin B-2 or riboflavin, the lack of which causes several symptoms comparable to those of thiamine deficiency; and the vitamins B-3, or niacin and niacinimide, which are found in liver and whole-grain cereals and are responsible for the regulation of several enzyme systems within the body.

Avitaminosis B-3 may cause pellagra, a disease that is manifested by red and roughened skin, diarrhea, motor disturbances, psychological depression and peculiar oral sucking movements. Pellagra is found most often in the United States among American Indians and farmers who eat large amounts of corn and little else. The hippies did not consume corn to the exclusion of other carbohydrates and therefore did not lack vitamin B-3 in their diets. But mild avitaminosis B-3 may have contributed to their many dermatological and gastrointestinal problems. This was suggested by the fact that these difficulties seemed to occur less frequently in those patients who told the Clinic doctors that they treated their bad trips with vitamin B-3.

One additional water-soluble vitamin in which these young people were commonly deficient was ascorbic acid, or vitamin C, found in citrus fruits and leafy vegetables. It is employed by the body in the formation and sustenance of such intercellular supporting structures as bone matrix, cartilage and the dentine of the teeth and is also used in the maintenance of blood capillaries. Avitaminosis C may lead to hemorrhages of the gingivae, or gums, porosity of dentine, and scurvy, the symptoms of which are pronounced hemorrhaging, loss of teeth, swelling and pain in the joints, resistance to healing, a marked bleeding tendency and anemia. Although it is now rare in nutritionally advanced areas of the United States, from two to ten cases of mild scurvy were seen weekly during the Summer of Love at 558 Clayton Street. Many patients who experienced less serious avitaminosis C nevertheless exhibited abnormal bleeding and dental problems. The only time these problems appeared to decrease in the district was shortly after the blue dot episode, when LSD was marketed on Haight Street in tablets of vitamin C.

The presence of scurvy and other avitaminoses partially explained the prevalence of disease in the Haight-Ashbury and also helped distinguish its two subcultures. Yet, although such distinctions did exist, there were many problems that the young residents of the district shared. The speed and acid abusers veered further and further apart over the summer of 1967, but they still infected one another through their mutual physical confinement and through their interaction at places like the Clinic. Because of this, the members of the new community and the new population were all exposed to such illnesses as upper respiratory tract infections. And many of them were susceptible to the mass infections which had prompted the organizers to conceive of 558 Clayton Street in the spring.

The Sickness They Shared

The first contagion to sweep the Haight during the Summer of Love was rubeola, or measles. This infection is caused by filterable viruses which are transmitted by droplet spray and result in high temperatures, nasal obstruction, sore throat, rashes, a lowering of the white blood cell count and/or a swelling of the regional lymph nodes. Over one hundred young people sought treatment for rubeola at the Clinic during July of 1967, where they managed to infect Dr. Smith and two dozen volunteers. Those physicians who did not catch rubeola themselves prescribed analgesics, bed rest, nourishing diets and isolation for the infected patients who came to them. Yet they were unable to combat the contagion effectively, and it passed from person to person along the street with every cough and sneeze.

Another illness the doctors could not control was mononucleosis, or mono. Mononucleosis is an acute viral infection that is transmitted primarily through droplet spray but is also spread from one person to another through an exchange of saliva, a fact which explains its nickname, "the kissing sickness." Its symptoms usually include fever, sore throat, rash, general malaise and enlarged lymph nodes.

Treatment is symptomatic, especially in those patients with secondary complications, and includes bed rest and the administration of analgesics and the appropriate antibiotics. Such medications were in constant demand during July of 1967, when mononucleosis appeared concurrently with the rubeola epidemic. Over seventy suspected cases were seen at 558 Clayton Street, but because the facility lacked the equipment necessary to make definite diagnoses, all were referred to the General Hospital for further tests.

The third contagion to hit the district was streptococcal pharyngitis, or strep throat. This is an acute infection that is caused by treptococcal bacteria, which are transmitted by respiratory droplets. It results in an abrupt fever that is often accompanied by sore throat, nausea, vomiting, headaches and abdominal pain lasting from three to seven days. Streptococcal pharyngitis is treated with bed rest, isolation and antibiotics such as penicillin. It was an extremely serious problem in the Haight, where isolating its victims was a virtual impossibility. Over one hundred patients were treated at the Clinic for its symptoms during July. Dr. Meyers, Peter Schubart and several other staff members had strep throats that summer. Twenty-seven volunteers were also infected.

Even more young people suffered from influenza, the flu, an acute infection caused by several types of virus and transmitted by the respiratory route. Influenza has an incubation period of from one to four days followed by a fever which persists for about four days. But for those weakened by age or the malnourishment and other illnesses so common in the Haight-Ashbury, it may lead to such secondary infections as sinusitis, otitis media and bronchitis or to a pneumonia which may result from either pneumococcal bacteria or the flu virus itself.

Although certain vaccines and drugs like amantadine offer protection against the influenza virus, they confer only a short immunity and are used primarily with older patients. Other patients generally require supportive treatment that involves the administration of analgesics, sedatives, cough medicine and bed rest to reduce the possibility of secondary infections. Such methods were often employed by the physicians at 558 Clayton Street, for over two hundred young people picked up the flu in a mid-July attack.

Influenza, streptococcal pharyngitis, mononucleosis and rubeola continued to flare up in the Haight-Ashbury during the next few months, but all ran their most severe course by the middle of July. Furthermore, although the potential for even more dangerous infections always existed in the district, meningitis, tuberculosis and plague were never seen there during the Summer of Love. This was a great consolation to the Clinic doctors. Yet they were given no permanent relief, for acute and chronic sickness continued to increase in the Haight.

As always, the most common illnesses were bronchitis, colds and other infections of the upper respiratory tract. Pneumonia was also a problem that summer, both because of the high incidence of influenza and because the Haight-Ashbury was frequently blanketed by fog. On one weekend night in July, for example, two adolescents who had tried to mask their symptoms with toxic chemicals stumbled into 558 Clayton Street and had to be rushed to San Francisco General. During the next week, three youths who had avoided treatment contracted pleurisy, an inflammation of the double-layered mucous membrane which lines the lungs, the diaphragm and the chest. Antibiotics were administered to these three patients, along with analgesics to relieve their pain. Two of the young people responded well to the medication. Neither had to be hospitalized.

The exception was Alan, whose chronic bronchitis enabled him to contract both pneumonia and pleurisy after he meditated through a rainstorm in Golden Gate Park. Alan was stoned on mescaline at the time and did not realize the full extent of his symptoms until he came to 558 Clayton Street to volunteer that evening and passed out in the waiting room. He was then rushed by Kurt Feibusch to San Francisco General, where he spent several days in an oxygen tent. Alan felt fine following his release from the hospital, but Dr. Dernburg and the other physicians familiar with his history of asthma feared that he might someday succumb to respiratory and pulmonary disease.

Less serious, but equally alarming to the doctors were the many skin problems they had to contend with over the summer. In addition to the cellulitis and abscesses seen in amphetamine abusers, these included eczema, impetigo, cold sores, athlete's foot and dermatophytosis, tinea corporis or body ringworm and tinea cruris, or jock itch, a fungal infection of the skin around the genitalia that is related to improper drying, to profuse sweating and to the wearing of tight clothes. This disease was treated with dusting powders and Tinactin solution at the Clinic. The same medication was used in treating the body ringworm that patients contracted from their domestic animals.

Along with ringworm, many young people picked up pediculosis and scabies in the Haight. Some of them also suffered from the bites of spiders and mosquitos and the fleas which lived in their beds and on the bodies of their pets. These bites were seldom serious, but many hippies scratched them so frequently that they developed purulent rashes which required antibiotics and cortisone ointment for relief. Cortisone was also called for in the case of patients who contracted poison oak from their animals or from playing, sleeping and/or balling in the park.

A more common skin problem seen in the Haight-Ashbury during the summer of 1967 was acne vulgaris. The Clinic physicians tried to educate adolescents with acne about proper hygiene and eating habits. They also prescribed haircuts and shaving for some patients who developed pustules under their long hair and beards. Others were urged to irradiate their skin with sunlight and to use antibacterial detergents and astringent lotions to counteract oiliness. The doctors often prevented extensive scarring through these procedures. Yet they could not reach those who were committed to eccentric diets or those who patronized the food stands on Haight Street.

This was unfortunate, for these young people sustained more than their share of dental problems. Because they seldom brushed their teeth or gums, many had halitosis. And because they often ate carbohydrates and sticky foods, they also manifested a great deal of tooth discoloration. Some who smoked incessantly and drank a great deal of coffee had yellow and brown stains on their teeth. Others had green stains because they scrubbed their teeth with clumps of grass. A few even had teeth which were motley-colored, such as one macrobiotic dieter who cleansed her mouth with a combination of salt, eggplant, and ground charcoal.

One common result of these unhygienic practices was trench mouth, which is known clinically as Vincent's infection, an acute inflammatory disease of the gums. Many patients exhibited caries, or cavities, because they allowed substrate and bacteria to accumulate on their teeth. In addition, four cancers of the lips were observed in patients at 558 Clayton Street, and over fifteen adolescents had infected and/or impacted wisdom teeth. Surgical excision was not required in all these cases, but many had to have their teeth removed at the Oral Surgery Unit at General Hospital. None could be afforded corrective dentistry on the Clinic premises, for although the former dentist's office had the plumbing and wiring necessary for such services, the facility lacked a dental chair.

Some corrective dentistry was done by sympathetic dentists like Dr. Charles Fischer at the University of California Dental Clinic. Dr. Fischer found that most of his patients sought treatment only when their agony became unbearable. He also learned that many had smoked marijuana before coming to the dental clinic, apparently to anesthetize themselves against their pain as well as the anxiety of seeking help there. And he realized that in addition to dental measures, most of these young people required education about the future consequences of their poor oral hygiene because they lived so totally for today.

Now-ness also accounted for a substantial amount of eye, ear, nose and throat infections, including laryngitis, sinusitis and allergic rhinitis, or hay fever. The most common eye affliction seen that summer was conjunctivitis, a bacterial or viral inflammation of the mucous membrane of the eyelids. One of the most widespread ear diseases was external otitis, a diffuse dermatitis of the ear canal which usually results from a fungal infection and may be precipitated by injuries sustained in attempting to clear the canal of earwax. Another was otitis media, an inflammation of the middle ear that often stems from upper respiratory tract infections which pass through the Eustachian tube. Otitis media occurs most commonly in young children and may lead to several complications, including perforation of the eardrum, infection of the mastoid bone and paralysis of the facial nerve. It was treated with penicillin and other antibiotics.

Antibiotics were also employed in the treatment of acute and chronic tonsillitis, a localized infection caused primarily by streptococcal bacteria, in which the tonsils become swollen and the tonsillar crypts often fill with pus. The symptoms of tonsillitis may also include sore throat, headache, fever, swelling of the regional lymph nodes and an elevation of the white blood count. Over sixty patients were given antibiotics for such symptoms during the summer of 1967. Surgical excision was also prescribed for twelve persons, ten of whom did not seek treatment until their throats swelled shut.

In addition to these and other eye, ear, nose and throat diseases, the Clinic volunteers were exposed to a great deal of gastrointestinal disturbance. Little or no dysentery was seen during the summer, but over six hundred patients did experience food poisoning, diarrhea and several other disorders. Over forty also suffered from peptic ulcers and/or from nonspecific ulcerative colitis, an inflammatory illness of the colon which is manifested by fever, abdominal tenderness, cramps and a persistent diarrhea that may lead to weight loss, malignant degeneration of the colon and deficiency disease. Colitis is a relatively common affliction in the United States and is believed to be a psychosomatic condition related to conflicts regarding the retention and expulsion not only of feces but also of aggression and other emotions. It was found in sixteen patients at 558 Clayton Street, eight of whom appeared at the facility in July. Four of these young people reported that they had been overwhelmed by hassles in the district prior to sustaining their symptoms. A seventeen-year-old summer visitor added that he had been robbed while intoxicated on acid two days before becoming acutely ill.

Another gastrointestinal problem which brought several patients to the Clinic was appendicitis. Appendectomies could not be performed on the premises, so the dozen patients suspected of having appendicitis were rushed to General Hospital, where they usually proved to be cooperative. One exception was an eighteen-year-old girl who was delivered twice in one night to Mission Emergency. This patient ran away from her attendants and hitchhiked her way back to 558 Clayton Street, where she sat in the waiting room writhing in pain. She was finally returned to the hospital by Laurel Rowland, who held her hand until she entered the operating room for surgery.

Surgery of a less ennobling nature was also required occasionally by those persons who contracted hemorrhoids, or the piles. These are dilations of the veins in or around the anus that are caused either by portal hypertension, local infection or by a straining at stools and appear as small, purplish tumors. Although the piles was never a widespread problem in the

Haight, its relative frequency did astonish the Clinic doctors, especially when they learned that many of their male and female patients had become afflicted after engaging in anal intercourse. Some of the younger adolescents seemed to view hemorrhoids as a necessary price to be paid in exchange for food and rent. Others stated that they were willing to try any and all sexual practices, the further out the better. Because of this, the problems they experienced became convenient symbols of the unbridled experimentation which characterized their life-style.

Other handy symbols were venereal disease, genitourinary-tract infections and hepatitis. Gonorrhea and hepatitis were extremely common in the Haight-Ashbury that summer, and although nonspecific urethritis, vaginitis, cervicitis and trichomoniasis were never as prevalent as they were a year later in the district, their incidence was steadily on the rise. Few of the young residents had ever incurred such illnesses before reaching the city, so that some of the younger girls remained oblivious to the cause of their discomfort until they began soiling their clothes with discharge. Furthermore, a number of boys came down with venereal complications that the physicians had never encountered in their professional careers.

One such problem was gonorrheal prostatitis, a bacterial infection of the prostate gland which is treated with sitz baths, massage of the gland via the rectum, and antibiotics. The disease is extremely rare among young people in the United States, and the only volunteers at 558 Clayton familiar with it were those military physicians who had previously treated American servicemen stationed in such areas of Southeast Asia as Vietnam. "Things like gonorrheal prostatitis were simply unheard of in adolescents in this country prior to 1967," one intern observed. "I knew coming to the Clinic would be an education, but I never thought I'd be learning how to administer a prostate massage."

Whatever his expectations, this intern also treated several cases of abnormal uterine bleeding, menstrual pain and other gynecological problems over the summer. In addition, he and his co-workers were often asked for abortions by female patients. The doctors generally felt that giving birth would be physically or psychologically hazardous to the young people, but no such operations could be performed at the facility. Because of this, the patients usually received letters recommending that their pregnancies be terminated and were referred either to Planned Parenthood or to the local therapeutic abortion society. And if they threatened to have themselves illegally treated, the physicians tried to warn them about complications like puerperal sepsis which often follow births aborted by criminal means.

Puerperal sepsis is a general term for any infection that occurs as a direct result of abortion or childbirth. It stems from the bacteria which inhabit the genitourinary tract and has been largely eliminated in medically advanced sections of the United States. But because of the unhygienic condition of some hospitals, the antiabortion legislation in certain states and the prevalence of criminal abortionists in low-income areas, it still ranks as a major life-threatening disease. Puerperal sepsis is sudden and therefore difficult to diagnose. It can bring on hypotensive shock, anemia and hyperthermia with temperatures that plunge and rise within a range of ten degrees.

No cases of puerperal sepsis resulting from criminal abortions were specifically treated at 558 Clayton Street during the summer, but the doctors there learned that at least eight young women who did not hear or heed their advice contracted the disease. Six of these were operated on by ghetto abortionists, while the others had their abortions at the hands of witch doctors or gurus in unsanitary crash pads. Although five of the patients recovered spontaneously, three had to be taken to Mission Emergency and subsequently came to the Clinic for postabortion care. All survived their infections, but their physicians doubted that two of the three could conceive again.

Children of the Future

Word about these postabortion patients spread quickly at 558 Clayton Street among the volunteers. Yet few of the summer hippies voiced great concern about their future infertility. These adolescents did not plan to have children that summer and were often too young to appreciate the consequences of infertility. But this was not the case with those older and more mystical hippies who looked on infants as magical beings. Babies had always been revered in the new community, and as the summer progressed and the community disintegrated, its members became even more determined to bear offspring. Dr. Dernburg saw two reasons for this behavior. He thought that the young people wanted to reconstitute their own narcissism by creating self-images which they could then care for as they wished they had been cared for themselves. He also felt that they hoped to expand their subculture and perpetuate their spiritual line.

Since primitivism was integral to their philosophy, the hippies often desired to experience natural childbirth like the Indians they so ardently admired. Such events were eagerly anticipated within the tribes, so that although some mothers bore their children in relative privacy, many did so as the climax to communal celebrations which were held either in or out of doors. In certain cases, their desire to share the beauty and mystery of birth prompted them to visit companions who had already left the city. In others, they merely sent word for departed commune-mates to join them in town.

Alan and other local astrologers were often invited to interpret the heavenly forces impinging upon the gatherings, while other participants were sometimes urged to help select the infants' names. The hippies seldom used conventional first or family names for their children. Instead, they christened them with such appellations as Zodiac, Krishna, Gypsy, Christ, or Frodo, after a character in Tolkien's *Lord of the Rings*.

Toxic chemicals also played an important part in these ceremonies, contrary to the Clinic's advice. Several scientists outside the Haight-Ashbury had published statements linking hallucinogenic drugs to chromosomal damage by this time, but although they and the media had all but equated thalidomide and acid, most of the doctors working at 558 Clayton Street remained unconvinced that genetic defects were commonly caused by LSD. Dr. Smith, for one, studied over two hundred hippie babies and found only one deformity — a boy with a sixth finger on his right hand. He did not consider this significant, since the incidence of deformity is two in every one hundred infants in the population at large.

Nevertheless, he and the other physicians regularly posted drug information at the Clinic and urged their patients not to use acid, particularly during the first trimester of pregnancy. Some actually suspended their drug-taking because of this counsel. And although most rejected the chromosomal damage thesis, a very few were receptive to the sound physical and psychological arguments against LSD.

In most cases, however, the young mothers continued to drop acid and smoke marijuana throughout their pregnancies. These drugs also assumed a role at their birth celebrations, where marijuana was used as a sedative and the hallucinogens were employed to help participants "merge their consciousness" with the fetus. The precise moment of birth was often marked by chanting and music making. Several babies were born to the beat of conga drums, and on at least one occasion, the participants passed the infant among them and then consumed his afterbirth.

Aside from indigestion, there were many obvious medical dangers in such practices. Puerperal sepsis and gonococcal conjunctivitis were a constant threat to hippie mothers, and although the young people thought of themselves as hardy primitives, their physical health was often abysmally low. Furthermore, although they claimed to be open to life, many of the mothers had difficulty in relaxing their cervical muscles due to chronic tension or suffered severe local pain because of genital infections or venereal disease.

Yet in spite of such complications, they usually refused to have their children by any but natural means. Some sought advice on hygiene and muscle relaxant techniques at 558 Clayton Street; others were prudent enough to have physicians in attendance at their deliveries. A dozen or so even changed their minds at the last moment, such as one twenty-two-year-old mother who called the Clinic from a phone booth when she began to experience extreme labor pains. After being given a proper sedative at 558 Clayton, this patient was rushed to San Francisco General. There she gave birth on a cart outside the delivery room.

Because this patient had her baby in a hospital, the child received a birth certificate and was immunized against measles, tetanus and other forms of childhood disease. Yet many mothers who held to the natural method avoided such inoculations and refused to register their children because the infants would then become part of straight society and subject to taxes and the draft. The Clinic doctors warned against such practices, urging that the children at least be inoculated. Yet because the young people so seldom followed their recommendations, they were often forced to vaccinate the babies themselves.

The physicians also offered free advice on how the infants might be brought up, but the mothers usually wanted to raise their children within the subculture and on their own terms. Although these hippie child-rearing practices varied, most of the parents granted total permissiveness to their offspring, ostensibly to undo the damage their parents had done them. They also showed a pronounced emotional inconsistency and would either smother their babies with affection or totally neglect them.

Furthermore, they rarely gave the infants a point of reference in the adult world, treating them not really as children but as miniature adults or cuddly toys. The young parents often appeared more zealous than their offspring while playing in the Panhandle and sometimes completely monopolized the infants' games. In fact, they frequently competed with their children. This supported Dr. Dernburg's observation that they wanted to be children themselves.

The hippie infants were invariably breast-fed and were weaned only when they tired of that type of feeding or when their mothers could no longer lactate. In addition, the children were rarely cleaned or disciplined, even when a father or father figure was present in the home. Toilet training was performed on an impromptu basis, sometimes not beginning until the infants were three or four years old and after they had been introduced to marijuana. As the children grew they became community property and were often shared. They were allowed to romp on Haight Street, were always present at such tribal gatherings as the Summer Solstice Festival and the be-in, played in places like the Psychedelic Shop and the Print Mint, and were exposed to the supposedly educational environment of their free school. The infants also came to 558 Clayton Street with their parents, so that although many were referred to the Well-Baby and Pediatric clinics at the Medical Center or to Children's and San Francisco General Hospital, they afforded the physicians a long look at their general lack of physical and psychological well being.

The doctors found that many of these infants were unwashed and in relatively poor health, despite the fact that some hippie parents took better care of their offspring than they did of themselves. Several of the children were seriously malnourished, for example, and some seen at 558 Clayton Street showed cracks at the corners of their mouths and other symptoms of vitamin deficiency. Red eyes, runny noses and soiled diapers were seen often, while the older children usually wore sparse and unwashed clothes. Furthermore, most of those who lived in communal settings were extremely susceptible to measles, influenza, upper respiratory tract infections and other forms of communicable disease.

Because of their low resistance and constant exposure to contagion, the children understandably suffered from many of their parents' own physical problems. Eczema was seldom seen in those babies who were breast-fed, but a significant number did sustain rhinitis and other allergenic reactions with psychological and/or genetic origins. Asthma was observed in at least seven children, four of whom were brought to the Clinic at the time of acute attacks and required emergency injections of epinephrine.

Conjunctivitis, tonsillitis, bronchitis, and external otitis and otitis media were also common, and two patients were found to have mastoiditis and ruptured eardrums as well, as a result of untreated ear infections. In addition, several of the younger infants contracted croup, a viral infection of the throat which causes coughing and difficulty in inspiration and may be accompanied by secondary bacterial infections. Three patients with such secondary complications had to be hospitalized during the summer, although ten others were treated in the Haight with antibiotics and hot-steam therapy to facilitate their breathing.

At the same time, many hippie children sustained skin infections as a result of parental neglect and improper hygiene. Impetigo and other staphylococcal infections were widespread among these patients, as were tinea corporis, tinea cruris, dermatophytosis and similar fungal irritations. Poison oak was seen in several of the infants, along with the bites of such insects as bees, lice, mosquitos and the infamous San Francisco flea. And because they often ate with their parents, the children were also threatened with gastrointestinal disorders from rancid and/or nutritionally deficient food.

An even greater threat to the infants was the ingestion of toxic chemicals and caustic poisons. Since the hippies often left drugs lying around their residences, some of their children accidentally swallowed dangerously high doses of aspirin, antipsychotic medication and LSD. Others were intentionally introduced to acid as well as marijuana by their parents, so that a total of fifteen infants, ranging in age from six months to five years of age, were treated for bad trips at 558 Clayton Street in the month of July alone.

The doctors chose to keep most of the children and their parents together in the calm center rather than sending them to impersonal hospital settings and, whenever possible, treated them in the familiar surroundings of their homes. Many of the infants were terrified by their perceptual distortions and by the monsters they "saw" swarming around them, so the doctors tried to distract them with music and candlelight. They also relied on verbal techniques, mild sedatives and, in three cases, Thorazine administered rectally. In one instance, Dr. Dernburg used building blocks and other toys which he employed in his private practice to gain the attention of a four-year old patient whose mother was unable to calm her. The children responded well to these various types of treatment, and all fifteen treated at the Clinic went home unaided after their encounters with LSD.

Although no follow-up studies could be done on these patients, their facial expressions and erratic behavior offered mute testimony to the psychological agony which accompanied their adverse reactions. This fact was generally discounted by the hippies, most of whom insisted that because their infants received a great deal of sunshine and acid they would grow up to be natural, joyous and free. But most of the physicians took a different view. In their experience, the children gained little in the way of health and mental alertness. They did not acquire much happiness, either, and many seemed depressed because of inadequate mothering.

Furthermore, Dr. Dernburg felt that their freedom was largely an illusion and that the infants appeared to have plateaued in their development, like their parents. They could play anywhere in the Haight-Ashbury, but their independence was clearly circumscribed by the geographic and psychological boundaries of the new community. Because of this, the children were unprepared for any but hip society. They were generally undisciplined and exhibited an extremely low level of tolerance to frustration. Some seemed to be seriously disturbed by their parents' emotional inconsistency. Others were hyperactive and confused.

As Dr. Norman Sissman said during the summer, "the present is bad enough for these kids, but the saddest thing may be their future. We have no way of telling what drugs and exposure to an environment as disorganized as this is going to do to them. Yet one thing is certain: in spite of their desire to create superior children, the hippie parents are raising their offspring to be exactly like themselves."

Dr. Sissman was not alone in his fears for the infants, but there was little that he or anyone else at 558 Clayton Street could do for them. Most of the long-haired volunteers saw nothing wrong with the hippie child-rearing practices and few would have criticized the parents even if they had wanted to. The doctors found themselves in a different dilemma, for although intervention was difficult with older patients, it was virtually impossible where children were concerned. Because of this, they could only hope for the best and try to help the children survive.

Growth

The physicians were far from pleased by this policy of nonintervention, but it did bring more hip parents and infants to 558 Clayton Street. A number of older white, Negro and Indian alcoholics, some of whom Dr. Smith recognized from the Alcohol and Drug Abuse Screening Unit, also came to the facility. In fact, by the end of July, the only members of the waning new community and the waxing new population who did not use the Clinic were those hoodies and bikers who refused to admit their sickness and those young blacks who resented its efforts to aid the hippies and therefore stayed on the street.

This absence of Negro patients was regretted by the doctors, particularly Dr. Bertram Meyer. Yet the influx of other patients created new problems which demanded their attention. This was especially true in the calm center, whose delicate equilibrium was upset by the changes in drug-taking in the district. The tiny storeroom was once geared primarily to treating adverse hallucinogenic reactions. But the volunteers now had to contend not only with children dropping acid but also with patients of all ages using alcohol, STP, barbiturates and amphetamines as well as LSD.

They also had to work in the worst possible conditions. Over one forty-eight hour stretch in July, for example, Al Rose, Kurt Feibusch and others detoxified fifty-two patients, ranging from eighteen months to sixty-one years of age. Two days later, after the fuses blew once again, Dr. Dernburg had to counsel two boys on packing crates. He was then assaulted by a thirty-year-old French sailor freaking out on speed.

Given such circumstances, no records could be kept on those who sought treatment for drug reactions or psychological difficulties during the early summer. But a list of patients with physical problems was drawn up in response to Dr. Ellis Sox's request at the Haight-Ashbury Roundtable. It revealed that over nine hundred females and twelve hundred males, with an average age of twenty and one-half years, had been seen at 558 Clayton Street in the month of July. Over one thousand of these young people gave addresses in the Haight at the time of their treatment. Most of the rest came from wealthy San Francisco neighborhoods or the Tenderloin.

This list was forwarded to Dr. Sox after its completion, at which point the organizers hoped to be reimbursed for their efforts and to receive additional financial aid for the future. But they soon realized that the Public Health Department had no intention of helping them. Dr. Smith learned from a local realtor that the department had not purchased a site for its proposed regional health center. And Dr. Sox told Dr. Morris that because the Clinic did not meet Public Health Department standards it could not count on his support. The organizers argued that such standards could never be met without the city's assistance. But Bob Conrich was tired of arguments, of drug-taking and of difficulties with his girl friend. He therefore resigned in July from his position as administrator, "out of a combination of mental exhaustion, physical fatigue and moral disgust."

Conrich's action was not taken lightly at 558 Clayton Street. Indeed, several staff members insisted that the Clinic should be closed to dramatize his departure and because it was seven hundred dollars in debt. But closing was out of the question to the organizers, so they resolved to give their program in the Haight-Ashbury another chance. Peter Schubart agreed to fill Conrich's position, and several people offered to organize a dance-concert benefit at which the new community might provide an alternate source of financial aid.

The Clinic's first benefit was held at the Fillmore auditorium on the evening of July thirteenth. It was made possible by Bill Graham, who donated his staff and facilities for the occasion, and by an emcee at the Avalon Ballroom who publicized the event. Volunteering their talents that evening were the Charlatans, Blue Cheer and Big Brother and the Holding Company. Big Brother was perhaps the most popular rock group in San Francisco at this point, and its members, including Janis Joplin, were regular visitors at 558 Clayton Street. It was therefore fitting that over two thousand young people came to hear them at the Fillmore. Five thousand dollars was collected, and Lowell Pickett was so impressed by the turnout that he volunteered to organize a second benefit for mid-August to raise additional funds.

Don Reddick anticipated an even larger crowd at this second benefit, so he decided to expand the Clinic's medical services with the proceeds from the first. His first act was to lease the second seven-room office behind that already used at 558 Clayton Street; combined with that of the first office, the rent was now three hundred dollars a month. He and other staff members then created a passageway between the two offices and turned one of the recently acquired rooms into a pharmacy to replace the broom closet in which medications had previously been kept. Shelves were installed, new procedures were inaugurated, and the volunteer pharmacists and nurses started stamping prescription envelopes with the blue cross and white dove of peace.

After the pharmacy was outfitted, the organizers converted another large room into a laboratory. Reddick and his business partners then donated a microscope, a sterilizer and a centrifuge so that volunteer lab technicians could check vaginal smears and urine samples and make blood tests. The third new room, a bathroom, was used as a detoxification area. The fourth became Lowell Pickett's office. The fifth room was converted into a new calm center. The sixth and seventh were used as offices and storerooms. These connected with the old calm center, which became part of the waiting room. Paint and dance-concert posters were applied throughout the seven-room addition. By the time Reddick and his co-workers were finished, 558 Clayton Street, which would henceforth be called the Medical Section, was one of the most fully equipped facilities in town.

It was still the most chaotic, a fact that was causing friction with the volunteer counselors and psychiatrists. Professor Wolf was also eager to move his educational program from All Saints' Episcopal Church by this time, so he and Dr. Dernburg began to look for a separate location which would serve their mutual purposes. After considerable searching, they found a pale blue Victorian at 409 Clayton Street.

This residence was leased for three hundred dollars a month and registered, as the Medical Section was, as the private office of Dr. Smith and as a field project of Youth Projects. Professor Wolf offered to pay half the rent on the facility, moved rugs, chairs and a paperback-book library onto the first floor, and turned it into a classroom for his Happening House. Encounter groups, gestalt therapy sessions and courses on cooking, natural childbirth, candlemaking and Russian orthodox music were offered there during the summer, along with shorter seminars covering such topics as how to avoid pregnancy, malnutrition, robbery and rape.

After Happening House was in order, Dr. Dernburg, Stuart Loomis, and others converted the second floor of 409 House into a Psychiatric Section. They were assisted by Trina Merriman and Charles MacGuillamay, a twenty-five-year-old history teacher from a local high school who served with Miss Merriman as co-administrator of the facility. Tables, couches and other pieces of donated furniture were used to decorate the second deck, and a reception desk was placed at the top of the stairs. Dr. Dernburg and other psychiatrists began treating their regular patients at the Psychiatric Section in August, while Stuart Loomis and others provided counseling and crisis intervention for the psychedelic syndrome.

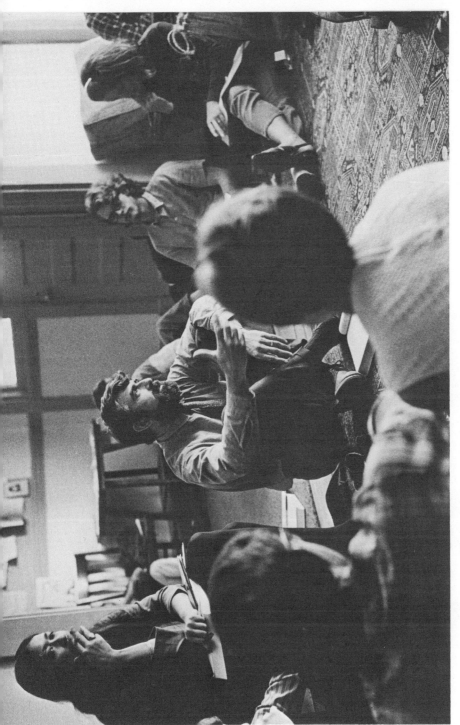

409 Clayton Street: Professor Leonard Wolf conducts a class at Happening House.
(Jim Marshall)

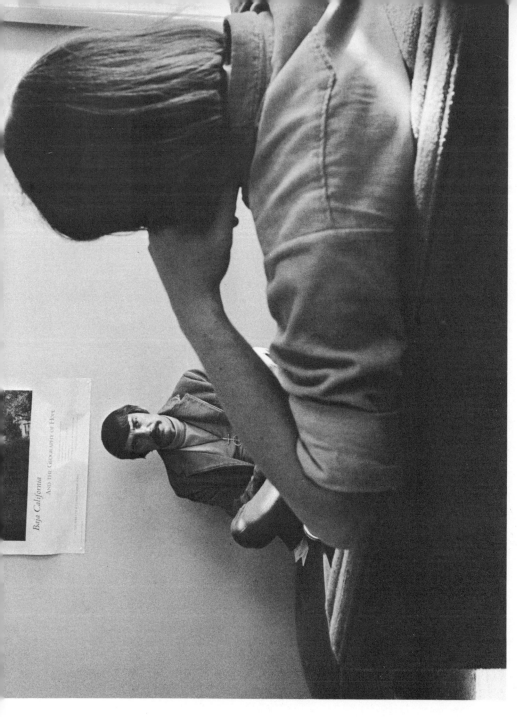

409 Clayton Street: Professor Stuart Loomis, chief psychologist, with a patient.
(Elaine Mayes)

Professor Loomis was ideally suited for this purpose; he cared for his patients and spent most of this free time with them. Long active in the civil rights movement, he was motivated by a belief in the concept of counterculture — and by a desire to help it grow. Professor Loomis did not dissuade his patients from staying in the Haight. Instead, he became involved in their struggle for self-assertion and tried to enable them to work through their problems within the new community.

Dr. Dernburg disagreed with this approach and those of the Clinic's gestalt therapists and encounter group leaders for professional reasons. Yet he admired Professor Loomis's dedication, valued his contribution, and never attempted to impose his psychiatric theories on the volunteer counselors. This was in keeping with the do-your-thing bias of the Clinic. It was necessitated by emergency conditions in the Haight-Ashbury. And it enabled Dr. Dernburg to eventually recruit over one hundred volunteers.

Meanwhile, the third-floor space at 409 Clayton Street which housed Dr. Smith's personal office was turned into a Publications Section through which the staff could disseminate health information and distribute the Clinic's *Journal of Psychedelic Drugs,* a compilation of papers delivered at conferences it was co-sponsoring at the Medical Center with the Psychopharmacology Study Group. Another room on the top deck was used to isolate and detoxify speed freaks. Thus, although adverse LSD reactions were still treated up the block, the physicians had a place to help violent amphetamine abusers and long-term patients and could thereby reduce the traffic at 558 Clayton to a more manageable flow.

Visitors

As it turned out, the opening of the Annex could not have happened at a more crucial time. Speed had increased in popularity by early August, and although *Time* continued to call the district "the vibrant epicenter of the hippie movement," the immigration of bikers, hoodies and mulitiple drug abusers was squeezing true hippies out of the Haight.

Several articles on Dr. Smith and the Clinic had appeared in national magazines by this point. These articles proved to be beneficial in terms of fund raising and also brought a number of visitors to 558 Clayton Street, some of whom wanted to serve the district. One was Frederick Shick, a twenty-three-year-old medical student from the University of Indiana. Others came to study. Among them was Dr. Kay Blacker, a psychiatrist from Langley-Porter, who drew from the Medical Section's patients and personnel for his investigation of hallucinogenic drug abuse.

Senator Charles Percy of Illinois also stopped by the facility, as did Dr. Lewis Yablonsky, a sociologist who reported his findings in *The Hippie Trip*. And several journalists also used 558 Clayton as a reference. Among them were Nicholas von Hoffman, author of *We Are the People Our Parents Warned Us Against,* and William Hedgepeth, a young *Look* writer wearing hippie garb, who hoped to interview Dr. Smith but was given an examination for skin cancer instead.

Hedgepeth's tumor proved to be benign, but he was shaken when he left the Clinic. The same was true of Dr. James Goddard, then director of the Food and Drug Administration, who was first taken on a tour of the Haight by Dr. Smith. Dr. Goddard started his inspection at a local coffee shop, where he was lectured by Ron Thelin on the virtues of organic vegetables and was advised to pour as much money as he could into a study of "brain food." Dr. Goddard then proceeded to the Medical Section, where he was met by a welcome committee of volunteers and patients who accused him of being hostile toward hallucinogenic drugs. The organizers in turn applauded his stands against the unethical practices of the American pharmaceutical industry, and an impromptu debate ensued in the calm center. But Dr. Smith called off the meeting after intercepting a cup of coffee prepared by a patient for Dr. Goddard that contained a king-size dose of LSD.

Dr. Goddard left later that evening, praising the efforts of the Clinic, puzzled by the volunteers' vehemence, and unaware that he had been but one sip away from his first acid trip. Yet conditions never returned to normal after his departure, for doctors from as far away as France continued to seek information at 409 and 558 Clayton Street. A number of teachers and even athletic coaches, most of whom assumed that they too would be dealing with drug abuse when school reopened in the fall, came to the Medical and Psychiatric sections. Physicians from throughout Europe, Japan and the United States consulted with the organizers about starting similar programs in their own communities. Several middle-echelon members of the San Francisco Public Health Department also studied its procedures, but no top-level administrators ever appeared.

Yet the Clinic *was* flooded with phone calls and letters from young people and parents across the country. Over fifty thousand requests were made for drug information and for *The Journal of Psychedelic Drugs*. Some six thousand people with abuse problems inquired about psychiatric advice or referrals to understanding physicians in their own areas. Seven hundred and thirty people from outside the city volunteered their services to the Medical and Psychiatric sections. One sixty-three-year-old migratory worker offered to hitchhike from Kansas to San Francisco but was cautioned against coming because of his age.

Although many of the calls and letters which arrived in August were dispiriting because of the desperation of their senders, only one caused any permanent regret. This came two days after Luce's article in *Look,* when Dr. Smith was notified by a medical protection association in Fort Wayne, Indiana, that his malpractice insurance would soon be canceled because he was "working with all those weirdos in the Haight."

The cancellation could have closed the Clinic, for its volunteers and staff members had heretofore been covered under Dr. Smith's personal policy. Yet that eventuality was averted by Dr. Morris, who suggested that he apply for group insurance under the auspices of the San Francisco Medical Society. Dr. Smith was not optimistic about being accepted by this organization, which he assumed was opposed to his free treatment philosophy. He was therefore surprised when the Medical Society not only granted him membership and group coverage but also endorsed the operations at 409 and 558 Clayton Street.

These actions forestalled the Clinic's closing, yet problems continued to mount at the Medical Section. The first were caused by a number of bogus doctors who used forged or stolen medical licenses to gain access to patients. One of these well-dressed impostors worked at the facility on three successive evenings with a license which said he was an anesthesiologist at the University of California. He was apprehended only after he referred two patients to the physician whose license he had stolen at the Medical Center.

At the same time, 558 Clayton Street had to deal with the Thelin brothers and the Diggers, whose hostility seemed to mount as their influence in the Haight-Ashbury decreased. Arthur Lisch and Emmet Grogan also wanted to close the Clinic in August because they feared its patient histories would be turned over to or impounded by the police. Dr. Fort talked them out of this action, but they continued to inspect the Clinic during the summer and urged young people not to go there lest they contribute to Dr. Smith's alleged ego trip.

Dr. Smith was disappointed by this vendetta, particularly because Lisch, Grogan and the Thelins had originally encouraged him to become active in the Haight. But these new enemies had little power over the patients. And while they were attempting to undermine the Clinic's good name in the new community, Dr. Smith and the other organizers were trying to repulse a more serious challenge to its standing in the person of Papa Al.

Papa Al was a familiar yet mysterious father figure in the Haight-Ashbury. He carried a thirty-eight revolver, traveled with a burly hoodie named Teddybear, owned a palatial estate in Berkeley — and had no visible means of support. But in spite of these factors, Dr. Robert Morris and many young people in the district considered Papa Al a Good Samaritan because he maintained a facility for amphetamine abusers called Masonic House. Others claimed that he used the center as a place to train drug salesmen. Still others swore that he was a prosperous speed dealer who protected himself either by killing off his competitors or by turning them in to the police.

These latter reputations never preceded Papa Al at the Medical Section, where he and his lieutenant were allowed to do their thing alongside the other volunteers. They actually proved to be quite useful in early July and were thanked for recruiting patients and personnel on several occasions. But Don Reddick and Peter Schubart learned that Papa Al and Teddybear were passing themselves off as full-time staff members toward the end of the month. They then realized that the two were trying to turn the facility into their base of operations in the Haight.

This became evident on the evening of July twenty-second, when word was circulated that the blacks were going on a rampage in the district later that night. The rumor was not entirely groundless, for there had been a minor flare-up in the Fillmore a few days earlier. But by the time it passed down Haight Street, the speculation about a possible disturbance was escalated into a riot scare. Some H.I.P. merchants then brought in pickup trucks to transport their stock out of the Haight-Ashbury, while Mnasidika's and the Print Mint offered space for homeless adolescents inside their stores.

The Clinic would also have remained open to receive riot victims had Papa Al not stormed up the front steps of 558 Clayton Street, swearing that he had seen "dozens of spades with shopping bags full of knives" and insisting that the facility be closed. He then sent several patients for reinforcements and turned the Medical Section into a command post. Blankets and bandages were distributed to all present; frightened young people were stationed with axe handles behind the front door. Meanwhile, Papa Al positioned himself on the stairway, brandishing a forty-five caliber automatic in addition to his thirty-eight.

Teddybear raced in a few minutes later, reporting that he had observed "carloads of spades with machine guns" cruising the street. Don Reddick arrived, totally unaware of the impending riot. After being briefed, Reddick voted to contact Park Police Station. But before he could, Teddybear grabbed the phone, placed a call to a Hell's Angel named Chocolate George, and announced that the bikers were coming in force to protect 558 Clayton Street.

Reddick remained unconvinced, however, and decided both to call the police and to inspect the street himself. He did find a few drunken Negroes, but when a single carload of patrolmen arrived a half hour later, order was readily restored. The Angels, who were partying that evening, never did show up. Yet by the time Reddick returned, Papa Al and Teddy-bear were crediting themselves with having saved the facility from a race war.

Several additional encounters with the two men followed, each more fantastic than the first. A few days after the alleged siege of the Medical Section, for example, Teddybear and the Hell's Angels almost lynched a bogus doctor with forged credentials whom they caught examining a female patient. Then, one night in early August, Papa Al confronted a young Vietnam-bound psychiatrist from Stanford and told him that he was no longer welcome at the Clinic. An argument followed and Don Reddick escorted Papa Al down the front steps. Papa Al returned to upset operations several times during August until an anonymous story documenting his history as an informer to the State Narcotics Bureau was printed in the *Berkeley Barb*.

Although his presence was not felt again in the Haight for almost a year the district was still deluged by older criminals. This was reflected in three killings, all of which occurred in the month of August. The first involved the Hell's Angel named Chocolate George, who was run over by a tourist while joyriding on Haight Street. The second was a murder committed on a twenty-five-year-old speed seller whose life and right arm were cut off by a long-haired biker wielding a carving knife.

The third killing involved Superspade, a black dealer whom Matthew O'Connor described as "the closest thing to a Mafia type ever seen in the Haight-Ashbury." Superspade lived at 848 Clayton Street until July 1967, when he moved to the Mission district. Rumors then spread that he, like Papa Al, had remained in business primarily by informing on other dealers. One of them apparently caught up with him in August, for Superspade drove across the Golden Gate Bridge to consummate a sale and was found stuffed in a sleeping bag at the base of a Marin County cliff.

As word of these killings spread through the new community, those hippies like Alan who had lingered in the Haight through the summer naturally longed for the shelter of Morningstar and other rural retreats. But conditions at these communes were no better, both because of local straight opposition and because a few hoodies and bikers had followed the more peace-loving young people out of the Haight. Morningstar was raided several times by the police during early August, and five members of the Gypsy Jokers motorcycle club raped seven girls there in one week. In Big Sur, the Monterey County Sheriff's Office and the Public Health Department were harassing long-haired adolescents and threatening to condemn their tent cities to protect local property owners from "the steadily rising tide of vandalism and venereal disease."

These incidents too were well publicized, yet some of the remaining hippies still preferred the possibility of being hassled in the country to watching their community collapse. Their departure in turn created a vacuum, especially as more of the summer visitors also left. Some simply swallowed their pride and went home to their parents, convinced that they had finally had enough. Others looked for space in the rural communes or settled in outlying sections of San Francisco. But several thousand stayed in the Haight-Ashbury, where they spent more time indoors and clung to the surviving service agencies for support.

This meant more problems for the Clinic, as the adolescents asked for any employment which would keep them off the streets. Both the Medical and Psychiatric sections were low on funds by this time, but jobs were found for some of the summer hippies. Others began hanging out in the waiting room at 558 Clayton Street, forcing the physicians to post a Patients Only sign. Yet this gesture was futile, for as the Haight grew more dangerous, it became increasingly difficult to differentiate between patients and paramedical volunteers. The Clinic had evolved into a sanctuary at this point in its history. It was not only a health center for the sick, but was also a haven for the helpless, the frightened, and the weak.

A Free American

One person who embodied all these characteristics was Jackie, a nineteen-year-old girl who had been an occasional patient at 558 Clayton Street since the start of the summer. Although she was not actually ethereal, Jackie's fragile smile and long brown hair helped her fit the mold of a flower child established a year earlier in the Haight-Ashbury. She was somewhat of a hippie, but she shunned the Jesus and Indian costumes of young people like Alan in favor of blue jeans, peasant blouses and other articles of clothing which gave her an air of perpetual springtime — and peace.

Peace was not a part of Jackie's background. She came to the Haight by way of suburban Detroit, where her father was a prominent neurosurgeon. He was apparently a better physician than a father; from what his daughter said he seemed to use his profession as an excuse to stay away from home. Her mother, a shrewish individual given to irrational tantrums, ruled the family as a result. Jackie expressed little love for this woman; she preferred her grandmother to her mother, cared strongly for her younger brother and sister, and described her home life as "a total hell."

One probable reason for this situation was that Jackie's mother saw her not as an autonomous being with feelings and interests but as an extension of herself. She constantly berated her daughter for not fulfilling her own social ambitions and also made many covert references to her alleged sexual promiscuity. Jackie did have intercourse with three young men before her eighteenth birthday, yet this behavior was far from excessive by contemporary standards. And it was actually less an indication of promiscuity than a reflection of her desire to gain the love and involvement she never received from her family.

There was also some spite in Jackie's sexual activity, for she reasoned quite rightly that her mother was trying to keep her and her father apart. Such intercession increased after she turned eighteen, at which point she decided to move away from the house. But she did not make the break entirely; instead of going to an Eastern college she enrolled at nearby Wayne State. She continued to see her father occasionally but was never allowed, by him or her mother, to become too close. Competition between the two females kept increasing, and Jackie apparently found some outlet for her anger and resentment by finding a regular lover and taking marijuana, LSD, and other readily available hallucinogenic drugs.

Jackie's mother strenuously objected to this boyfriend, so much so that she threatened to withhold her daughter's college tuition. In retaliation, Jackie introduced her younger brother to marijuana and started to mock her mother for being so straight. Yet these overt expressions of anger only made her more depressed. In the spring of her freshman year, she and her lover broke up. A week later, her grandmother, who had lived on and off with the family for several years, was sent to a nursing home. Two weeks after this, Jackie finished her first year of college with a C-plus average. She then left Detroit with a carload of classmates bound for the Haight-Ashbury.

Jackie was originally enthralled at becoming a part of the new community. In fact, when she first came to the Clinic during the measles epidemic, her doctor said that she "seemed to be in love with love." But as the summer wore on, Jackie smiled less and less. She was separated from her original companions in early July and had to attach herself to a number of lovers to find housing and to remain fed.

Her chemical consumption increased in the process; she experimented with acid, STP and oral amphetamines and smoked marijuana to anesthetize herself against loneliness. Then, as her life-style degenerated, she began to experience several physical problems, including irregular menstrual bleeding and a chronic bronchial cough. On one occasion, Jackie wrongly feared that she was pregnant. On another, she contracted trichomoniasis and VD.

It was primarily because of these genital infections that Jackie was attracted to the Clinic. She had also been abandoned by her latest old man and rousted from her commune by early August and thus had two more reasons for spending time at 558 Clayton Street. Jackie needed the Medical Section, but she minimized her dependency by trying to become indispensable as a temperature-taker and volunteer clerk. As she proved her competence, she was encouraged to work on the fund-raising benefit that Lowell Pickett and other staff members were organizing at Longshoreman's Hall on August fifteenth. This gave her an opportunity to make new friends, whom she invariably greeted with an embrace. She showed the same warmth and enthusiasm toward the Clinic patients, adopting a maternal attitude toward every new surrogate brother and sister she met.

But in spite of these signs of buoyancy, Jackie continued to get depressed. She also began to depend more on the Medical Section as a place of security and on the physicians as father substitutes. She sometimes wanted the doctors to scold her for her actions, although they were never as harsh as she was on herself. At other moments, she used them as sounding boards, particularly when she sensed the disparity between the safety she had once known and the danger she saw daily in the Haight. Jackie said that she was not ready for psychiatric counseling during the summer and insisted that the Clinic provide her with sufficient occupational therapy. But she did discuss her feelings with Dr. Smith on several occasions, one of which caught her in a characteristically ambivalent state.

Jesus, there sure are a lot of screwed-up people coming through here lately. I pulled the charts on three speed freaks this morning you wouldn't believe; you know, one of these guys lived in the Tenderloin and has been shooting up for eight months. I don't get it; that's how the whole Haight-Ashbury is going. Like, wow, these three chicks I was living with, really beautiful people; did they get burned the other night. They were going to front a hundred dollars — Vicky's dad sent it to her for her birthday — to score some weed and get this car to go up to Mendocino with, but this cat burned them. Then these two other cats, friends of Superspade they said, started hanging around trying to get them to whore. They kept coming around, saying that it was the best way to make money, that it'd be no sweat. So they just, like, split; left their stereo and everything and just took off to stop the hassle. So now I'm out of another place.

But it's cool: I've been without a bed before, so there's no reason to get up tight. Everybody's so strung out these days about having a place of their own

— it's the same old story about property rights. You can't blame the spades; the Man gave them the shaft from the first day.

And you know, it's not just happening here; she's been up to Morningstar, and they're taking the worst kind of hassles there. Her old man — you know, the guy with that groovy camper truck — he got cut up with a wine bottle. And to think he came here so his draft board wouldn't find him; it just shows you can't be safe.

You know, sometimes I just wish I was back in kindergarten, doing what I wanted with no one hassling me. It used to be like that here, like when I first came — people giving away flowers, sharing their food. Hell, you never had to buy acid; you could just stand on Haight Street and somebody'd walk up and lay it on you. Now, this shit they're selling; you know we had a chick in the calm center yesterday who looked like she'd swallowed rat poison. It's turned into a big ego trip; nobody smiling, nobody sharing anything. People locking themselves inside and the speed freaks fucking it up for everyone.

But what are you supposed to do? Go home? Man, you know that scene is worse than it is here. Oh, I dig staying warm and not worrying about people like Superspade, but it's worse where I come from. I mean look at how they're screwing up my brother and sister. You think I'm crazy; wait till you see them. Are they ever going to need a shrink!

Either that, or they'll leave too, just like I did. My brother Jerry wrote me through the Switchboard that my old lady is on his back all the time, just like she was on me. She even went through his clothes and found some grass. And you won't believe it, but she wanted to turn him over to the police! My father finally put a stop to it — I guess he's worrying about what they'd say at the hospital. But can you imagine what's going to happen when Jerry refuses to go in the army? My parents will positively flip.

The thing is, they just don't understand what's happening. They can't begin to figure out why Jerry shits on the war, and they think that only heroin addicts use drugs. My father will sit there with his martini and my mother with her diet pills, telling me I'm some kind of freak. You know, when I said I was going to the Haight-Ashbury my mother started screaming and called me a dope fiend to my face! Man, if she only knew the half of it. You can buy grass and acid around every college in the country, even in Detroit. They haven't heard much about speed there, but if the Haight's any example, they sure will.

Don't get me wrong: I'm not hot for all this. Sure, I've tried dexies a few times but that's enough. There've been times I wanted to shoot speed to see what it's like, but right now I don't need that for my head. Anyway, I'm too busy working here. I guess the Clinic — I don't want to get all mushy, Doc, but this place means a lot to me. Before I was just hanging out, trying to get together, but hung up.

Al Rose says there's no money, and I know you're worried about having to close down, but we'll make it. This benefit, we're really giving our best. Laurel and some of the kids are hanging posters, and the deejays are giving all kinds of plugs. It'll help. It's got to. I really dig the Clinic, and I'm sure not going home yet. Man, this is my home now. I don't know what I'd do if we ever had to close.

From New Community to New Population: The Death of Hip

Jackie and the other volunteers worked their hearts out for the second benefit, but their efforts were not enough. Both the Fillmore Auditorium and Avalon Ballroom were booked on the night of August fifteenth, and without Bill Graham to supervise their preparations and publicity, they could not draw a full house. The Charlatans and Quicksilver Messenger Service performed capably at Longshoreman's Hall, yet only five hundred of their fans attended the fund-raiser. By ten that evening, it was obvious that the second benefit would be a complete bust.

This became clearer three weeks later, when Lowell Pickett reported at a staff meeting that the Clinic was two thousand dollars in debt. Dr. Meyers and several others wanted to close 558 Clayton Street at this point, but the volunteers, who had already treated ten thousand patients during the summer, asked for another chance. The organizers were unable to refuse them. They therefore dipped into their pockets and came up with enough money to lengthen the life of the Medical Section by almost a month.

The younger volunteers and staff members then began another desperate drive for funds. Some painted signs, refurbished the donation can, and started begging for spare change on the street. Jackie and others went door to door through the Haight-Ashbury, soliciting gifts. Laurel Rowland and Lowell Pickett called a number of friendly physicians and sent out a plea for assistance on the mailing list. But the contributions they received were negligible, for San Francisco was becoming tired of hippies and fed up with the Haight.

While this was occurring, Dr. Smith and Robert Laws called on Jack Morrison, the supervisor who had helped them open the Medical Section. He was willing to approach his colleagues, yet the Board of Supervisors could not save the facility. Peter Schubart turned to Joan Baez, with whom he had once been arrested. She drove up from her Institute for the Study of Nonviolence in Carmel Valley, filled out charts, and sang for donations in the waiting room. But few patients could pay for Miss Baez's singing, and less than fifty dollars was raised at 558 Clayton Street.

After exhausting every conceivable resource, the organizers finally decided that they would have to limit their operations in the Haight-Ashbury.

409 Clayton Street could stay in business because it did not dispense medication and because half of its rent was paid by Professor Wolf. But the Medical Section, whose overhead was approximately five times that of the Psychiatric Section, would have to close.

The volunteers were notified of this decision, and positions were found for a few at 409 House. The rest, including Alan and Jackie, were informed that 558 Clayton Street might reopen sometime in the future and were advised to stay in touch. Dr. Morris then prepared a press release, which David Perlman of the *Chronicle* used to write the Clinic's first obituary. On the morning of September twenty-second, the release was posted outside the Medical Section. That afternoon, the door to 558 Clayton Street was shut.

Although news spread quickly about the Clinic's closing, it was not accepted at first. In fact, the front steps to the Medical Section were crowded for several days with patients waiting to see their physicians. Most of the young people scattered eventually, but a few remained there until the end of September, when the national media, which had all but vacated the district, once again descended on the Haight. Some of the reporters and television cameramen focused on 558 Clayton Street as a symbol of the end of summer in the Haight-Ashbury. Other people arrived with a different intention, for although the Summer of Love was certainly over so far as the Clinic was concerned, the new community had not had the last word.

It did in early October, when Emmett Grogan, Arthur Lisch and the Thelin brothers, whose Psychedelic Shop was now bankrupt, decided that their community could be restored if the press was bucked from their backs. They therefore met at Happening House and agreed to bury the hippie label and replace it with that of the Free American at a Death of Hip funeral on October sixth.

The funeral itself was scheduled for midafternoon, but the Death of Hip festivities started at sunrise, as several dozen young people assembled at Buena Vista Park. After chanting in the new day, they proceeded down Haight Street to the Psychedelic Shop and gathered under a sign urging all present to Be Free. The Thelins opened their store and invited the young people to take what was left of their merchandise. But the doors soon had to be closed to silence the screams of a twelve-year-old girl on a bad trip.

After the girl was given medication, the Thelins and their companions walked to Fell Street in front of the Switchboard. Waiting for them was a long coffin stuffed with crumpled dance-concert posters and surrounded by young people and an almost equal number of representatives of the press. Some of the mourners hoisted the coffin to their shoulders, while others, including Alan and Jackie, serenaded them with tambourines and Hare

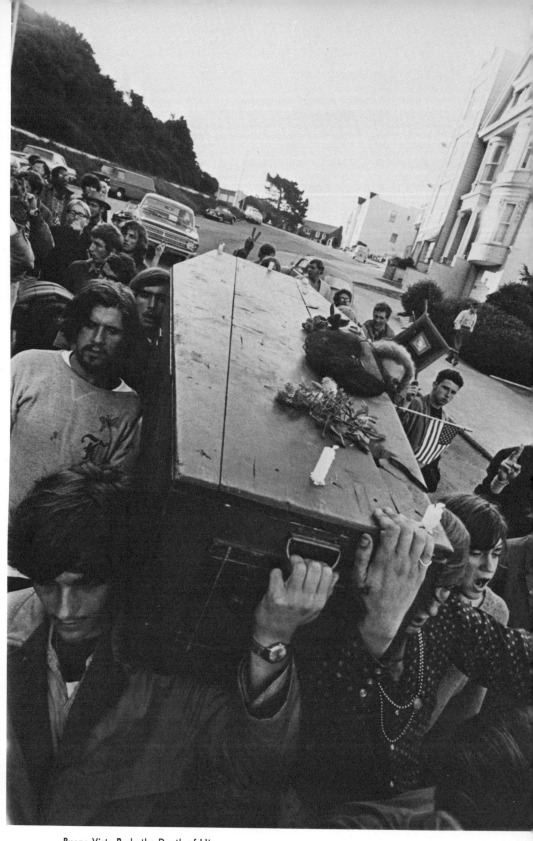

Buena Vista Park: the Death of Hip.
(Michael Alexander)

Krishna chants. The procession then set off across the Panhandle, marching to a cadence provided by Arthur Lisch. It circled the district and picked up a number of stragglers, including Randy, other speed freaks, and older alcoholics who were shaken from their slumber by the passing parade.

The mourners returned to the Panhandle an hour later. A torch was held to the coffin, and some of the hippies leaped through the funeral pyre. Others joined hands and snake-danced, stopping occasionally to drop clothing, cigarette papers and capsules of acid into the flames. A truckload of firemen then arrived, along with two squad cars from Park Police Station, and the young people, now Free Americans, dispersed. Most returned to their residences, but a half dozen of the mourners stopped outside the Medical Section. Among them was Jackie, who took a stub of crayon from her pocket and scribbled a message above the Clinic steps. "The Haight Was Love Once," she wrote; "Now, Where Has All the Love Gone?"

Part IV

After

Love

Has Gone

Hell hath no limits, nor is circumscribed
In one self place; for where we are is Hell,
And where Hell is there must we ever be.

Christopher Marlowe, **Doctor Faustus**

I have been a stranger in a strange land.

Exodus 2:22

But Annie kept on speeding, her health was getting poor.
Saw things at the window, she heard things at the door.
Her mind was like a grinding mill, her lips were cracked and sore.
Her skin was turning yellow, I just couldn't take it no more.

Canned Heat, "Amphetamine Annie"

The Front of
the Storm

Jackie may have been emotional when she crayoned her message above the Clinic steps on October sixth, but she was correct in noting that little love was left in the Haight-Ashbury after the Death of Hip ceremony. Most of the reporters and television cameramen who worked the Haight had apparently come to the same conclusion long before October, and those who returned to cover the funeral service packed their gear soon after the festivities were over and abandoned the area. A few street preachers stayed to do battle with sin in the district, but other members of the clergy were beginning to avoid the Haight-Ashbury. So were most of the social scientists who had completed their research by the end of the summer and the tourists who had contributed to the congestion there.

Also vacating the district were many homeowners and merchants who had belonged to its old community. FOR SALE signs began appearing in ever-increasing numbers after the symbolic burial in the Panhandle, as property values plummeted faster in the next three months than they had during the previous five years. Over one hundred and sixty members of the Neighborhood Council had been burgled by the young people whom they gave shelter to over the summer. More than two dozen straight proprietors on Haight Street were now trying to find buyers for their stores.

Father Leon Harris had been forced to call off his housing program, and although he still maintained a free bakery and a Community Affairs Office for the Diggers in the basement of All Saints', half his bakery equipment had been stolen and his office had been repeatedly robbed. The Diggers themselves had suffered losses in their numbers and self-esteem over the summer, and were now through with peace, acid and love. Like New Left radicals across the country, they were turning to confrontation and violence in direct proportion to their frustration and political impotence. Some were even attempting to overcome their powerlessness with speed.

A more common tactic for the hippies was withdrawal. Jefferson Airplane, Quicksilver Messenger Service, Big Brother and the Holding Company, and the Grateful Dead had all become nationally famous by the fall of 1967, along with the Steve Miller Band and other new groups, but only the Dead still considered the Haight its home. Many poster artists had also left the district. The Council for the Summer of Love had been disbanded, as had H.I.P. and Allen Cohen's *Oracle*. Only the Switchboard and the Straight Theatre were still functioning. So was Alan, who began spending more of his time at 409 House after the door to 558 Clayton Street was closed.

Although the psychedelic movement had actually swelled with the addition of thousands of summer hippies, its geographical center was no longer the Haight-Ashbury. Several hundred Free Americans stayed in the district after the Death of Hip ceremony, including Jackie, who managed to find another bed and a new old man. Yet many of her former companions had either returned to their parents, reenrolled in school, or left the Haight like the beats and hippies before them.

Some who could still stomach urban and suburban life had followed their spiritual elders to San Francisco's North Beach and Mission districts or to Berkeley and Marin County, thereby helping the Bay Area maintain its reputation as the national mecca of alienation. Others were going to India, Europe or Canada, hitchhiking around the country, or drifting up and down the West Coast in their camper buses. They adopted a vagabond code system comparable to that employed by hoboes during the depression and marked their passage with warnings for fellow travelers. Included were ↓ for "Down on Longhairs," ⬆ for "You Can Crash Here" and T for "Diggers in Town."

While nomadism was increasing, many of the more passive young people were emulating their forefathers in returning to the land. Thousands of refugees from the Haight-Ashbury passed through such early communes as Morningstar after the summer or went on to join newer centers in Mendocino County, in the hills behind Big Sur and in the distant mountains of northern California. Some of them lived on the fringes of rural communities and found friendly neighbors for whom they could work in exchange for free meals. Others existed on subsistence stealing, horoscope casting, Tarot card reading, begging, and other techniques used by gypsies for centuries. Many were more modern and scavenged their suppers from garbage cans.

But most of the young people were so fearful of conflict and rejection that they wanted no contact with society. They therefore retired further into the wilds, where they bought or borrowed property, built shacks and lean-tos, and tried to live on what nature might provide. Because they had left clothes, books, language and such philosophic contaminants as the media behind them, they assumed they could perfect the loose structure of the new community. Thus, they created alternative institutions, while continuing to engage in their drug-taking, natural child-rearing practices and so called therapies. As winter approached, some of the modern "Indians" were completely isolated on the reservations they had created to escape the White Man.

Yet, in spite of their efforts, others who sought safety outside the city could not avoid intrusions. The press was still after these young people, and local sheriffs hounded them. In addition, the public health departments of several northern California counties followed the pattern set earlier in San Francisco by raiding the settlements using the excuse of their lack of sanitation and their high incidence of hepatitis and venereal disease. Some of the inspections were necessary for the health of the hippies and their surrounding neighbors. But from the stories that reached the Haight-Ashbury, it appeared that most were punitive attacks designed to drive the young people from their land.

Many adults seemed to approve of such wholesale retaliation against the young people, whom they blamed for the deterioration of the Haight and equated with gypsies as inveterate thieves, parasitic vagrants, seducers of innocent children and carriers of disease. The hippies certainly encouraged this attitude, for the summer had left many of them without any apparent goals other than self-perpetuation and survival. But they were neither so intrinsically evil nor so responsible for what happened in San Francisco as the public contended. In truth, although they generally avoided trouble, they were taking the blame for everyone in America with long hair.

This was unwarranted, for shoulder-length locks, along with beards and sideburns, were common to almost every metropolitan area of the country by this time. Those hip communities founded in other cities around the start of the summer had grown immeasurably by the fall of 1967, and other subcultural enclaves were springing up in places as unlikely as Hawaii. Furthermore, many of the young people who had visited the Haight during its heyday and then returned home were now regarded as heroes. They were therefore evolving into local gurus and keeping the concept, if not the name, of hippie alive.

Concomitant with this diaspora was a steady proliferation of the psychedelic lore. Almost every city in the United States had its own superamplified groups, hip shops and underground newspapers by this point in history. Light shows, dance concerts, Day-Glo paint and mixed-media environments were everywhere. Bill Graham, whose Fillmore West now housed a huge straight audience, was about to open Fillmore East in New York City, while Denver had already acquired its version of the Avalon Ballroom under the aegis of Chet Helms and the Family Dog. The advertising industry had appropriated phrases like "far out" and "groovy" for its own commercial purposes; products ranging from detergents to hair sprays were touted as being out of sight; and doing your thing was becoming as American as violence and apple pie.

A second aspect of the cultural diffusion lay in the nation's unprecedented preoccupation with sensory stimulation. Just as young people in San Francisco once signaled their presence with patchouli and incense, so were adults now attracting attention with fruit-flavored perfumes, aftershave lotions and colognes. Miniskirts, bell-bottomed trousers, Nehru jackets and the American Indian Look were sweeping the fashion world and people from all walks of life were sporting plastic love beads and paisley flower decals. As advertisers emphasized Now-ness in their commercials, Dr. Dernburg and the authors felt that the psychological propensity to avoid frustration that once seemed common only to the children of affluence was now being catered to everywhere.

At the same time, the country was showing an intense interest in the alternate therapies and the communal spirit on which the new community was founded. Fraternities and sororities were dying on the college campus, their places taken in some instances by coeducational living units that bore a striking resemblance, at least in principle, to the Haight-Ashbury's early tribes. Experimental free schools were being developed; encounter groups and gestalt therapy sessions were gaining in popularity; the Esalen Institute was inspiring over fifty imitators across the country; and the straightest possible people were participating in the square games at Synanon.

In addition, the nation was seeing a steady growth of techniques like yoga, Transcendental Meditation, and Krishna Consciousness, which promised instant psychic release and personal enlightenment. As the Summer of Love faded into memory, it became quite apparent that the eupsychic ethic spelled out by Norman Mailer and then applied by beats and hippies in the Haight was being increasingly accepted by the population at large.

Drugs had always been an important part of eupsychia, so it was inevitable that they too were being assimilated by society. Here again, American advertising was setting the pace of public acceptance by promulgating a casual attitude towards all kinds of chemical consumption. The pharmaceutical industry was coming out with its regular raft of products alleged to relieve tension and help regulate external and internal stimuli, and was also adopting the hip jargon to sell everything from so-called tranquilizers to diet pills. Even the National Dairymen's Council was joining the act by trying to convince young and old alike that "milk turns you on."

A few people may actually have tried to alter themselves with milk, but more established psychoactive agents were in much greater supply and demand. Marijuana use had increased dramatically by the fall of 1967, with some investigators estimating that over fifteen million Americans, some of them enrolled in grammar school, were now experimenting with grass. The hallucinogens were also winning a wider audience, set by Dr. Timothy Leary at four million souls. STP and the psychotomimetic amphetamines were popping up in Eastern cities. And, as Jackie predicted, the country was starting to hear about underground speed.

In the Midwest, for example, the captain of a high-school basketball team was found dead after overamping on amphetamines. In San Francisco, a report prepared by the Office of Economic Opportunity indicated that one-hundred-thousand-dollars worth of speed had been purchased during September in the Tenderloin district. No one had made as thorough a financial breakdown in the Haight-Ashbury, but a poll taken by Drs. Joel Fort and Richard Blum at a Berkeley high school revealed that over twenty percent of the eleventh and twelfth graders had sampled oral amphetamines.

As such statistics mounted, more and more people were seeing the need for programs modeled after those which had been founded to help the new community. Over thirty service agencies patterned after Huckleberry's and the Switchboard were established in California during the fall of 1967, thirty of them in the Bay Area alone. Several doctors began studying Dr. Harry Wilmer's Youth Drug Unit, and medical leaders everywhere became interested in the Mendocino Drug Abuse Program and Family.

Over six medical and drug-abuse clinics modeled after the Haight-Ashbury Free Medical Clinic were also either opened or contemplated across the country during this period, most of them following the Clinic's acceptance philosophy and employing its techniques of amphetamine and hallucinogenic drug detoxification. Los Angeles had its first facility by October and three more by December of 1967; the Open Door Clinic was started in Seattle; and Dr. Joseph Brenner, a professor of psychiatry at the Massachusetts Institute of Technology, was visiting San Francisco and formulating plans for a volunteer-operated center in the Cambridge-Boston area.

"This is only one indication of the future," Dr. David Breithaupt of the Clinic predicted. "Our experiences show that the Summer of Love was the most intense period of chemical experimentation in the history of the United States. But it's important to realize that drug and health problems were not and are not isolated to the Haight-Ashbury. For all its publicity, the Haight was and is no more than a microcosm of the entire country. The summer may be over, yet as far as speed is concerned, the Haight-Ashbury is only the front of the storm."

America's First Teen-age Slum

Dr. Breithaupt's clinical observations were given additional validity by a research project that was completed at 558 Clayton Street while the Medical Section was closed. This survey of drug practices in the district was conducted by Dr. Meyers, Dr. Smith and Frederick Shick, the medical student from the University of Indiana who came to the Clinic after reading about it in *Look* magazine. Shick worked at 558 Clayton Street for a month before preparing a questionnaire that was distributed in late September to over four hundred young people at the facility and within a twenty-block surrounding area. He then collected the forms and ran them off on a computer when he returned to school.

After collating his results, Shick found that forty-six percent of his respondents were female and fifty-four percent were male, with a median age of twenty and one-half years. Eighty-six percent identified themselves as Caucasian. Most came from middle- or lower-middle-income families, and almost twenty-four percent had fathers in professional fields. Although only seven percent were college graduates, approximately forty percent had obtained some education past high school.

Shick considered it significant that less than twelve percent of the respondents came originally from the Bay Area. Over thirty-four percent were raised in such large metropolitan centers as New York, Chicago and Los Angeles, while another twenty-six percent were from urban or suburban communities with populations of one hundred thousand or more. An additional fourteen percent of the sample were from smaller suburbs; only eight percent were from rural areas.

Regardless of their point of origin, the respondents exhibited an almost universal acceptance of drug use and abuse. Ninety-one percent took marijuana for social and/or medicinal purposes, and eighty-four percent had also tried LSD or another hallucinogen — a finding that came as no surprise. But their high level of acquaintance with other toxic chemicals *was* surprising. Although most of those questioned praised the hallucinogens for their mind-altering qualities, as many who used these agents were also familiar with alcohol, while fifty percent had employed barbiturates and other sedative-hypnotic-general anesthetics to change their moods.

Almost sixty-eight percent had also sampled what they thought to be opium, and thirty-five percent claimed to have experimented with cocaine. Twenty-four percent had tried heroin on at least one occasion, although only a very few were addicted to the drug at the time of the survey. Furthermore, sixty-nine percent of the respondents had tried oral amphetamines. Thirty-four percent had taken the compounds intravenously, and over ten percent could be considered habitual abusers of speed.

These latter respondents fell into many different categories. Some alternated between amphetamines, acid, and other drugs and could therefore be considered multiple, as well as habitual, abusers. Others took speed only and said that they preferred stimulants to the hallucinogens and to such depressants as barbiturates and heroin. Still others insisted that amphetamines were inferior to downers but much more available.

A fraction of the true hippie types and a much larger percentage of the hippies who had come to the district during the summer stated that they had taken LSD until they became depressed and switched to speed. Almost all of these respondents praised acid for its eupsychic properties, although they still considered amphetamines their chemicals of choice. As a result of their preference for speed, these hippies shared with the other respondents the suffering which stemmed from their speed-based life-style.

Further observation indicated that this suffering would increase, for amphetamines and other powerful drugs were becoming ever more available in the Haight. Several additional speed laboratories had begun operating by the end of the summer, most of which cut the LSD they made with inert substances or amphetamines. Thus, although hallucinogens could still be had on Haight Street, only intimates of Owsley and the few other remaining hippie chemists could purchase pharmacologically pure LSD. Because of its scarcity, many who craved the hallucinogenic experience were continuing to switch to substitute compounds, while those who stuck to the street drugs were becoming more dependent, whether they wanted to or not, on the central effects of speed.

Although this shift had serious repercussions across the country, it was especially harmful in the Haight-Ashbury. Hallucinogenic drugs and the nonviolent philosophy had hitherto reinforced the unaggressive aspects of the hippies' behavior and thereby allowed them to sustain a delusion of peace and love. Yet the new population was growing in a philosophic and pharmacological vacuum now that the new community had all but quit the area. The last thing it needed was encouragement to shy away from acid in preference for speed.

This was particularly true for those younger and more ingenuous adolescents who were still arriving in the district. Most of them partook of the hippie modality, but they generally came from homes that were less affluent and more disturbed than the homes of the original hippies. They also arrived at a time when most of the communes had been turned into crash pads and when even the older homosexuals were leaving Haight Street because of the violence there. They were therefore more helpless than the summer visitors and more vulnerable to the amphetamine-oriented subculture which was now assuming control.

Because of this, the new arrivals usually became members of the subculture themselves. Roger Smith noted that some began experimenting with what they hoped were hallucinogens, as many respondents to the Clinic survey had done, and then turned to stimulants to overcome their depression. Others started directly with speed when they were faced with their environment and their own lack of self-confidence. They usually began with oral amphetamines before trying intravenous drugs, at which point they frequently experienced acute adverse reactions. But they gradually assimilated the lore of the subculture, became habitual abusers, and were then identified as speed freaks who followed the cyclical swing between euphoria and despair.

In the course of their new acculturation, a very few of the young people became manufacturers of amphetamines. But most never approached such prominence. Because they were unable to compete with the older hoodies in alley smartness, they evolved into middle-echelon distributors, or, more likely, nickel and dime bag dealers who were so desperate for stimulation that they sniveled over used cottons employed to strain the impurities out of street speed, and tried to augment their incomes with rip-offs and burns. Many eventually learned how to succeed at burglary, hustling and petty thievery. Yet in the meantime, they turned to prostitution and other trades. Their LSD-oriented counterparts once freely shared their bodies in the name of universal brotherhood, but love now carried a price tag in the Haight-Ashbury.

Some of these young people carried guns and knives to obscure their helplessness. Others, like Randy, had to prove how stoned and sick they could get and still stay alive. But their recognition was nominal when compared to that of other drug abusers. As Roger Smith said, "The speed freak is regarded as a fool by heroin addicts, as insane and violent by those using hallucinogens, and as a bust by nondrug-using hustlers. In many ways, he is an outcast in a society of outcasts."

Smith also believed that the amphetamine abusers exiled themselves from one another. They frequently substituted drugs for interpersonal relations and experienced a complete isolation reinforced by their paranoia and psychotic behavior. They sometimes had sex, but their lives were ego trips dominated by speed. A twenty-two-year-old needle freak named Terry later described this state to Roger Smith.

It's a very personal thing to me. I always used to refer to myself as we, in the third person, and when I did that, someone would say, "What do you mean, we?" I said I'm so great that I can consider myself more than one person. The "we" was essentially the needle, like, we're going to go home and enjoy ourselves, aren't we?

It's a real party. You find with speed that you're your own best entertainer. To me it was a love affair. I was in love with shooting up; I was in love with myself. At times I would think of these sexual acts, like, female, come in here and let me do all these weird things to you, but when the final orgasm takes place I don't want you here — I want it all for myself. I want you to help anoint me in oil and prepare me for this, except that you rarely find a chick that will prepare you for this thing and then let you kick her out. I reached orgasms by myself at times under meth, but I didn't realize it until I took my pants to the coin-op laundry.

The press would never report it, but thousands of people like Terry would pass through the area within the next year, as the Haight entered a new stage in its development. The district would now continue to be a Fort Lauderdale, particularly during vacation periods. It was not yet a ghetto, but it was established as the national center of multiple and habitual drug abuse and as America's first teen-age slum.

As such, the Haight-Ashbury had the same lack of food, employment, housing and health opportunities that the Diggers once hoped to remedy in all of America's marginal areas. It also exhibited a typical inability to solve these problems, for while many of its former residents were slumming for the fun of it, those left after the summer of 1967 had little experience in utilizing public services because they had been denied access to them for most of their lives. Like most ghetto dwellers, they were incapable of community organization and had neither the economic means nor the political muscle to improve their welfare.

Yet the Haight differed from traditional ghettos because it was dominated by hallucinogens and stimulants instead of opiates, barbiturates and other depressants. Downers were available there in the fall of 1967, as Shick's survey revealed, and would become even more so in 1968. But in the meantime amphetamines were setting the drug tone of the district and helping to turn it into the type of behavioral sink that can be created by crowding laboratory animals.

At a certain level of population density, these animals undergo biochemical and psychological changes which are manifested as a stress syndrome and, in some cases, as a physical degeneration that is called "shock disease." Experiments with mice, rats and bobwhite quails have indicated that density per se is not the crucial factor initiating the stress syndrome. It seems instead that an excessive number of encounters with unknown individuals — which naturally increases in direct proportion to density — sparks the response. Environmental restriction is therefore harmful because of concurrent emotional buffeting. This in turn results, in lower animals, in a lowering of the birthrate, in disease susceptibility and mortality and in a dramatic increase in homosexuality, incest, cannibalism and infanticide.

Not all the young Haight-Ashbury residents were restricted in their environment, and some did leave the district over the coming year. Yet others were trapped — by alienation from their parents, by their lack of education, income and self-sespect, and by their drug dependence. These people and their counterparts in other urban areas would henceforth be called street people, because they used the street as a place to live, eat, sleep, barter and entertain themselves. But their lives were not entertaining. Cut off from the straight world, crammed together in inhuman conditions, and controlled by chemicals that probably exerted an aggregate toxic effect on their functioning, they behaved quite naturally like rats in a cage.

The city treated them accordingly. San Francisco had long been hostile toward the Haight, but it became even more antagonistic after the Summer of Love. Park Emergency Hospital, which had never been sympathetic towards the new community, was all but off limits to the new population by the fall. The police from Park Station had grown increasingly desperate in their methods and were now patrolling the district in heavily armed paddy wagons and squad cars. They had also escalated their sweeps of Haight Street to the point that one hundred and fifty young people were rounded up during the second week of October alone.

At the same time, the city had begun to harrass those private social agencies in the Haight-Ashbury that had been founded to aid the new community. The police searched both the Switchboard and Huckleberry's in mid-October, ostensibly to find runaways. They also cruised by 558 Clayton Street continually and chased several dozen people off the front stairs. Park

Station had not yet moved against the Clinic annex, but the volunteers at 409 Clayton Street were certain that their turn would come.

They also had to contend with a great deal of anxiety while the Medical Section was inoperative. 409 House was one of the Haight's only surviving sanctuaries at this point, and as the streets became increasingly dangerous, more and more young people began looking for safety inside. There was ample space for several hundred within the three-story Victorian, but its legitimate occupants were neither equipped nor willing to accommodate an influx of such size.

To complicate matters, the volunteers could not distribute medication in the Psychiatric Section as they would a year later, when 558 Clayton Street was once again closed. Most of the summer physicians were on hand in October, but they were too swamped with adverse speed and acid reactions to help young people with less pressing problems. Dr. Dernburg was tied up with long-term patients like Alan, leaving only Professor Loomis and a few other counselors free for crisis intervention. Charles MacGuillamay, Trina Merriman and several paramedical volunteers from the Medical Section were doing their best to refer patients to outlying facilities, but in many instances they could do no more than send the young people to Happening House downstairs.

Although it was often overcrowded as a result of this procedure, Professor Wolf's educational project was operating more efficiently than ever before. Happening House was now one of the only productive social centers left in the Haight-Ashbury. Professor Wolf had given over fifty separate classes there during the summer. He had also invited mayoralty candidate Jack Morrison to 409 Clayton Street to lecture on political reform in San Francisco and peace in Vietnam. But peace had become a rather inappropriate subject in the Haight, by this point, and the continual deluge of alienated adolescents to the district was pushing Professor Wolf towards a debacle that would spell the death of Happening House and seriously threaten his academic career.

This occurred on Wednesday, October eighteenth, when he sponsored a conference on runaways at the Straight Theatre. The ancient movie palace had been turned into a community town hall for the evening, and a crowd of over one thousand young people was assembled to discuss survival. The discussion remained scholarly for three hours, at which point Professor Wolf retired momentarily to 409 Clayton Street. When he returned to the theater he saw six young men and women dancing nude on the stage. Professor Wolf tried to halt the performance, only to find that the police had beaten him to the punch. After clearing the theater, they arrested him for

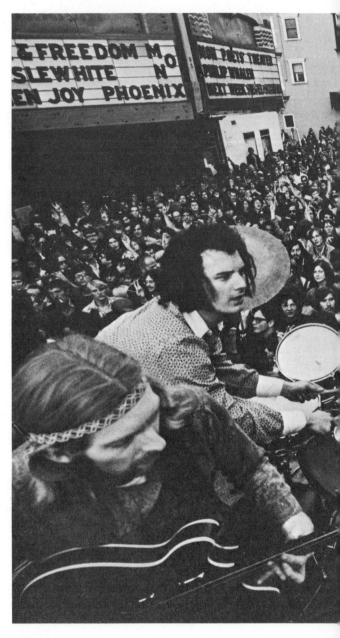

Haight Street: The Grateful Dead entertains in the behavioral sink.
(Jim Marshall)

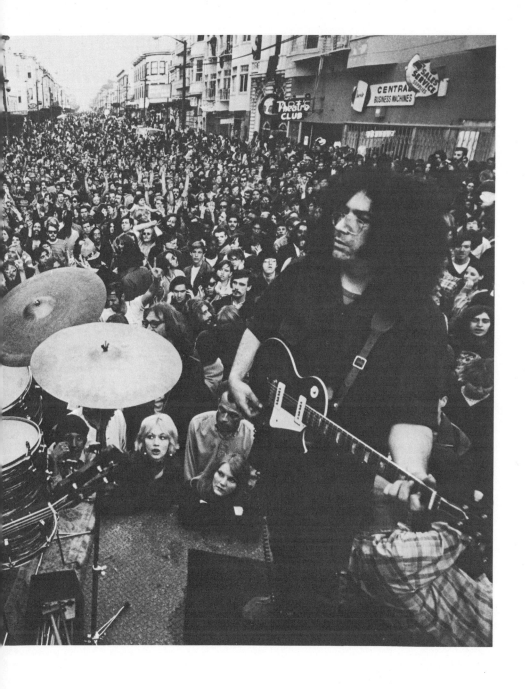

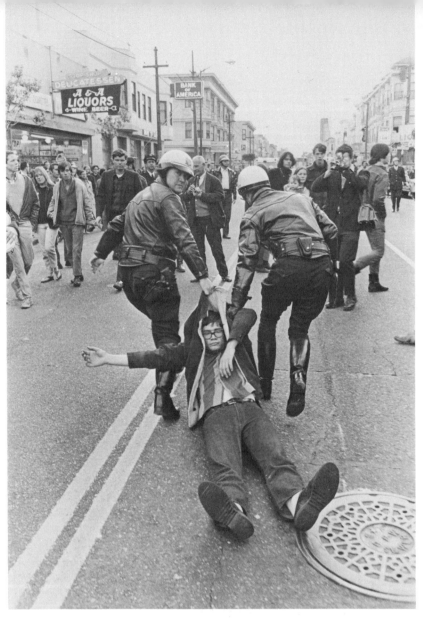

Haight Street: caught in a sweep.
(Michael Alexander)

contributing to the delinquency of the minors in attendance and for allowing the public disrobing to occur.

The Straight Theatre bust was both damaging in itself and also the signal of an equally disastrous event to come. Two nights later, a patrolman from Park Station entered Huckleberry's and inquired after a fifteen-year-old runaway. A director of the organization then told the patrolman that the boy was not present, although he was actually hiding upstairs. The boy's mother, who apparently knew his whereabouts, had signed a warrant which allowed the police to search the premises and arrest her son, nine other residents, the director and two additional aides. An attorney representing one of the plaintiffs contacted Father Larry Beggs the following week and told him that all charges would be dismissed if he would close his facility. Father Beggs inferred from this that Huckleberry's had been set up in advance for the arrests. He therefore refused the offer and was ordered along with Professor Wolf to stand trial.

Huckleberry's stayed open after the incident, but the program at Happening House was brought to a standstill while Professor Wolf fought for his academic standing and started collecting the witnesses and the capital necessary to prepare his legal defense. Furthermore, those patients who once depended on his hospitality reasoned that society was now totally against them. Some of the young people who had previously hung out at Happening House returned to the streets after they were deprived of their only refuge. Others began asking if and when 558 Clayton Street would open again.

Reorganization

The organizers had been meeting regularly to arrive at an answer, but they too were uncertain about the future of the Medical Section. Many were disheartened by the Death of Hip ceremony, and there was a great deal of factionalism among the staff. Yet the city's action against Father Beggs and Professor Wolf did serve to unite most of the disparate elements in their determination not to be driven from the district. And the organizers were given another good reason to resume operations now that Happening House was virtually closed.

As always, the most important reason concerned the needs of their patients. When the organizers first conceived of their facility, they and the others who worked there shared a sympathy for and an identity with the beats and hippies, an enthusiasm for the ideals of the psychedelic movement, a dissatisfaction with current medical practices and a vague desire to do something in the community health field. While implementing this desire over the summer, they learned how difficult yet personally rewarding it was to provide alienated young people with some semblance of proper care.

Now, the organizers did not want to waste that education. Theirs was still not a neighborhood center, for they were unable to reach all of the new population or any of the old. But they felt a strong commitment to community medicine, even though the new community they had once hoped to help had all but disappeared. At the same time, Dr. Smith thought that some members of the community might return to the Haight-Ashbury now that the media had abandoned it. He had kept in touch with a number of young people who had moved to the country or to other parts of the city and believed that the beats and hippies would continue to use 558 Clayton Street, especially those with children who were treated there during the Summer of Love.

Another reason for reopening related to the myths which had evolved about the Clinic. Dr. Smith and the facility were now known throughout the country, partially because of John Luce's *Look* story. But because Luce and others never documented the Clinic's trials and tribulations, most people outside San Francisco assumed that the Medical Section was a well-financed and smoothly run operation with a large, professional staff. Some also believed that it was a hip organization which had outlived its usefulness now that most of the hippies were gone.

Nothing could have been further from the truth. The Clinic had more than its share of problems and amateuristic procedures, and the organizers had sanctioned many improper medical practices during the summer. Illegal chemicals had been sold and used at the Clinic; Dr. Smith and others had failed to adequately supervise the facility; some patients had received only minimal treatment; and many records, donated drugs and boxes of medical equipment had been lost or stolen in the confusion. The organizers were not eager to advertise these deficiencies, but they did want to improve their facility and let others learn from their mistakes. Many also felt that a free health center with a nonviolent bias was more needed in the Haight than ever.

In addition, even those who suspected that their efforts would soon be irrelevant in the Haight-Ashbury wished to extend their influence beyond the immediate area. Dr. Smith and other physicians at 558 Clayton Street were now lecturing at colleges and consulting with medical associations, educational groups and community leaders in many American cities. They were also being asked to treat people of all ages who were fearful of being denied public service or who were intimidated by private doctors. Over fifty letters were still arriving daily from housewives, students and professional people who had suffered bad trips or were strung out on diet or sleeping pills. Dr. Dernburg and Professor Loomis were running an LSD rescue service for the entire Bay Area out of 409 House. Other psychiatrists and counselors were making house calls outside of the Haight and lecturing at local colleges and high schools.

Finally, the Clinic was taking an active part in the planning of other free medical facilities across the country. Some volunteers were advising in Los Angeles, Seattle and Cambridge, while others were working with physicians like those of the Salud Clinic in Tulane County, who were founding centers for minority groups in other deprived areas. The organizers agreed that the United States was just beginning to experience drug problems. They needed the Medical Section as an experimental model, as well as a base to operate from.

As a case in point, Drs. Meyers and Smith had recently been asked to head a Drug Abuse Information Project for the state of California, which had allocated thirty thousand dollars to them to collect information on research and service projects related to drug abuse and to provide advice with respect to fields in which research was needed. Dr. Robert Morris was still working with the San Francisco Medical Society to amend the legislation covering the treatment of minors. After drawing its philosophic orientation from the new community, the Clinic had been conceived as an alternative — and hopefully an inspiration — to the San Francisco Public Health Department and medical establishment. Most of the organizers and volunteers hoped the Medical Section would fulfill this function if it were opened again.

Most, but not all. Bob Conrich was long gone from 558 Clayton Street by this point, and Peter Schubart had left to study biochemistry at the University of California at Santa Cruz. Fred Shick and the other medical students had also returned to their classes. Kurt Feibusch had become involved in the San Francisco Gestalt Therapy Institute during the closing of the Medical Section. Laurel Rowland had gone to Mexico, as had several other original hippie workers, including Doc and Superguru.

At the same time, Dr. Smith was encumbered by a variety of professional commitments. After dividing his time between the Clinic, the Alcohol and Drug Abuse Screening Unit and the University of California Medical Center during most of the summer, he was now under fire from Dr. James Stubblebine, head of mental health services, for neglecting his duties with the Public Health Department. Dr. Arthur Carfagni had defended Dr.

Smith by saying that his work at 558 Clayton Street served a public health function. But Dr. Stubblebine insisted that he cut back on his commitments, particularly since he would soon be involved with the Drug Abuse Information Project.

Also torn between his many responsibilities was Dr. Meyers. He had spent much of his spare time at the Medical Section over the summer, but was now hard pressed to handle his independent research, his classes at the University of California and his future role in the Drug Abuse Information Project. Furthermore, Dr. Meyers deplored the drug use and lack of supervision at the Clinic and did not share Dr. Smith's belief that the new community could be reestablished in the Haight-Ashbury. Although still concerned with its members, he thought that the hip subculture had died in the Haight and predicted that the district would experience an increase in violence at the hands of the police and the new population during the months to come.

Because of this, he feared that the Clinic might become a victim of its environment and urged that its policy of complete acceptance be abandoned in favor of more assertive intervention designed to dissuade new arrivals from the district and its prevalent life-style. Dr. Meyers still wanted to collect and help identify the new drugs that he assumed would appear on Haight Street and was especially anxious to launch an in-depth study of amphetamine abuse. He was therefore willing to retain his title as research director, although he could not give 558 Clayton Street the same attention as before.

This was a severe loss to the Clinic, but although a few other medical staff members also had to leave or limit their activities, over fifty nurses and physicians, including Peggy Sankot, and Drs. Richard Gleason, Norman Sissman, Alan Matzger, Bertram Meyer and David Breithaupt, remained. Dr. Robert Morris and Dr. William Nesbitt were ready to resume work and were also interested in establishing executive and advisory committees to lend additional respectability to the facility and provide more structure for its staff.

Equally concerned with structure was Don Reddick, who believed that the Medical Section might have survived the summer if its clinical and fund-raising activities had been better organized. After making an extensive inventory at 558 Clayton Street after its closing, the administrative director and his business partners concluded that new accounting and budget procedures were indicated for the future. Reddick also felt that the facility could cut back on its hours of operation somewhat but would have to offer additional services to help its patients. He was seconded by Alan Rose and several other people who had arrived during the latter part of the summer and were anxious to become full-time members of the staff.

One of these volunteers was Judy St. Onge, a twenty-two-year-old from Northeastern University in Boston, who came to the Bay Area by way of Berkeley and became a resident of the Haight-Ashbury because she was offered free housing there. Miss St. Onge originally visited the Clinic to be treated, but ended up serving at the facility out of a need for involvement. She had been put in charge of writing referrals in August, and was now ready to augment these duties with supervision of the paramedical volunteers.

Interested more in business was a thirty-five-year-old ex-biker named Jerry Read. Read was a prescription amphetamine user and the manager of a rock group called The Initial Shock. He was also a close friend of Janis Joplin. Read wanted to strengthen his position in the music world by holding nighttime benefits and outdoor concerts for the Clinic in Golden Gate Park with the local bands. Because he believed that the Public Health Department would never support the facility, he advised the organizers to call on the former leaders of the new community and on liberal elements in San Francisco for future funds.

Few of the organizers could argue with Read's belief about the city, but the *San Francisco Chronicle* was not similarly inclined. Shortly after David Perlman prepared his obituary, the *Chronicle* endorsed the Medical Section's activities and then editorialized that the Clinic should be financed by the Public Health Department. Herb Caen and others wrote statements of support in their columns, but although Dr. Ellis Sox, Mayor John Shelley and Chief Administrative Officer Thomas Mellon remained unmoved, those persons whom Read had urged the organizers to approach started coming instead to them.

The first was Bill Graham, who visited 558 Clayton Street and told Dr. Smith that he wanted to make a donation. "These kids have made my business possible," Graham said as he looked out the front windows at a police sweep of Haight Street. "They don't deserve this treatment. Now, I want to do something for them. I'll help you with another benefit at the Fillmore: a big one, but it'll have to be my last. There are lots of good causes in this city, and we gave over fifty fund-raising events last year. But we need the Clinic. It's humanity — and the least I can do."

Graham's least was more than enough to insure a completely successful affair. He provided his auditorium and staff and also talked Blue Cheer, the Charlatans and the Jefferson Airplane into performing on the evening of October sixteenth, thereby guaranteeing a gross of five thousand dollars. In addition, Ralph Gleason of the *Chronicle* covered the preparations for the event in his music column. His support created an atmosphere of anticipation in the city, gave the organizers a new optimism, and prompted several others to host benefits of their own.

Among them were the proprietors of the Straight Theatre, who sponsored a Mixed Mediathon on the weekend of October fourth, fifth and sixth at which hundreds of local performers appeared. Next in sequence was Dr. Sunday's Medicine Show, an afternoon concert on October eighth which was given at the Family Park in San Jose. It was organized by Dr. David Breithaupt and by Ron Polte and Julius Karpen of West Pole Productions, who helped obtain Big Brother and the Holding Company for the occasion, along with several other bands. Nuns were used in place of the more traditional long-haired ushers and ticket-takers to set a peaceful tone at the benefit. Eight thousand dollars was raised for the Medical Section, and after the event was over, Dr. Breithaupt held a dinner for Big Brother and the paramedical staff.

Ralph Gleason reacted to the Medicine Show by writing in his *Chronicle* column that "it is a strange world indeed when such a valuable public service as the Clinic should have to go to an adjacent city to, quite literally, beg for funds." This in turn inspired John Bolles, a local art dealer, to sponsor a twenty-four hour benefit sale of paintings, prints and drawings at his gallery. A champagne reception was held prior to the event, at which Alton Kelly, Rick Griffin and other poster artists donated their material. Over fifteen hundred dollars was raised, some of it from unexpected sources. One case in point was an irate patron who mailed back the invitation she received with "shame on dirty hippies — shame on your gallery" scrawled across it. Lowell Pickett had the invitation matted and framed, and the choreographer of the San Francisco Ballet bought it for ten dollars.

Another person who responded to Gleason's column was Norman Stone, the thirty-year-old son of a wealthy and conservative Chicago insurance executive. Stone was studying at the San Francisco Art Institute when he read of the Clinic's financial difficulties and offered to make a substantial donation. Dr. Smith was initially suspicious of this offer, for an older man had walked into 558 Clayton Street a few days earlier and donated a bad check for a somewhat smaller sum. But he subsequently determined that Stone was in a position to follow up on his intention. Stone did — by giving thirty thousand dollars.

These several gifts were enough to provide for a budget of approximately four thousand dollars a month for the coming year. This was all the organizers needed to resume their operations. Yet, now that they had finally attained solvency and were not faced with so extreme an emergency as that which existed in the summer, they took time to make several important changes in the Medical Section.

Dr. Smith, for example, resigned from his position with the screening unit (which subsequently was taken away from the Center for Special Problems and then dissolved), and took a part-time job as a consultant on drug abuse at the Public Health Department while lecturing to support himself and raise funds for the Clinic. He and Dr. Meyers then began organizing the Drug Abuse Information Project. At the same time, they opened negotiations with the National Institute of Mental Health for the thirty-seven-thousand-dollar grant that would allow Roger Smith to begin his study of speed.

Although they continued to work together, Dr. Smith and Dr. Meyers gradually strained their friendship. This resulted in part from Dr. Meyers's dissatisfaction with the Clinic and from his belief that Dr. Smith was too permissive in his approach towards drug abuse. Yet the most basic reason was the disruption of their teacher-student relationship. Dr. Smith had been Dr. Meyers's protégé six months earlier, but he established his own reputation during the Summer of Love.

Dr. Smith welcomed the attention he had gained for political reasons. He still saw the Clinic as a symbol whose influence was disproportionate to what the facility really was. But Dr. Meyers did not value this symbolic function. He felt that Dr. Smith was advancing himself as a symbol and saw the Clinic as the means to his personal, as well as political, ends.

This attitude was held by several of Dr. Smith's associates, including John Luce, who was only tangentially involved with the Clinic. But although Luce feared that the facility might yet collapse without a strong, full-time leader, he appreciated Dr. Smith as an educator and inspirer and as the one man whose vision had kept the Clinic going. He therefore urged him to increase his public speaking. At the same time, he began counseling young people, assisting Dr. Smith on several research projects, and taking a stronger advisory role.

Dr. Morris was installed as head of the Executive Committee and set out to establish an advisory committee of prominent local physicians. Robert Laws expanded his legal referral service. Don Reddick and his partners instituted a revised schedule whereby 558 Clayton Street would be open six days a week from two to eleven P.M. After purchasing and donating new medication and equipment, they ended up with an unprecedented budget surplus which would allow the Medical Section to pay a few members of its staff.

Because of this, Alan Rose took over Peter Schubart's office and began serving as administrator at a salary of two hundred and fifty dollars a month. Peggy Sankot was appointed head nurse at a five hundred dollar a month salary, while Judy St. Onge and Jackie were assigned to supervise the paramedical volunteers. Lowell Pickett, who had been drinking more since the summer, was asked to leave the Clinic; he began producing erotic films. Jerry Read, the new business manager, moved into Pickett's office and decorated it with the business cards of visiting dignitaries, with *Chronicle* columns and with a poster from a local bondsman who offered free bail for the Clinic. By the end of October, the facility was ready to resume operations. On November first, its front door was finally opened again.

The Florence Nightingale of the Haight-Ashbury

Most of the volunteers were too busy to notice at the time, but they soon realized that this second opening was different from the one before. Much less publicity surrounded the second event, a fact which was related to the media's declining interest in the Haight-Ashbury. The patient load was also lighter; only one hundred and twenty-five young people came to 558 Clayton Street on that afternoon and evening, one-half the number present on the seventh of June.

The lessened load meant that those who did seek help at the Medical Section received more attention. And because the staff members were more familiar with each other, they lent a feeling of intimacy to the facility. At least five physicians were scheduled to be on hand daily, most of them on a regular basis, so the patients had a better chance of seeing the same doctor on each visit and a better reason for spending some time there. Because they did, the Clinic underwent another change in its development. It was already a sanctuary by the end of the summer. Now it resembled a loosely structured family as well.

This family had as many father figures as there were physicians, but its mother was Peggy Sankot. Although she was a shy and straight woman when she first appeared at 558 Clayton Street, Miss Sankot adopted many hippie values over the summer. But unlike some people who became involved in the Haight, she never sacrificed her professional competence in the name of love. Miss Sankot had a mission. "I agree with a lot that the kids are saying," she said. "I appreciate their need for community, their search for new institutions, their interest in spirituality. And I believe in real love, a commodity sorely needed in medicine, which can be so mechanical and cold. But my place is between hip and straight worlds. I want to help the kids appreciate what's good about the Establishment and vice

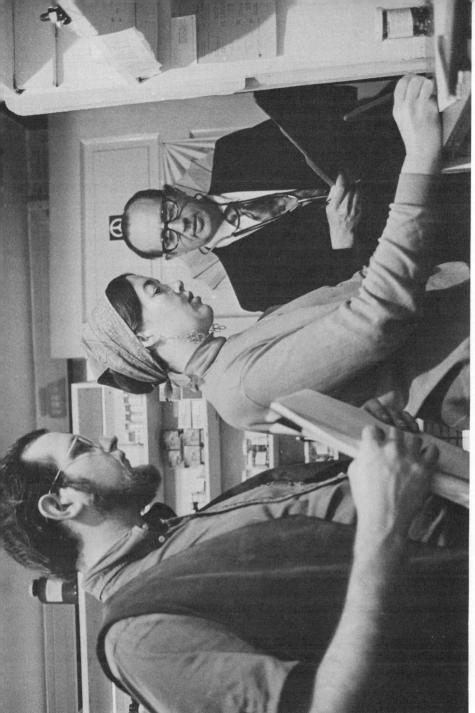

558 Clayton Street: Alan Rose, Peggy Sankot and Dr. William Nesbitt in the Clinic pharmacy.

(Elaine Mayes)

versa. And I want both sides to realize the one thing that working here has taught me the most: sick and confused people need care and human contact, not computerized medicine or pills."

Miss Sankot never stopped furnishing medication during her involvement with the Medical Section, and as head nurse she often assisted the volunteer pharmicists in filling prescriptions in the Clinic pharmacy. Although she utilized modern treatment methods, she never tried to supplant the meaningful interaction of the doctor-patient relationship with medication alone. She resisted turning 558 Clayton Street into a dispensary and made every possible attempt to talk personally with the patients. Her influence was not all that Dr. Meyers wanted in the way of intervention, but it set a positive tone.

It also caused some difficulties within the medical profession, for the idea of a highly personalized approach to community health ran counter to the standards of medical piecework and mass production prevalent at the time. Peggy Sankot had little use for such standards. She found it amusing that the Medical Section, which was once criticized for offering free services to its patients, was now being accused of coddling them.

Although some members of the San Francisco Medical Society made formal complaints about the new arrangement, the society never retracted its initial endorsement. In fact, Miss Sankot's personal touch actually seemed to appeal to more people than it offended. It was especially attractive to medical students, to young physicians and to those older doctors who considered themselves overspecialized and therefore came to 558 Clayton Street to volunteer.

Her philosophic leadership also made a profound impression on the clerical and paramedical workers. The younger volunteers were relieved to be able to spend more time now with the patients. They were also pleased with the new familial atmosphere because it allowed them to become closer to the many surrogate parents at the facility. Jackie, for example, was so inspired by Miss Sankot that she outgrew some of her defensiveness and eventually asked Dr. Dernburg for psychotherapy. "I was trying to prove I didn't need parents," she told him. "It took Peggy to show me that I had to have a family, too."

While Jackie and the other staff members profited from Peggy Sankot's presence, the greatest beneficiaries were the patients. Most of these young people needed considerable nurturing, and many were afraid of rejection. But for all their protective toughness, some of them appeared to mellow under Miss Sankot's influence. Alan was so comforted by her that he began to divide his time between the Medical and Psychiatric sections, while Randy offered to sweep the floor at 558 Clayton Street after she took him under her wing. Even the more unruly hoodies and bikers reacted positively to her strong but unobtrusive maternalism. Violence was usually lessened at the Clinic whenever the Florence Nightingale of the Haight-Ashbury was there.

Yet neither Peggy nor the other staff members could ever achieve total peace at the facility. Fights flared up often at the Medical Section, and for every person who was receptive to her approach, there were dozens who simply could not and would not respond. In essence, the distance between the volunteers and their patients was steadily increasing because of changing conditions in the Haight. Peggy and the staff members did their best, but they could not possibly bridge the void.

Nor could they begin to meet all the medical needs of the district. Almost every infection which had existed during the summer was still present in the Haight-Ashbury after November, and although new arrivals tended to experience acute difficulties at first, those people who had been in the area for several months were now quite debilitated by chronic disease. Some could be taken care of at 558 Clayton Street, yet so many required referrals and/or transportation to other facilities that in certain cases the Clinic could only diagnose their problems and give them first aid.

At the same time, the patients frequently got lost, misplaced their referral slips, were mistreated or rejected by public health workers, or refused to continue treatment at agencies like the city Venereal Disease Clinic after leaving the Haight. The street people were less transient than their counterparts over the summer, but the volunteers could not keep track of them because they had no adequate follow-up procedures or posttreatment care.

Finally, for all of Peggy Sankot's philosophic strength, she and the staff members were unable to combat drug abuse in the district. Some young people took their advice and were helped into Mendocino and the Youth Drug Unit, while others seemed to transfer some of their dependence on chemicals into a dependence on the Medical Section. But many came to 558 Clayton Street merely for medication and retained an absolute faith in the healing power of pills.

Randy, for one, never cut his drug consumption during his association with the Clinic, and too many other speed freaks used the facility only when their pain became too much to bear. The same was true for the hundreds of young experimenters who suffered acute reactions to LSD and to the impurities in street acid. It applied to older people like Clifford, a fifty-year-old American Indian who stumbled into the Medical Section almost daily complaining that he was "on a bad trip from booze." And it also applied to those adolescents who were so eager to obtain hallucinogenic experiences that they tried any number of substances in place of LSD.

New Chemicals

The most unexpected substitute seen during the fall and winter was catnip, a plant of the mint family which contains alkaloids that are alleged to possess hallucinogenic properties. The nation's largest manufacturer of catnip reported that his sales doubled after the underground media praised the substance in 1968, while the cat population did not appreciably rise. One Midwestern legislator took this situation seriously enough to introduce a bill imposing a fifteen-year sentence on anyone caught smoking catnip. Similar legislation was considered in California, but although catnip smoking was rather common in the Haight-Ashbury, no adverse reactions were observed either in human patients or in felines.

Other substitutes which did pose a problem were the halogenated and unhalogenated hydrocarbons found in petroleum distillates, cleaning fluids and model airplane cement, or glue. These compounds can exert a sedative-hypnotic-general anesthetic effect if inhaled in sufficient quantities by depressing the central nervous system. They can lead to liver damage, bronchial inflammation, chemical pneumonia and potentially fatal illnesses like aplastic anemia, a condition characterized by bone marrow depression with subsequent reduction in certain blood cells that results in tachycardia, excessive bleeding and lassitude. The hydrocarbons can also cause physical addiction, as evidenced by those recorded cases in which people have become addicted to gasoline. No gas or glue addicts were ever seen at the Clinic, primarily because more esteemed chemicals were available in the surrounding area. But over two dozen patients from nearby suburbs were treated at the facility after inhaling model airplane cement and carbon tetrachloride, two of whom required transportation to Mission Emergency. In addition, the physicians were asked to consult in the case of a seven-year-old glue sniffer who developed aplastic anemia and was subsequently hospitalized at the Medical Center.

This boy was the son of a prominent local banker and had two older brothers, aged eighteen and thirteen. The older brother, a college student, took LSD ritualistically and then told the middle brother about his experiences. The thirteen-year-old was unable to purchase any righteous acid, so he settled for marijuana and model airplane cement. His seven-year-old younger brother followed suit until he wound up in the hospital. The patient eventually recovered, but his case served as a reminder of both the extreme to which youthful drug experimentation had progressed and the complications that often resulted from the unavailability of pure LSD.

Along with this case, the doctors observed many other bizarre reactions to the shortage of acid. Some young people said that they had taken methysergide, the expensive ergot alkaloid employed in the treatment of migraine headaches. Others were interviewed after eating ground-up morning glory and baby rosewood seeds, which contain lysergic amide. Two nineteen-year-old girls were given medication for acute gastritis after they each chewed up over two hundred seeds in one hour. MDA, MMDA and other psychotomimetic amphetamines were also used by patients, as was DOM, or STP.

STP made its first postsummer appearance on the afternoon of November 11, 1967, when a tablet called the pink wedge was hawked on Haight Street as a superior chemical containing fifteen hundred micrograms of high-quality LSD. Since the fifteen hundred microgram dose was approximately five times that found in the blue dot and other early acid preparations, most of the young people who purchased these wedges ingested only a fraction of the tablets. But in spite of their general caution, dozens of the buyers began freaking out because of panic and perceptual distortions.

Eighteen patients were treated at 558 Clayton Street that afternoon and evening, eight of them suffering from hallucinosis and paranoia as well as extreme anxiety. After being talked down or given small doses of Thorazine, seventeen of the patients recovered as the tablets they consumed were eventually metabolized. But one girl who swallowed a whole wedge was so disturbed she had to spend the next week at San Francisco General Hospital.

This new wonder drug also presented serious patient management problems. One volunteer nurse was struck by a thrashing boy on the evening of November eleventh, and several other patients became so violent that they had to be quarantined in the Psychiatric Section. Furthermore, such physical agitation was so widespread that the physicians realized that the pink wedge could not contain only LSD. They collected a sample for Dr. Meyers to forward to the Food and Drug Administration, which found it to consist of two hundred and fifty micrograms of acid and nine hundred milligrams of STP.

This chemical analysis was posted at the Clinic, and the pink wedge, like so many street preparations, gradually passed into oblivion. But the staff members had to live through eight more kinds of wedges before the end of 1967. And they had barely recovered from this first episode when they were hit with a rash of reactions from compounds alleged to be THC. THC, or tetrahydrocannabinol, is the active component in marijuana, hashish and other cannabis drugs. Since marijuana was a focal point of alienation and a commonly used medicinal and social drug by 1967, the synthesis of tetrahydrocannabinol was reported with great jubilation in the underground press. Rumors then started sweeping the Haight-Ashbury that the compound would soon be widely available.

These rumors were unfounded. A seventeen-stage synthesis is required to manufacture THC, at a cost of approximately fifty dollars per psychoactive dose. The compound is also stable only under liquid nitrogen, while the finished product is foul-tasting and not sufficiently soluble to be put in a pill. Such investigators as Dr. Leo Hollister have determined that genuine tetrahydrocannabinol may produce hallucinogenic effects comparable to those of lysergic acid when taken in doses as small as seventy milligrams. But until further research is conducted, the United States will never experience wholesale consumption of THC.

Some of the Clinic doctors informed their patients of this fact as early as the summer of 1967, but expectations of an increased availability of synthetic tetrahydrocannabinol continued to mount. Drugs alleged to be THC were even passed out on the street occasionally, yet all were found to consist of talcum powder, amphetamine and/or insecticide. Then, in December of 1967, the *Berkeley Barb* heralded the emergence of peace pills, capsules containing a white powder which was supposed to be synthetic marijuana. The capsules appeared on the street shortly thereafter, where the dealers made a killing on adolescents who purchased their products at two dollars and fifty cents apiece. The customers in turn learned that the peace pill, like STP before it, produced nothing resembling peace at all.

It did cause an intoxication that the physicians at 409 and 558 Clayton Street considered one of the worst trips ever. The young people who came to them appeared to be drunk immediately after ingesting the drug, but they then slipped into a stupor, began vomiting, and lashed out furiously. One eighteen-year-old boy picked up a chair and attacked a fellow patient in the calm center. Another took out after Peggy Sankot with a wastebasket. Three patients had to be restrained at the Psychiatric Section in the course of one afternoon. The oldest, twenty-eight years old, was sent to the Immediate Psychiatric Aid and Referral Service, where he threw a bedside table, a bed and its occupant against the wall.

Because of such incidents, some of the Clinic doctors reasoned that the peace pill might be either a psychotomimetic amphetamine or a central nervous system stimulant and were therefore tempted to treat their patients with sedatives. But in keeping with the general procedures established before the summer, they did not administer any drugs until the exact composition of the chemical was determined. This proved to be fortunate, for although the patients pleaded for medication, all survived their experiences. But a physician at a local hospital who failed to take a detailed history of the peace pills' effects from one of his patients assumed that he was faced with a THC reaction and gave the girl in question a sedative and a high dose of Thorazine. The patient did calm herself somewhat when the sedative took effect, but an hour later she stopped breathing and died.

This death could have been predicted, for as the doctors learned later, the peace pill was actually a depressant whose effects were intensified by the sedative administered by the attending physician. Dr. Meyers ultimately determined that the drug was phenyl-cyclohexyl-piperdine, the chemical name for phencyclidine, or Sernyl. Phencyclidine is a sedative-hypnotic-general anesthetic which was once tested in human medicine as a tranquilizing agent but was rejected in part because it caused nausea, hallucinations, delirium and unconsciousness if taken in high doses. Other than its use in the Haight-Ashbury, the compound is employed solely to knock out rhinoceroses and elephants in zoos.

Dr. Meyers posted these facts on the Medical Section bulletin board on December twentieth, 1967, after which a flyer was distributed on the street. Both actions were beneficial, but young people continued to take the peace pill. Over sixty patients were treated at the Clinic for adverse reactions to the drug during December and January, as phencyclidine was sold on certain occasions not only as the peace pill, but also as mescaline, MDA and methamphetamine. The compound gradually passed into disuse, only to return in the spring of 1968 as one component in a concoction called the hog. And long before it did, the Clinic doctors had to deal with several parasympatholytic agents that were also used in place of LSD.

The parasympatholytic agents are so named by Dr. Meyers because they prevent the action of acetylcholine, a substance which transmits nerve impulses along the parasympathetic nerve system to smooth muscles, glands and the heart. Since the drugs' primary actions are qualitatively similar to those of the best-known member of the atropine group, they are often referred to as atropinelike substances. They are also called antispasmodic agents, although this term is somewhat misleading. These compounds do prevent muscle contractions when taken in small doses, in addition to causing a dilation of the pupils and a slight tachycardia and stimulation of the nervous system. But high doses can bring about an extreme stimulation which is followed by central nervous system depression, hallucinations, delirium and death.

Delirium may be undesirable in hospital settings, but in the Haight it was very much in demand. For this reason, atropine, scopolamine and other parasympatholytic agents were sometimes used by young people in the district, especially during LSD dry spells, to obtain legal and allegedly hallucinogenic highs. Particularly popular was Dr. Schiffman's Asthmador, which caused serious overdosage problems because the individuals who used it never knew how much atropine they consumed.

Other difficulties arose from the ingestion of Sominex and Sleepeze, two nonprescription sleep-inducing medications that contain scopolamine, and the so-called tranquilizer, Compoz. Although the manufacturers of these compounds imply that their products are sleeping pills and mental relaxants, they actually produced a state of mental disturbance and physical agitation in those who used them in large doses in the Haight-Ashbury. So did Jimsonweed, which contains both atropine and scopolamine. This substance is known as loco weed for its toxic effects on cattle. It apparently caused similar reactions in those who took it while living on rural communes.

No Jimsonweed reactions were ever treated at the Clinic, although several hippies were known to have become disturbed from the substance when it was distributed at a funeral celebration for Neil Cassady that was held in the spring at Big Sur. But the doctors did see over forty patients who were intoxicated from Sominex, Sleepeze, Compoz and/or Dr. Schiffman's Asthmador during late 1967 and early 1968.

Since most of the physicians had either lived through or heard about the STP episodes early in the summer, they did not administer Thorazine to these young people because of that drug's atropinelike side effects. They therefore used Librium, phenobarbitol and other long-acting sedatives in small doses so as not to send their patients through the excitation phase of their intoxication into respiratory arrest. Atropine and scopolamine caused several close calls at the Medical Section, but there were no fatalities. Furthermore, most of the patients indicated that they would never again use the parasympatholytic agents because their experiences were so devastating.

In spite of this, the doctors also had to deal with several cases of accidental atropine and scopolamine poisoning. Especially vulnerable to these drugs were infants living in the Haight-Ashbury, ten of whom, ranging in age from twenty months to seven years, were treated at 558 Clayton Street. All were delirious on their arrival at the Clinic, and some exhibited widely dilated pupils and temperatures as high as one hundred and six degrees. The children were given artificial respiration on the premises and rushed to General Hospital, where their symptoms eventually subsided. Most were still quite psychologically upset after being released, but none seemed physically the worse for wear.

Yet the very fact that ten infants were even exposed to atropine or scopolamine indicated the increasingly confused and destructive conditions in the Haight. Some of the physicians at the Medical and Psychiatric sections were depressed by the evidence that parents had left the drugs lying around their residences, while others were struck by the desperation and naïveté of those who employed the compounds to intoxicate themselves. Thus, the use of parasympatholytic agents became a symbol to the doctors of the amateurism which characterized so many experimental drug-takers in the Haight-Ashbury. At the same time, the professionalism that existed in drug use in the district came to be represented by the occasional abuse of cocaine.

Cocaine, or benzoylmethyleogonine, is an alkaloid obtained from *Erythroxylon coca,* a small tree or shrub indigenous to Peru and Bolivia, where its leaves have been chewed by local natives for centuries. It is classified pharmacologically as a local anesthetic because it can block conduction when applied to nerve tissue. The drug also produces a profound stimulation of the central nervous system which is comparable to, and the direct historical precursor of, the amphetamines. Because of its central effects, cocaine can cause an elevation of mood, a decrease in appetite and a feeling of increased strength, self-worth and mental capacity. Because of its high abuse potential, the drug is not prepared commercially in injectable form.

In spite of this fact, cocaine is still illegally imported to the United States by way of Florida and can be obtained through drugstore and pharmaceutical company robberies. It is therefore available in the underground, where it is called coke, candy or snow because of its white, powdery appearance. Several abuse patterns have developed around the drug, which can either be sniffed or injected. Sniffing is hazardous, for cocaine constricts the veins on the surface of the nose and can cause nasal septum perforations. The compound is also shot by heroin addicts, as amphetamines are, either as a substitute for the opiate or as a medication to ward off depression. It is similarly employed along with opiates and barbiturates in speedballs.

Such preparations were known in the Haight during 1967 and 1968, but cocaine was usually too difficult to acquire and too expensive to ever compete favorably either with street acid or with amphetamines. Furthermore, although many respondents to the Clinic's end-of-the-summer survey claimed to have taken the substance, the physicians never treated a single adverse cocaine reaction. They therefore assumed that its use was limited in general to blacks, to prominent candymen, or dealers, from the Fillmore and to members of the more successful San Francisco rock bands.

The doctors also felt that cocaine was a professional's chemical and interpreted its presence as an early indication of the prevalence of older and more experienced criminals in the area. They were supported in this belief by Randy, who said that all the cocaine in the district could be linked to representatives of semiorganized crime. "Coke is too good for the amateurs out here," he stated. "You just can't find it easily. But let me tell you, it's worth the hassle. I'll take candy any time I can get it. Man, that shit is the speed-freaks' caviar."

Another hors d'oeuvre the amphetamine abusers sampled was amyl nitrite. This is a so-called coronary vasodilator which is used medically to treat angina pectoris, a throttling pain in the chest that stems from occlusion of the coronary arteries. Amyl nitrate is obtainable without prescription as a volatile liquid in easily crushed ampules which resemble smelling salts. These ampules are known as poppers in the underground.

Poppers were popular in the Tenderloin district before 1968, where they were inhaled by some people to attempt to enhance their orgasms. The drugs were also widely available in the Haight during that year and were employed to provide a temporary stimulation and relief from depression, as well as for sexual purposes. As such, they served as regular addition to many street people's chemical regimens.

Their staple, though, was speed, which was sometimes mixed with strychnine to increase its flash effects. Impurities, as well as poisons, were also found in the street preparations, a fact that caused severe problems for inexperienced adolescents injecting the drugs. Because of this, well over one thousand acute amphetamine reactions were treated at the Clinic during 1967 and 1968, until the abuse of the compounds peaked in the fall of the latter year.

At the same time, both 409 and 558 Clayton Street started to see many more chronic speed difficulties as the year progressed. Some of the experimental and periodic users turned into habitual abusers during this period, and depressions, exhaustion syndromes and paranoid-schizophrenic reactions were extremely common as a result. This was particularly true for users like Randy, who developed such a tolerance to amphetamines that he required five times the normal dose of antipsychotic medication when he became strung out from his extended speed runs.

Randy's reputation was boosted by his incredible amphetamine consumption, but his psychological condition, like that of so many abusers, deteriorated with every injection of the drug. These young people stormed into the

Psychiatric Section by the dozen, demanded treatment, and caused such overcrowding that they often had to come down in the bathtub. The psychiatrists and counselors could sometimes help those younger adolescents who wanted to cut their speed dependence and were willing to leave the district. But they could only detoxify the older and more confirmed abusers and then send them to the Medical Section for treatment of their physical difficulties.

More Disease

The most superficially obvious of these problems were traumatic injuries which were attributable either to personal neglect or to interpersonal violence. The amphetamine abusers invariably overlooked their symptoms and continually cut themselves up while stoned. They were also subject to a wide range of accidents: some fell out of windows or off motorcycles, while the Clinic physicians treated over one dozen male and female patients in the single month of December, 1967, for infections incurred after the young people had used contaminated ice picks, safety pins or switchblades to pierce their ears.

The doctors saw four persons during the same period who had damaged their genitalia as a result of gang rapes, knife fights and robberies. They also had to intervene in the case of a nineteen-year-old hoodie who had been given a silver ring by his girl friend as a token of her affection. Finding the present much too large for his finger, the boy slipped it on his penis, which swelled until he had a permanent erection. The couple made the most of this state for several hours, until the boy arrived at 558 Clayton Street in agony. Detumescence was eventually achieved with the aid of a ring cutter, but the patient left the Clinic swearing that he would soon acquire a new and less demanding girl friend.

Along with these and other injuries, the speed freaks also suffered from the same general debility, protein and vitamin deficiencies, gastrointestinal difficulties, muscle cramps, tachycardia and dermatological and dental problems that were categorized as the amphetamine-abuse syndrome during the summer. The physicians treated over two thousand patients for one or more aspects of this syndrome in 1967 and 1968. They also saw over fifteen hundred cases of severe tooth discoloration, caries, trench mouth, periapical abscesses and periodontal disease.

In most cases, the doctors gave oxygenating mouth rinses to these patients and then referred them to Dr. Charles Fischer at the University of California Medical Center Dental Clinic, to the Oral Surgery Unit at San Francisco General or to a few private dentists who would treat long-haired young people. They also did what they could for those others who were afflicted with the general syndrome or who manifested more uncommon problems which were aggravated, if not caused directly, by speed.

One such difficulty was rheumatic fever, a systemic illness that may either be self-limiting or may lead to kidney impairment or to severe cardiac deformity. Rheumatic fever reaches a peak incidence in children between the ages of five and fifteen years and is thought to result from an allergic-type response to such streptococcal infections as tonsillitis, pharyngitis and scarlet fever. Its initial symptoms include a tenderness and inflammation around the joints, along with fever, the skin nodules of erythema nodosum, and nosebleed. It can best be prevented by avoiding strep infections or by treating them promptly with the appropriate antibiotics if they occur.

Such infections were extremely common in the Haight-Ashbury, and although rheumatic fever was never diagnosed in any children living in the district, it was a constant threat to many infants. It was also a potential problem to older adolescents, four of whom were seen at the Medical Section with the symptoms of rheumatic fever. One patient, a thirteen-year-old female, had apparently contracted the disease after developing chronic tonsillitis and streptococcal pharyngitis over the summer. The three others had incurred the illness and subsequent heart damage during childhood. All four were worsening their already weakened condition by regularly injecting amphetamines.

More common, and much more serious, was epilepsy, a cerebral dysfunction that is often precipitated by emotional disturbances and is manifested by periodic seizures or fits; it was once referred to as the falling sickness for this reason. Although all types of epileptic seizures are discomforting, grand mal is particularly dangerous because fractures and injuries to the soft tissues may occur when patients lose consciousness and fall. Treatment of epilepsy includes the suppression of general symptoms and the relief of individual attacks. Sedatives, anticonvulsants and true antispasmodics are sometimes administered in the latter situation, while such objects as tongue depressors are placed in the mouth to prevent the patients' tongues from falling backward in their throats and obstructing their breathing. In addition, people who are susceptible to seizures most often receive anticonvulsant therapy with agents like Dilantin and/or phenobarbital on a daily basis throughout life. They should also be urged to avoid hazardous occupations, driving, drinking and other forms of drug abuse.

Such urging was all but ineffective in the Haight, where the incidence of epileptic seizures was increased by overcrowding, by the emotional problems of young people and by the street chemicals they used. The hallucinogens were especially harmful in lowering the seizure threshold of those with convulsive tendencies. Dr. Dernburg interviewed three patients at 409 Clayton who had experienced only one or two epileptic attacks before reaching the district and had sustained an average of nine seizures per month after taking LSD. He also spoke with five patients who had sworn off acid because of its threshold-lowering effect but had nevertheless continued to trigger seizures by injecting amphctamines. He was eventually so impressed by the prevalence of such attacks that he had the Psychiatric Section stocked with tongue depressor blades.

The doctors at 558 Clayton Street were equally concerned with epilepsy, particularly because all of the eighteen young people they treated for the condition were low on, or out of, medication at the time. The Clinic could rarely afford the drugs these people needed, and although the physicians managed to secure samples of Dilantin and other agents in a few instances, they could usually do no more than give their patients sedatives at the Medical Section or help them during house calls. On one such occasion, Dr. Smith visited a run-down crystal palace in which four young people were fixing up in the living room. He was then beckoned to the back of the residence, where he found an unattended seventeen-year-old girl who had begun writhing in epileptic convulsions on a filthy mattress after shooting speed.

Along with epilepsy, the physicians also had to deal with several other serious complaints in those who abused amphetamines. One of the most common of these was migraine, a paroxysmal disorder that results in recurrent attacks of piercing, pulsing, one-sided pain in the head which may be accompanied by flashes before the eyes, double vision, drowsiness and nausea. Although psychotherapy may be indicated in the treatment of chronic migraine, such agents as the ergot alkaloid methysergide, which was employed more commonly as a substitute for LSD in the Haight-Ashbury, have proven to be useful in controlling the condition. Acute attacks may be eased either by sedatives or by the alkaloid ergotamine.

Patients should rest in a quiet setting until these drugs become effective, as they did in the calm center or at the Psychiatric Section when space was available. Over forty patients with migraines were treated in the Haight during late 1967 and 1968, some of them members of the new population who had asthma, allergenic reactions, ulcers, colitis and other psychosomatic difficulties as well. Furthermore, in addition to these young people who sought help at the Clinic, there were hundreds more who medicated themselves with black-market sedatives that the local dealers prescribed.

Although migraine and certain other illnesses were found most often among the speed freaks, other problems could not be linked to one specific group in the Haight-Ashbury. Those hippies who remained in the district suffered a wide variety of difficulties, as did those new arrivals who borrowed from both extremes in creating their own life-style. Various groups differed in their backgrounds, their drug abuse patterns and their physical conditions. Some seemed to come to 558 Clayton Street daily, for example, while others asked merely for psychiatric and medical examinations which they could then forward to the Welfare Department or to their local draft boards.

Furthermore, although the Haight had become less of a gypsy encampment now that most of its former gypsies were camping in the country, the behavioral sink was still characterized by overcrowding and contagious disease. Because of this, many young residents shared certain health problems in spite of their personal dissimilarity. Measles and mononucleosis were not so common in the area after the summer, and neither meningitis nor any other extremely serious contagions were seen at the Medical Section. But strep throats, colds and other upper respiratory tract infections often afflicted anyone who ventured onto Haight Street; dysentery could never be contained to the amphetamine-based subculture; and the entire area was hit by several sieges of the flu.

Gynecological complaints also continued to mount in the Haight-Ashbury after the summer, while the Clinic saw an increasing amount of obstetric problems as well. Many of the hippies stranded in the district wanted to bear offspring like their contemporaries in the country, and although the summer hippies had shown little interest in infants during the summer, some of those who stayed in the Haight started asking for information about natural delivery. Jackie, for one, still seemed unwilling to have a baby, but as the Haight-Ashbury grew drearier, she admitted that the thought of having a child to nurture appealed to her.

The same was true for certain members of the new population. Although few of the female hoodies, bikers or overtly psychotic persons valued infants as much as the original hippies did, some unwittingly became pregnant through their indiscriminate and inordinate sexual activity. Thus, while most of them merely asked for contraceptive advice or for free birth control pills, over one hundred and fifty were either referred to the therapeutic abortion society, counseled against going to ghetto abortionists, or given postabortion care.

In general, those young people who did have children before or during their stay in the district appeared to mother them insufficiently. The infants were often in poor shape when they reached 558 Clayton Street, while their parents were sometimes too intoxicated to care. Just as the hippies accidentally or intentionally introduced their offspring to LSD and marijuana, so did the members of the new population leave street compounds lying around their premises and occasionally gave their babies speed. Eighteen acute amphetamine reactions were treated in these children during late 1967 and 1968, emphasizing the fact that many parents seemed to subject their progeny to the same neglect and overstimulation they had received themselves.

At the same time, these parents exposed their infants to a great deal of contagion. Many of the children exhibited the same symptoms seen earlier in the district, and their parents manifested a wide variety of genitourinary tract infections and a surplus of venereal disease. Gonorrhea was particularly common among members of the new population, many of whom refused to seek help and rarely completed treatment even when it was afforded them. Nonspecific urethritis and vaginitis also persisted in the young people, as did cervicitis, condyloma acuminata, trichomoniasis and several other infections which were previously rather rare.

One of these disorders that became more common during the fall and winter was moniliasis or candidiasis, an infection of the genital region which is caused by the fungus *Candida albicans. Candida* is a sporiferous organism that resembles yeast and displays its presence by white, cheesy spots on the vulva, in the vagina and in the cervix, along with a thick, watery discharge. The disease appears with comparative frequency in those female patients who have been overtreated with antibiotics, which can kill off the native protective bacteria in the vaginal area. Treatment involves the administration of such vaginal suppositories as Candeptin over a three-to-four week period and the use of vaginal douches to restore the proper acid balance in the vagina.

Treatment was difficult in the Haight-Ashbury, where many patients were afflicted with disorders like trichomoniasis and bacterial vaginitis as well. Since many of these young people received antibiotics for these other ailments, they could be cured of vaginitis only at the risk of exacerbating their fungal infections. One twenty-five-year-old female carried drugs to treat not only candidiasis but also cervicitis, the clap and the crabs.

In addition to these disorders, dozens of the patients also suffered from cystitis, an inflammation of the bladder which is caused either by physical trauma or by the many organisms that can enter that organ by way of the urethra. Its symptoms may include a burning sensation in the urethra during urination, a feeling of fullness in the bladder that leads to a need to urinate without being able to do so, and sharp lower abdominal pain. Acute cases of cystitis often remit either in response to decreased sexual activity or after the application of lubricants which decrease pressure on the bladder during intercourse. But if bacteria are responsible for the condition, it should be treated with antibiotics, in addition to thorough cleansing of the urinary and genital area. Such hygiene was extremely rare in the Haight, whose young residents had little respect for their bodies and would not abstain from intercourse in spite of the discomfort it caused.

Yet, for all this evidence of erotic activity, there were many individuals in the Haight-Ashbury who preferred drugs to sex. Because of this, hepatitis was an even more appropriate index of the physical degeneration in the district than either genitourinary tract infections or venereal disease. This illness did not reach epidemic proportions until the fall of 1968, when amphetamines were established as the area's chemicals of choice, and when 558 Clayton Street was closed. But it was still the most crippling adolescent health problem as early as December of 1967, at which point the Medical Section was seeing an average of from four to six infected patients a day.

Although a few of these patients were hippies with infectious hepatitis, the great majority were young people with serum infections who had been shooting speed. Furthermore, although many of the latter patients exhibited intermittent symptoms which were suggestive of specific viral infections, Randy and others appeared to follow such a regular and progressive course of deterioration that the Clinic physicians suspected they were not plagued by hepatitis alone.

Dr. Dernburg, for one, believed that some were also suffering from primary sclerosing cholangitis, a diffuse inflammatory process which produces a scarring of the liver tissue, a blocking of the biliary tract and a subsequent backing up of bilirubin and liver bile. Biopsies were needed to determine the full extent of scarring in these patients, and no one could tell how much their organic deterioration was directly influenced by the behavioral sink. But Randy and his jaundiced companions were obviously reinfecting and/ or destroying their livers with every new injection of amphetamines.

Given this situation, the doctors did what they could to treat those patients known to have hepatitis and tried to segregate others from the infection. Cortisone, which is used along with surgery to treat cholangitis, was administered to some young people on an experimental basis, while most were merely sent to San Francisco General Hospital for isolation and convalescence. The physicians also gave gamma globulin shots to those who had been exposed to hepatitis. And they made every possible attempt to dissuade their patients from taking the toxic drugs that seemed to intensify the disease.

In spite of their efforts, the doctors could not begin to check hepatitis in the Haight-Ashbury. Few of their patients could or would forego chemical stimulation, and the Clinic constantly ran out of gamma globulin and other supplies. In addition, many young people who were willing to be helped in the Haight discontinued treatment when they were forced to use — or prevented from using — facilities elsewhere. Because they lacked proper follow-up procedures, the physicians had no way of telling how extensively their patients infected others and reinfected themselves.

They did have several indications, though. Nearly one thousand cases of hepatitis were reported in San Francisco during 1967, many, if not most, of which occurred in and around the Haight-Ashbury. Some one hundred serum infections were also noted in patients who had received whole blood or plasma in local hospitals during the same period. These statistics were undoubtedly underreported, yet one Stanford doctor was so alarmed by the probable incidence of hepatic infections that he urged a ban on all commercial blood banks in the Bay Area. Many young residents of the Haight sold their blood to these institutions, and it was reasonable to assume that they were at least partially responsible for the spread of the disease.

Several public health officials supported this inference, for they, too, were aware of the dramatic rise in serum hepatitis. So was Dr. Charles Fischer, who reported that it was becoming increasingly difficult to sanitize needles used to inject anesthetics in hippie and hoodie patients at the Medical Center Dental Clinic and at the Oral Surgery Unit. Several of Dr. Fischer's colleagues were so impressed by this fact that they wanted to create special and isolated services for long-haired patients at the two facilities. Dr. Fischer favored such segregation, in spite of its philosophic implications. Like most of the Clinic organizers, he had come to look on serum hepatitis as a symbol of the social consequences, as well as the personal self-destruction, which resulted from the speed-freaks' life-style.

Riots and the Return of Papa Al

Another symbol was crime. Although the amphetamine abusers were not a numerical majority in the Haight-Ashbury during December of 1967, they were responsible for much of the violence there. Seventeen murders, one hundred rapes, two hundred and ninety cases of assault and over three thousand burglaries were reported at Park Police Station by the end of the year, and many local merchants and property owners were so terrified by the sickness and criminality they saw around them that they began lobbying for antiloitering ordinances as a solution to the new population. The more liberal Neighborhood Council members were also frightened, yet they hoped to close Haight Street to traffic on weekends and thereby ease tensions in the district, instead of forcing the old community and the new population into a showdown.

Both groups were trying to win Mayor Joseph Alioto's support, but San Francisco's new chief executive seemed unable to reach a decision. The mayor had promised an "all-out war on crime" before he defeated supervisor Jack Morrison and another candidate in November, and was now meeting regularly with Haight-Ashbury residents. Yet, for all his promises, Alioto would urge only further study of the difficulties of the district. Meanwhile, Leonard Wolf, who had once attempted to solve those difficulties with education, was preparing his defense in order to stand trial.

Before Professor Wolf could come to court, he had other problems to contend with. These new problems had started shortly after his arrest, when the resident manager of Happening House took her first LSD trip and invited more than a dozen homeless young people to create a commune with her on the first floor. They accepted her offer and began taking acid in the building and balling in the halls. Professor Wolf confronted the resident manager and talked her and the others into vacating 409 Clayton Street. But they returned in December, declared that they had liberated Happening House, and prompted Dr. Dernburg to erect a barrier leading to the second deck to keep them downstairs.

Further negotiations followed, but the young people refused to leave on the grounds that they were now an inseparable unit bound by cosmic energy. Then, in late December, unity proved to be their undoing. On the twenty-first of that month, shortly after Professor Wolf threatened to call in the police if 409 House was not immediately vacated, Dr. Smith visited the facility and found that its occupants had been felled by food poisoning and were in no position to leave. Several were lying in pain in the front hallway, while almost a dozen others were clutching their stomachs and vomiting in the living room. None mentioned cosmic energy after their bowels brought them back to earth, and all abandoned Happening House by Christmas, allowing Professor Wolf to redirect his own energy toward his forthcoming trial.

The proceedings formally began on January 27, 1968, with the city trying to convict Professor Wolf of contributing both to the delinquency of minors and to the deterioration of the Haight-Ashbury. He held his own at first, but as his case seemed more uncertain, his attorney started arguing that no single individual or group could prevent public nudity in the city. This point was dramatically brought home shortly thereafter, when two dozen adolescents — who were not called by the defense — took off their clothes and swam in the fountain across from city hall.

In spite of this stroke of good fortune, the trial dragged on for several months, at considerable expense to both sides. Finally, in early March, all charges against Professor Wolf were dismissed. But he was financially and emotionally drained by the experience and was also convinced that he had almost become the scapegoat for an increasingly repressive and desperate society. He therefore closed Happening House, finished a book entitled *Voices from the Love Generation,* and took a sabbatical leave from San Francisco State College.

Father Larry Beggs was also found innocent a few weeks later, but although Huckleberry's remained in the Haight-Ashbury for several months, there were no festivities to mark its survival. A great deal of spirit seemed to have evaporated from the district by the disbanding of Happening House. The speed freaks became even more sullen after they were deprived of the facility, whereas the police appeared to step up their sweeps, as Dr. Meyers had predicted. The Clinic was also shaken by Professor Wolf's departure. A dozen volunteers quit after Happening House was disbanded, and the organizers regarded his treatment as one more reminder of the city's failure — and the failure of most cities — to act constructively in meeting social problems. They therefore considered it appropriate that the Haight should experience the first riot in its ninety-year history as Professor Wolf and Father Beggs were standing trial.

The new population was initially responsible for this disturbance. But, like the disorder at the Democratic Convention in Chicago, it might never have escalated without the interference of certain members of the San Francisco Police Department. The incident began on the afternoon of February eighteenth, a Sunday, when a stray tourist ran over a dog on Haight Street and the ensuing clamor brought several hundred young people to the scene. A spontaneous street dance then started, until the patrolmen from Park Station quietly disbanded the crowd. But the quiet did not last, for Mayor Alioto chose the occasion to introduce his new Tactical Squad. Some members of the thirty-eight-man special unit marched down the street with their faces concealed under Plexiglas helmets, spraying tear gas and Mace before them. Others mounted motorcycles and roared down the sidewalk, scattering street people like bowling pins and clubbing them with riot sticks, cowboy style.

The young residents resisted this onslaught momentarily and then scurried to get inside. The Medical Section was closed that afternoon, but Peggy Sankot and a number of staff members were on hand to administer emergency first aid to over one hundred young people, most of whom had scalp lacerations or needed to have Mace and/or tear gas washed out of their eyes. Don Reddick was called to the facility around five o'clock and managed to drive two adolescents with broken arms to Mission Emergency.

Dr. Smith, who had spent the weekend lecturing at Joan Baez's Institute for the Study of Nonviolence, was driving back to San Francisco on Sunday afternoon when word came over the radio about the riot. He rushed to the Clinic and pitched in to help the patients. But the casualties kept mounting, and he could hardly breathe for all the Mace and tear gas in the air.

This fog finally lifted after dusk, when the Tactical Squad took over the street and imposed a curfew. Then, around eight o'clock, after a small band of curfew violators clustered outside the Clinic, a gas canister was suddenly lobbed into the crowd. Don Reddick and several staff members leaned out the front window and urged the young people to come into 558 Clayton Street instead of retaliating. But they were ordered by the police to lock the front door and to close the window. They had no sooner done so than a canister was hurled at the Medical Section. It hit the windowsill and bounced back onto the sidewalk, where it was retrieved by an officer in the Tactical Squad. He shouldered his riot stick, gave the finger, and spat out, "Too bad we missed — but we'll get you assholes next time."

This threat would be acted upon later, but in the meantime little damage was incurred by the Clinic, save for the permanent retirement of three members of its staff. Yet, although the incident was not serious enough to call for another closing, it did serve as a further validation of Dr. Meyers's prophecy. Most of the volunteers were extremely depressed by what was happening in the Haight-Ashbury, and the violence seemed to intensify their increasingly stoical attitude. They therefore reacted almost apathetically to the return of Papa Al.

Papa Al had not been heard from since the late summer, when the anonymous article documenting his activities as an informer was printed in the *Berkeley Barb*. But in March, shortly after Professor Wolf's trial was concluded, Papa Al and Teddybear arrived at 558 Clayton Street and declared that they had returned to the district to clear their names. The two demanded that Dr. Smith and Don Reddick close the facility or operate it in the future under their command. They then stormed out of 558 Clayton Street. Dr. Smith and Reddick were warned that Papa Al had issued a general murder contract on Haight Street for their lives.

The two intended victims were tempted to discount this threat at first. But they gradually realized that any enterprising speed freak could collect money and/or drugs for their scalps under the terms of a general contract. Dr. Smith then talked the matter over with Drs. Breithaupt and Sissman, who suggested he go immediately to the police. The police verified the possible danger but said they could do nothing until a specific crime occurred. At this point, Dr. Smith, who had been the target for several rightist political organizations since the previous summer, received an unusually high weekly number of death threats, including a postcard from a man who swore he had the doctor in his rifle sights. Dr. Smith began carrying a gun in the Haight, while Reddick hired a bodyguard.

This situation continued for a week, with Papa Al and Teddybear repeatedly stopping by 558 Clayton Street and restating their demands. Finally, after the tension became almost unbearable, a summit conference was called. Papa Al, Teddybear and several of their younger allies met with Don Reddick and Dr. Smith, who were backed up by Reddick's business partners and Dr. Robert Morris. Dr. Morris switched sides during the meeting and urged that Papa Al run the Medical Section. But Reddick refused, promising retaliation for any damage done him or the Clinic. Papa Al in turn decided to call it a day. He moved to the Tenderloin district, while Teddybear began to organize rock concerts with a communal group called the Thirteenth Tribe.

Life returned to normal after their departure, but not for long. Several of the younger volunteers had been quite intimidated by Papa Al's presence, and Dr. Morris cut back his involvement at 558 Clayton Street and established a private pathology lab. The staff members were next harassed by three young Negroes who threatened to burn down the facility because it did not do enough for black patients in the Haight-Ashbury. And no sooner had the Clinic family put out this potential conflagration than it had to deal with Charles Manson, who had a rather unusual family of his own.

Stranger in a Strange Land

Although Charlie Manson would one day be an international celebrity, his life — which "stood as a monument to parental neglect and to the failure of the American correctional system," according to the *New York Times* — offered little indication of his future notoriety. He was born in Cincinnati, Ohio, in 1934, the son of a teen-age prostitute and one of her many boyfriends. His mother married an older man to give her son a name, but he left the scene shortly after Charlie's birth. Mrs. Manson was then arrested for robbery, at which point she sent her son to live with relatives in Wheeling, West Virginia. When the mother was released from jail, she retrieved Charlie and tried to make a home for him. Yet she drank heavily, exhausted a series of lovers, and continually abused her son.

After attempting to place Charlie in several foster homes, Mrs. Manson eventually sent him to a Catholic boys' school, where he was beaten repeatedly. He supported himself by pimping and petty thievery, lived in several reform schools, stole a car and was kept in jail until he was twenty-one. He then returned to West Virginia to marry but forged a check and was sent to the McNeil Island Federal Penitentiary in the state of Washington. This time he remained behind bars until he was thirty-two. Charlie received his most complete prison education to date at McNeil Island. Like most of his fellow inmates, he learned sexual perversions, socially obsolete labor and more useful criminal skills. But he distinguished himself by reading a number of books, including the Bible, Dale Carnegie's *How to Win Friends and Influence People* and a handbook on Scientology. He also trained himself to play the guitar and to compose songs.

Charlie was released from McNeil Island in March of 1967, when, as he later told the *Los Angeles Free Press,* "I still didn't know anything about marijuana or LSD or any kinds of drugs. In fact, I didn't really want to come out of jail — I was frightened and didn't know where to go." He went to Los Angeles and thereby missed the Summer of Love. But when the summer was over, he moved to Berkeley and signed in with his new northern California parole officer. This was Roger Smith, who was then starting to phase out of probation work in order to launch the Amphetamine Research Project in the Haight-Ashbury.

Although Smith was accustomed to dealing with confirmed felons by this point, nevertheless found Charlie to be "one of the most hostile parolees I've ever known." He also discovered him to be one of the most blunt, for while many of the men Smith had previously counseled promised to go straight after their stays in prison, Charlie insisted that he would soon be back in the joint because he could neither stand society nor keep the terms of his parole. "You know where I'm from?" he asked. "I'm from Juvenile Hall, I'm from the line of people nobody wants. I'm from the streets, from solitary confinement. I can't readjust to your society, and I'm content to walk around the yard playing my guitar like I did in the pen."

Charlie did appear eager to break into the music business in spite of his general pessimism. He also said that he wanted to make some money so that he could find his long-lost mother, so Smith helped him find work in a night club while also searching for a halfway house and a job training program that would accept him. But no one wanted Charlie, so he set out for San Francisco, where he met a person who made a profound impression on him.

"Nobody had ever given me love before," he told the *Free Press* in 1969, "but I met this boy and he was warm and friendly. He was sixteen and I was thirty-two, but he knew a lot about life I didn't know. I asked him what he did and he said 'nothing.' I asked him where he stayed, and he said he slept in the park. I asked him how he lived, and he said he bummed change. That's how I met the hippies in the Haight-Ashbury."

Charlie wanted to move into the Haight after this meeting, but Smith, who was then volunteering at the Clinic in order to make contacts for his speed study, initially said no. After further consideration, he decided that Charlie might be better off in the Haight-Ashbury than in the Tenderloin or another traditional criminal area. He therefore gave his assent, urged Charlie to stay away from Haight Street, and referred him to an ex-Catholic priest who was running a halfway house in the Haight. Charlie stayed with this person for a while. Then he sought out the few remaining members of the new community.

"They were wonderful people," he later said in the *Free Press*. "They'd give you the shirts off their backs if you were cold. I never knew love existed before, but I fell in love with the kids. I went to the Haight-Ashbury and we slept in the park in sleeping bags. I started playing music and people liked my music and people smiled at me and hugged me. It gobbled me up, man. Here I'd never been involved with dope, but we smoked grass and I took LSD, which finally enlightened my awareness. I remember the first time somebody took me to the Avalon Ballroom to hear the Grateful Dead. It was one of the first times I had ever been high. I had never seen a strobe light before, and the music was so loud! I just got frightened and curled up in the prenatal position and felt like I wanted to run back to the pen. But I stuck it out, and I changed."

This charge was the most abrupt Roger Smith had ever observed in his professional career.

Charlie never lost his touch as a con man, and you could always tell there was something manipulative going on in the back of his mind. But that was to be expected, considering his background. What I didn't expect was that he lost almost all of his overt hostility. Suddenly, this poor guy who had been kicked around all his life seemed to accept the world. He would say, "If you love everything, you don't have to think about what bothers you; whatever hand you get handed, you just love the cards you have."

At the same time, Charlie became more intense, more messianic. I ceased being his parole officer in 1968, when I started working at the Medical Section, so he had no real reason to spend so much time with me. But he came anyway, preaching about love. He began to speak about protoplasmic consciousness, the way so many acid users did. "We should have no possessions," he would say. "We are all we are." Charlie admired the gentler kids, but he still put them down as naïve dreamers now and then. Yet he adopted the same line they did with even stronger conviction. Suddenly, thanks to this most unlikely of people, it seemed like old times.

The most likely reason for this was LSD. Charlie was taking acid daily at this point and seemed to be dissipating his anger and resentment and to be escaping his underlying depression with a manic smile. He also appeared to be masking his own confusion with the drug, for he began to develop a number of delusions as his involvement with LSD progressed. He believed that the Beatles would one day accept him as a musical peer and comrade, for example, and also felt that a Day of Judgment would come on which the Negroes, whom he distrusted, would rise up and slaughter the white man. In addition, he started espousing a philosophy which bore a striking resemblance to that set forth in the book which interested Ken Kesey and so many other early leaders of the psychedelic movement. This was *Stranger in a Strange Land*.

Although Roger Smith was not certain whether Charlie read Heinlein's novel in prison or in the Haight-Ashbury, he was impressed by how closely he modeled his own fantasies to its plot. Charlie was deeply interested in Valentine Michael Smith's Christ-like character and was also in an excellent position to become a savior in the Haight because of his mystical aspirations, his musical ability, his avowed nonviolent attitude, his apparent tenderness and his admiration for the young.

As a result, he soon began collecting a number of impressionable, maternal and/or groupielike girls and creating his own kind of family. Some of the young women who joined the nest he patterned after that in Heinlein's novel were former amphetamine abusers whom Charlie, in a complete reversal of the customary sequential pattern, induced to take up acid and renounce speed. Others had long histories of delinquent activity. Although many came from affluent backgrounds, all shared Charlie's feelings of rejection and alienation from society.

Among the girls was Mary Brunner, a former University of California student, Patricia Krenwinkel, a twenty-year-old college dropout from Los Angeles, Susan Good, the daughter of a San Diego stockbroker who spent most of her life in boarding schools "while my mother tried to get on the society pages," and Susan Atkins, the product of a broken home in San Jose. Miss Atkins was a parole violator and topless dancer who was renamed Sadie Mae Glutz when she joined the family. Charlie described her as "my right-hand man."

Real men were also included in the family, but they always constituted a numerical minority. Furthermore, Charlie usually chose weaker people who could not and would not challenge his authority. This dominance was sexual in the case of the girls, but Charlie had a purpose which clearly exceeded mere physical gratification. Along with the original hippies — and with Valentine Smith — he believed that people were conditioned from birth by society but could be reprogramed if they used LSD and engaged in unconventional sexual practices, particularly those of the oral, anal and group variety.

When a potential female family member came to him, he would give her acid and initiate her sexually, lecturing in the mystical terms so long used to reinforce the hallucinogenic experience. "You have to negate your ego," Charlie would say, obviously making his greatest impact on those adolescents whose ego boundaries were temporarily suspended by the drug and/or who had poor ego functions to begin with. "Life means working through your hang-ups, throwing up the crap that society has fed you."

Many of the girls never felt competent before they were admitted into the family and were therefore appreciative when Charlie encouraged them to express themselves and praised their creativity. Yet, although he preached against possessions and told others to negate their egos, Charlie treated the young women like objects and taught them to submit totally to his will. The girls either never realized the price they paid for his protection or were too blinded by the immediate rewards. They never complained of mistreatment or resisted him.

This resulted in part from the fact that Charlie exploited their fears of rejection by constantly subjecting them to tests by which they were called upon to prove their loyalty. He broke down their resistance by cutting away their social props and turned the girls into self-acknowledged "computers," empty vessels that would accept almost anything he poured. The girls tended Charlie's sexual wishes and also serviced male members of the nest in addition to a number of "sympathetic cousins" who supplied the family with food, housing, transportation and other needs. "You could have any one or all of them if you wanted," one cousin stated. "Of course, you then ran the risk of becoming Charlie's slave, too."

Slavery was not Charlie's sole objective in acquiring a family. He was devoted to infants in principle and felt that the world would be saved by a Christ child. He therefore urged the girls to bear his offspring and to raise them naturally. Such an idea ran counter to the practice of abortion then accepted by many young people in the Haight-Ashbury, but the girls were only too willing to comply. Many had read *Stranger in a Strange Land.* Like their fictional and real leader, they believed that a child would lead them toward the creation of a worldwide family in which they would play prominent roles.

Charlie often spoke of establishing "subnests" in several American cities that would survive the black-white holocaust and then come together on the banks of the Snake River in Idaho. The young women apparently shared his delusion. They wanted to recruit and/or conceive new male and female members and thereby help the family grow. And grow it did, until by April, 1968, a nucleus of twenty people was sequestered in the main nest at 636 Cole Street near the Clinic. The family supported itself primarily through gifts from sympathetic cousins and used marijuana and the hallucinogens. Its lowest common denominator seemed to be sex, in marked contrast to other communal groups in the area. Charlie himself had intercourse with several of the girls daily, much to the chagrin of neighbors like Terry who either preferred chemicals to balling or were limited to one female at a time. He became as well-known as Randy was for his idiosyncrasies and lifestyle.

Charlie's fame had spread to the Medical Section by this point, for the family used the facility on several occasions. Its leader never sought medical attention; he seemed to be in good physical shape despite his LSD consumption and believed, as he told Dr. Smith, that "sickness is the product of an impure mind." The girls also held this attitude, but they were treated for vaginal infections and frequently asked for advice on natural delivery as well.

Another reason for their coming to 558 Clayton Street was to see Roger Smith, whom they called Jubal after the lawyer in *Stranger in a Strange Land*. Sadie Mae and her cohorts swarmed over Smith and often filled the reception room, bringing operations to a standstill. Smith himself was flattered by the attention, in part because Charlie frequently offered him the services of his harem. Yet he retained a professional distance and suspected that Charlie thought that seducing his former parole officer would be a major coup.

The family also visited 409 Clayton Street in April, but its members never asked for consultation because Charlie considered himself a therapist and disliked psychiatrists for allegedly representing and reinforcing conventional morality. Because of this, Dr. Dernburg never formally interviewed the group. Yet he did observe or hear about Charlie and his girls often enough to arrive at several speculative conclusions regarding their psychological makeup and the dynamics of their family.

At first glance, Dr. Dernburg was tempted to dismiss Charlie as yet another defeated and desperate individual who tried to become hip by eulogizing love and handing out flowers. The man was too aggressive to be a true hippie and manifested none of the Indian identity and overt passivity common to young people like Alan. In fact, he appeared to bear more resemblance to the hoodies in being a reasonably intact and cunning person whose only fear was that of the law.

Yet although he exhibited many hoodie characteristics, Charlie's hippie-type delusions hinted at a much deeper level of psychopathology. In the first place, he took as much acid as Alan ever did and seemed to be governed by the same primitive and regressive pull toward protoplasmic consciousness and infancy. His interest in children further indicated this, as did the desire to withdraw that he experienced on first reaching the Haight-Ashbury. Dr. Dernburg felt that Charlie had probably always yearned for the order and security that a family might have imposed on him. He may very well have found this in prison and might therefore have unconsciously engineered his arrests. He might also have sought this sense of structure in creating his communal family.

The same sense of structure was evident in his fantasies. Aside from satisfying his desire to dominate others and to reconstitute his own narcissism by having children, Charlie seemed anxious, as so many gurus did, to gather followers who would subscribe to his delusions and thereby convince him and others that he was sane. He was neither as disorganized and random in his thinking as Randy was, nor as ignorant of reality as were Alan and the original hippies. But although his delusions did not interfere with his survival, he was significantly disturbed.

The more Dr. Dernburg saw this, the more he suspected — as did the authors — that Charlie was a paranoid-schizophrenic with an encapsulated psychosis who denied reality by surrounding himself with others who were similarly, though perhaps not so extremely, inclined. Like so many Clinic workers and young people in the Haight, he was apparently trying to find his parents — and trying to overcome his history of deprivation by becoming a parent himself to younger and weaker people and thereby nurturing himself by proxy. In his girls, Charlie had "mothers" whom he could control for the first time. He also had a "father" in himself who could threaten to reject others as he had been rejected. And he had a sense of peace and security which could be sustained as long as he kept taking acid and prevented others from intruding upon his fantasies.

Dr. Dernburg decided that the girls were probably not psychotics but hysterical women who were prone to broad swings of emotion and who required constant stimulation to compensate for their underlying depressions. They were extremely suggestible and yet aggressive. They appeared to avoid real one-to-one intimacy in favor of the diffuse homosexual and heterosexual gratification they achieved by making love to each other as well as to several men.

The girls' extreme submissiveness may have been indicative of underlying characterological disturbance, but it was only an exaggerated manifestation of the wish for protection and nurturance seen in so many young people in the Haight-Ashbury. In this respect, they were not substantially different from many volunteers at the Medical and Psychiatric sections. But whereas Jackie and others had the Clinic and its physicians to cling to, Sadie Mae and her companions had only Charlie.

This was true on a real level, but their leader had a symbolic role as well. The girls apparently possessed a strong, protective and permissive father figure in Charlie who not only allowed them to play with him and with each other but also provided them with more passive boys whom they could seduce, administer LSD to, and thereby nurture in turn. The boys themselves shared in Charlie's supposed power through this and therefore also felt protected. At the same time, they could care for children whose very presence was proof of the parents' creativity.

Charlie had made this complicated Oedipal situation possible and could destroy the arrangement at will. Thus, the feelings of rejection that he played upon, consciously or unconsciously, were probably the source of his supposed power. By keeping intrafamilial friction and overt hostility at a minimum while continually referring to the possible results of his disapproval, he was not unlike many of the real parents whose children had come to the Haight or the Pied Pipers who helped attract them there. Charlie did not appear especially dangerous or dwell on the discorporation favored by Valentine Smith while he was taking acid. But there was no way of telling what would happen if he stopped using the drug, if his delusions of omnipotence were slighted, or if the attention of others was ever withheld.

Nor was there any indication of the future of the family. Charlie was becoming increasingly frightened by both the police and the new population by now, so in early May, he and several of the girls boarded a Kesey-like bus they had been given and headed for southern California. The nomads were arrested for indecent exposure near Oxnard and eventually settled in Topanga Canyon outside of Los Angeles, while Charlie alternately cut his shoulder-length hair and grew a beard and/or sideburns to confuse his new parole officer.

He and the girls stayed with Brian Wilson of the Beach Boys for several weeks and then were allowed to reestablish their nest at the Spahn Movie Ranch, a former Western movie location on the outskirts of the San Fernando Valley once owned by silent film star William Hart but now used as a riding stable. Roger Smith, who kept in touch with the family by letter and telephone, learned that Charlie and the girls had befriended Mr. Spahn and were living a peaceful and relatively stabilized existence. The Clinic staff members therefore forgot about the bizarre family, until Alan Rose came under its spell.

Although Rose had met Charlie and his girls earlier through Roger Smith, he maintained only a nominal contact with them until most of the family left town. But when the nest was closed on Cole Street, those male and female members who had remained in San Francisco began spending more time at 558 Clayton Street and subsequently asked Rose to help them find a place to stay. Rose was lonely and frustrated with the Clinic at this point, so he invited them into his apartment in the Haight-Ashbury to give himself a diversion from his duties at the Medical Section and a form of occupational therapy. The girls had their own therapeutic notions and were apparently under orders from their leader to boost Rose's spirits and seduce him into the family. Being well experienced in the bedroom arts, they succeeded in a matter of days.

Rose's involvement increased with the family after this point, until he was giving the girls most of his meager income and also keeping their male companions in clothes. Then, a few weeks after he fell in with the young people, they decided that the Haight was too dangerous and therefore set out for Mendocino County to sign up new recruits for Charlie. Rose was invited to join the caravan, but he carried out his Clinic responsibilities for about a week until he suddenly went north without alerting his staff.

When he reached Mendocino, Rose learned that the girls had been arrested for possession of marijuana. He also discovered that one of them had given birth to Charlie's first familial baby. The child was delivered in the back of a camper truck after its mother had smoked marijuana as a sedative. It was registered as Valentine Smith and was held by the authorities while the girls were in jail.

Rose could not arrange for the family's release, but he did continue in his role as a sympathetic cousin to the girls. After returning to San Francisco to pick up what was left of his belongings, he moved to Mendocino and acted as an intermediary between the local police and his incarcerated companions. He visited the girls daily, brought cigarettes and candy for them, and attempted to pacify the jail matrons, who were disconcerted because their prisoners went naked and sucked the breasts of Valentine Smith's still-lactating mother. He also helped the family find a lawyer and arranged to place the baby, which had contracted a candidiasis infection during its delivery, with Roger Smith and his wife Carol.

The charges were dropped against the family members in Mendocino in late June. They then chose to join Charlie on the Spahn Ranch, so Rose went south with them both as a sympathetic cousin and as a sociologically oriented participant-observer in the strange communal phenomenon. He and his companions lived in condemned quarters on the Spahn property and settled into a quiet routine that was livened by Charlie's peals of wisdom and by the twanging of his guitar. The young people gathered in an ancient movie set at night, smoked marijuana, and tried to grok one another while

Charlie tutored them in his philosophy. They then made love, usually in the same room.

Charlie himself was sleeping apart from the family at this point and staying in bed most of the day. He was also involved at night with the Beach Boys and was hoping to have Doris Day's son, Terry Melcher, make a recording of his compositions, one of which was called "The Ego is a Too-Much Thing." In the meantime, his followers were busy cleaning the stalls at the Spahn Ranch, exercising the horses, entertaining Mr. Spahn, and taking visitors on horseback rides.

"Ours was a comfortable, isolated existence," Rose recalled. "I was never so infatuated with the ranch as the others, probably because I was always more of an observer than a participant there. But it was a good life, and I could really be of help on health matters. Considering what I'd left in the city, I thought for a while that I had found the warmth and involvement that the new community could have had."

Rose's enthusiasm did not last, for friction grew between him and the family. Charlie had always found the former administrator too straight for his liking, and he soon began to resent his medical knowledge, his belief in proper treatment procedures and his influence over the girls. At the same time, Charlie's recording ambitions were apparently being frustrated by Terry Melcher, while his temper, which had once been mollified by acid, was beginning to show.

Two local girls were drummed out of the southern California nest in July, presumably because they withheld their possessions, their bodies and/ or their egos from Charlie. Rose himself was put to a test three days later, when the leader asked him if he would hitchhike to New York to prove his loyalty. Aware that he was living in a potentially explosive situation that could be touched off if Charlie were sufficiently rejected, Rose decided to leave the Spahn Ranch. But he neither went to New York nor returned to the Clinic and the Haight-Ashbury. Instead, he rejoined his parents in Cleveland, Ohio.

A House of Peace

In doing so, Rose avoided becoming either an observer of or a participant in Charlie and the girls' future activities. And he left the Clinic family in quite a lurch. 409 and 558 Clayton Street were running rather smoothly at this moment, but both were being besieged by an unusually large number of patients. Summer was approaching, and the Haight had just experienced a bout with the hog.

Although the hog had been heard of earlier, it was first introduced to San Francisco at a Hell's Angel's birthday party in May. Extravagant claims about the drug subsequently swept the city, until the *Chronicle* reported that several underground manufacturers had stockpiled over one hundred thousand pills with which they hoped to flood the Bay Area. Before actually doing so, the paper said, the so-called Hog People planned to give samples of their product to prominent distributors and dealers in the Haight and elsewhere. They would then launch an all-out sales campaign for the supposed THC-LSD substitute that would lead to its mass acceptance in July.

The manufacturers might have succeeded, had the *Chronicle* publicity not promoted them to release their product prematurely. This occurred on May eighteenth at a rock festival held at the Santa Clara County Fairgrounds in San Jose. Chet Helms of the Avalon was emceeing the event, when a couple identified as Mr. and Mrs. Hog leapt on stage, seized the microphone, and tossed some five thousand pills into the crowd. Before Helms could recapture the mike and warn his audience, hundreds of adolescents had gobbled up the drugs and began to suffer nausea, vomiting, hallucinosis, muscle cramps and blackout spells.

Dr. Smith was present at the festival, so he, Dr. David Breithaupt and John Vasconcellos, a local assemblyman who was acting as legislative liaison for the Drug Abuse Information Project in Sacramento, helped cart the young people to the Santa Clara Valley Medical Center. After urging the physicians there not to give sedatives to their patients, they rushed a sample of the hog to Dr. Meyers, who found that it contained benactyzine, a antipsychotic tranquilizer with sedative-hypnotic-general anesthetic properties.

The *Barb* and the *Chronicle* then reported the damage the drug did in San Jose, and the hog never fulfilled its manufacturers' expectations. But they did produce over ten thousand more pills containing benactyzine and phencyclidine that managed to bring four dozen residents of the Haight-Ashbury to the Medical Section. The patients all survived their symptoms, while the compounds they had taken eventually vanished from the district. Yet the Clinic was hard pressed to meet the new problem. It was already weakened by Alan Rose's departure and could not afford a further reduction in its summer staff.

Fortunately, the exact opposite occurred. Fred Shick and thirteen other medical students returned to 558 Clayton Street that summer, along with such physicians as Dr. Andrew Weil, the young marijuana researcher from Harvard. Over a half-dozen conscientious objectors also volunteered at the Medical Section. One was Carter Mehl, a guru-ish graduate student in psychology at Ohio State University. Mehl came to the Bay Area early in 1968 to complete his alternate service at the Veterans' Administration Hospital in Palo Alto. He then turned twenty-six and considered returning to school until he met Professor Stuart Loomis at a health symposium and applied to become Rose's successor. Three nights after he was selected, a biker who had been in a knife fight stormed into 558 Clayton Street to have his forehead bandaged. The biker complained that he was not being afforded enough special attention. He then started swinging on the staff members and almost fractured the new administrator's jaw.

Helping to treat Mehl's injuries that evening was a person who would one day share his administrative chores. This was Delores Craton, a twenty-two-year-old nursing student from Arkansas who first came to the Clinic after the Summer of Love. Miss Craton had acquired enough medical experience by the time she arrived in San Francisco to qualify for employment first at the Alcohol and Drug Abuse Screening Unit and then at the Immediate Psychiatric Aid and Referral Service. She began volunteering periodically at the Medical Section shortly after the November reopening and gradually phased out of her responsibilities with the Public Health Department to become a full-time member of the staff.

The third staff member recruited that summer was Renée Sargent, a shy and depressed young woman. Miss Sargent was born in San Francisco and had lived with her family in Panama until she entered the Mississippi State College for Women. She then became a civil rights activist but was forced to leave Mississippi because of death threats from rightist political organizations. She came to the Clinic shortly after returning to the city and helped organize its summer staff.

Thanks to her, Miss Craton's and Mehl's involvement, the facility was soon functioning as efficiently as it had under Alan Rose. The same was true of the Psychiatric Section, where Dr. Dernburg and Professor Loomis had enlisted additional psychiatrists and counselors to assist them as adverse amphetamine reactions increased. The Clinic organizers therefore decided to expand the educational efforts which were being conducted out of the Publications Section on the third floor of 409 Clayton Street. A local speakers' bureau was established to coordinate lecture engagements. Then the organizers assembled a library of educational films on which they had consulted and began work on two documentaries covering marijuana abuse and speed.

While this was occurring, they were gratified when the summer brought important results to their efforts to liberalize certain state legislation. Of greatest significance to the Clinic was the revision of the Civil Health Code for which Dr. Robert Morris and the San Francisco Medical Society had so long argued. Under its provisions, minors fifteen years of age and older who were living apart from their families could henceforth obtain diagnoses and treatment without their parents' or legal guardians' consent. Minors over twelve who had come into contact with serious communicable diseases could also receive care without the consent of the parents, so the patients at 409 and 558 Clayton Street no longer had to lie about their ages.

Another legal-educational effort was conducted at this time by Dr. Smith and Dr. Meyers. They had completed their first report for the Drug Abuse Information Project early in 1968 and were now working on a second study, due in December, that would criticize California for its woeful lack of research opportunities and treatment facilities. They were also advising the governor's office and working with several legislators to end the classification of marijuana as a narcotic and eliminate certain incomprehensible state statutes which obfuscated and/or complicated drug abuse problems.

One such law then practiced in California allowed the police to subject marijuana offenders to regular Nalline tests as a condition of probation or parole. Nalline is an effective heroin antagonist that can be employed to identify opiate addicts, but it cannot detect the presence of marijuana in users and also has extremely harmful side effects. Those counties which indiscriminately administered Nalline tests to marijuana offenders before the summer of 1968 were responsible for giving many young people their first narcoticlike high.

The legislature reacted positively to Dr. Meyers's and Dr. Smith's recommendation to curtail such testing, but the two doctors only incurred the wrath of the state attorney general's office in urging a revision of the marijuana classification law. Furthermore, neither they nor their counterparts throughout the state made any headway in persuading Ronald Reagan to abandon his punitive attitude toward drug abuse. The governor insisted that "professional criminals and outside agitators" were entirely to blame for the incredible rise in chemical consumption in California, and refused to provide funds for research and for treatment facilities.

The organizers had no recourse in the face of this public apathy but to launch several private efforts of their own. The first was initiated by Roger Smith, who was now operating under the National Institute of Mental Health grant that Dr. Meyers, as project director, had received in May. Smith had moved out of the Medical Section and into 409 House by this point, where he spent most of June cleaning out the basement and converting it into an office for himself and Gail Sadalla. When this task was completed, he began collecting formal interviews from Randy and other young people until their condition inspired him, Dr. Meyers and Father Frykman to create the Drug Treatment Program that would be crucial to the Haight-Ashbury when 558 Clayton Street was closed during the coming fall.

Another project that would assume future importance was begun in June in the first-floor space once occupied by Happening House. Its founder was Lyle Grosjean, a thirty-five-year-old Episcopalian minister. Father Grosjean worked in Berkeley prior to the fall of 1967, when the Episcopal clergy in San Francisco recommended that another priest be installed in the Haight to lighten the load of Father Leon Harris at All Saints'. He then moved into the district with his wife and children and became a social worker while recruiting his clientele from the Clinic and from the street.

Father Grosjean's case load swelled during the winter of 1968, until the Episcopal archdiocese offered him an eleven-thousand-dollar annual grant to create a center that might meet the spiritual and secular needs of young people in the Haight-Ashbury. He therefore examined Father Harris's and Howard Rochford's programs and concluded that he might actually be able to establish a religious community in the district. Father Grosjean set up a local ecumenical ministry to facilitate this and then approached the Clinic organizers and offered to pay one hundred and twenty dollars a month for the first floor of 409 House.

The organizers quickly agreed to this proposal. Father Grosjean cleaned up the mess left behind by the former resident manager and her commune-mates, and he and an assistant then outfitted the first-floor kitchen so that meals could be prepared. They next opened an office and counseling area behind the kitchen which housed the records of the Episcopal Peace Fellowship, a national organization of liberal ministers, and of the Peace Cross Project, a volunteer operation whose members raised money through the manufacture of brass peace symbols. After they had converted part of the basement into a shop area, Father Grosjean and his assistant distributed leaflets advertising their presence and posted a sign near the front door reading, "Please, No Weapons — This Is a House of Peace."

A few guns and knives were drawn in defiance of this policy, but most of the young people who came to the Episcopal Peace Center after the mid-June opening respected its founder's beliefs. The reaction to the opening was so enthusiastic that Father Grosjean never had to advertise again. Over one hundred young people were visiting the facility daily by the end of June, at which point he began to offer a variety of additional services. Visitors were afforded free draft and welfare counseling at the Center, for example, and the staff saw many individuals who had either gone AWOL or were experiencing acute crises with the military.

Father Grosjean started coordinating draft physical and mental examina-

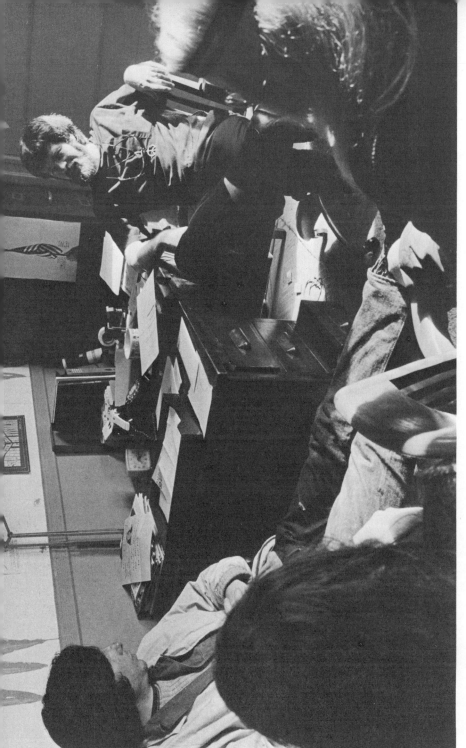

409 Clayton Street: Father Lyle Grosjean of the Episcopal Peace Center.
(Elaine Mayes)

tions with the Medical and Psychiatric sections and utilizing Robert Laws's legal referral program to avoid such crises. He also started a housing service and managed to find accommodations for dozens of young people who needed beds. By July, Father Grosjean was counseling over seventy-five people weekly, many of whom "came to me because they could talk easier to a priest than to a psychiatrist. We never did achieve a religious community, which was not surprising considering the condition of the Haight. But we did do a lot for the young people, and so many returned to us that we eventually had our own family too."

The Flight of the Flower Children

While Father Grosjean was emerging as a father figure in the Haight-Ashbury, Dr. Smith, Jim Sternfield, a young criminologist from Berkeley, John Luce and several Clinic staff members were launching another project outside of the immediate area. They had kept in touch with the psychedelic movement and were now eager to examine the living conditions of the hippies residing on urban and rural communes. They also wanted to determine the health needs of the former members of the new community and to design some method of delivering medical services to them.

This determination was no simple matter, for although some young people who lived in the Bay Area were easy to locate, others who had retreated into the wilds after the previous summer were accessible only by jeep trails. Futhermore, in spite of their respect for 409 and 558 Clayton Street, the hippies were fearful of public knowledge of their whereabouts. But the Clinic researchers did manage to visit over seven dozen communes in California, Oregon and other states during the summer and were thereby able to piece together a composite picture of the present status of the tribes.

A few of these communes contained SDS members and other leftist radicals, but most were apolitical structures that could be divided into the same categories previously applied to the Haight-Ashbury. The researchers saw several drug-oriented and nondrug-oriented family communes and group marriages with male or female leaders, for example. They also found crash pads which were dominated by sexual promiscuity and chemical abuse.

The crash pads contrasted sharply with the large, self-contained rural communes. These aggregates were comparable to the new community itself, and were made up of many young people who had banded together to protect themselves. The communal members often referred to their organizations as schools. They usually lived in teepees, tents, lean-tos or in more permanent buildings like the geodesic domes designed by Buckminster Fuller. These were situated around central lodges in which they socialized, took chemicals, gave classes, held rituals, and ate group meals.

In some cases, such as the Six Day School in Napa County, thirty residents were limited to a small sleeping space around a wooden dining and meeting area. In others, such as the Wheeler Ranch near Morningstar, forty people, some of them veterans of the Krishna Consciousness Temple, were scattered in teepees and huts over twenty acres. The largest self-contained commune visited by the Clinic researchers that summer was located near the California-Oregon border, where over one hundred and fifty modern "Indians" occupied a single two-hundred-acre plot of land.

Some of these communes were led by chiefs, gurus and other presumably benevolent dictators, but most had established rudimentary governments and were led by formal or informal councils of tribal elders. The larger communes also frequently functioned like small societies with their own divisions of labor. Included in these occupational breakdowns were craftsmen, carpenters and masons; farmers who planted vegetable gardens and harvested fields of wheat and grain; shepherds who tended sheep, cattle, goats or chickens; food gatherers who picked wild plants or stored provisions; teachers who cared for the tribal children; former medical students, nurses or witch doctors who practiced folk medicine; and the elders themselves, who often served as spiritual advisers and/or medicine men.

Along with this social specialization, many of the larger communes also contained such conveniences as group bathing spots, saunas, recreation rooms and small huts for meditating and taking hallucinogens. Water was usually obtained from nearby streams, lakes and rivers where the females did their washing, or was shipped and/or stored in rain barrels or in fifty-gallon drums. Sewage disposal facilities ranged from crude septic tanks to rather sophisticated pipe systems, while in several cases the communal members merely relieved themselves in nearby streams.

Although living patterns varied somewhat from one residence to another, the hippies still shared approximately the same life-style. Toxic chemicals were seen at every commune, and a peace offering of marijuana was usually enough to provide entry into even the most fearful tribe. Drug- and non-drug-oriented religious rituals were common, while prayer, meditation, magic and astrology sessions often preceded communal meals. Little reading or television-watching was practiced, but parents and children alike did spend a great deal of time eating, chatting, taking care of one another and attending school.

This preoccupation with education resulted in part from the fact that few of the hippies knew much about nature or were familiar with tools.

Although some had taken courses in survival, natural childbirth, and nutrition at Happening House and the free school in the Haight, most were learning these subjects only by experience and welcomed instruction in the outdoor arts from more knowledgeable hippies who belonged to neighboring tribes.

Educators were therefore in great demand at the communes, as were books on free learning. A popular text was the *Whole Earth Catalogue,* an illustrative manual modeled after the Sears, Roebuck and L.L. Bean mail-order catalogues. The first issue of this survival, ecology, plumbing, tool-making and carpentry handbook was assembled in the spring of 1968 by Stewart Brand, a former Merry Prankster and co-creator of the 1966 Trips Festival.

The modern "Indians" faced a number of problems that were not covered in the *Whole Earth Catalogue.* They were constantly visited by police and public health officials, and were besieged during the summer by homeless adolescents who wanted to camp or create crash pads on their property. They also had the elements to contend with. Some young people reported that they had sustained frostbite, sunstroke and heat prostration during their time in the country. Others said they suffered from extreme cold in the winter and had been all but washed away after they let in the rain by opening their teepee flaps to disperse smoke from cooking and heating fires.

The commune dwellers also had a host of internal enemies. Although most of their primitive villages contained passable sanitary facilities, some were noticeably unhygienic and had been hit by several kinds of contagious disease. The hippies' diets had not improved appreciably since they left the Haight-Ashbury, and since they still ate communally, their residences were frequently swept by food poisoning, strep infections and the flu. Animal bites, oak poisoning and traumatic injuries were common to all. The researchers saw a number of improperly set fractures in the parents and heard of worms afflicting the children of more than a dozen communes.

Furthermore, as observed earlier at the Medical Section, many of the young people took their previous infections with them to their new encampments. Over half of the approximately six hundred communal residents the Clinic researchers interviewed during the summer of 1968 had contracted hepatitis during the winter, while all the occupants of certain crash pads had picked up VD. Dermatological difficulties, upper respiratory tract infections and dental problems were widespread in the country, as were measles, mononucleosis, pneumonia and other infections for which herbs and incantations were not effective antidotes. The young people would not discuss the casualties within their ranks any more than they would in the city. But the researchers were certain that some deaths due to pneumonia, puerperal sepsis and other causes must have occurred. In the course of their travels, they noticed over a half-dozen freshly dug graves.

Although these burial grounds were probably reserved for older and more chronically ill tribal members, they may have housed some babies as well. A clear majority of the approximately two hundred infants the researchers saw that summer had health problems comparable to those previously observed at 558 Clayton Street. The children were usually unregistered and thereby deprived of inoculations, and many had either suffered generally uncommon childhood illnesses or were certain to contract them if they ever returned to the city for any length of time. The parents usually denied the fact, but pediatricians were sorely needed at most of the communes.

Yet the hippies had few people to turn to even if they did admit their dependence on society. Some had found friendly general practitioners who would treat them and their offspring, often in exchange for handicrafts or communal meals. Others lived with semiexperienced ex-medical students or used the state-sponsored clinics for migratory workers in the Sacramento Valley. Many had no access to medical services and asked the Clinic researchers for health information materials.

Finally, the rural residents also required assistance in the general education of their children. Although they had supposedly avoided social contamination by moving to the country, their offspring appeared, as expected, to be quite psychologically disturbed. This was documented in part by Pamela Hudson, a former psychiatric nurse at the Langley-Porter Neuropsychiatric Institute who had once worked in the Haight and was now helping out at a free school in Mendocino County and trying to establish a health clinic there.

"These kids aren't learning much of anything," Miss Hudson said. "Their parents can't give them a sense of structure or identity because they want to be children too. They tell the kids to be nonviolent and keep them from playing sports and using war toys, but my first day here I found a group of six-year-olds ganging up on some younger children and playing a game they made up, called 'slavery.' I've also seen a number of children who come to class on acid. The hip parents say how much better things are in the country. But as far as I've seen, nothing has really changed."

Indeed, the only difference in the now scattered new community was its numerical increase and its anticipated longevity. Although the Clinic researchers never conducted a formal head count during the summer, they estimated that over ten thousand young people were living either permanently or periodically in urban and rural communes in northern California and southern Oregon. Dr. Smith was told by Dr. Timothy Leary and others that the hippies had both proliferated and remained philosophically committed since they left the city. And John Luce came to the same conclusion when he visited Ken Kesey on the farm near Springfield, Oregon, to which he had retired after spending five months in jail.

Luce expected to interview the Chief for a literary journal, but he was equally interested in the farm. Kesey's eighty acres were as yet unproductive. They were dotted with abandoned camper buses, huts, a Day-Glowed barn and a log cabin cookhouse, as if a clutch of psychedelic Okies had settled there. The Chief himself watched television, listened to the Grateful Deal in a specially constructed sound chamber, and supervised twenty-five Merry Pranksters and other residents who made their living by picking crops and taking odd jobs. He also worked on a cartoon book recounting his adventures at the La Honda prison camp. But Kesey did not want to discuss his or anyone else's writing. Other than Tom Wolfe's *Electric Kool-Aid Acid Test,* the only reading matter on his property were manuals on irrigation and beekeeping and a copy of *Zap* comics prepared by the San Francisco poster artists.

The Chief was also unwilling to talk about his role in or the future of the psychedelic movement. Instead, he ushered Luce into a geodesically domed greenhouse and answered with a parable. "We watered the tomato plant on the left with STP," he said, pointing to a wilted green stalk. "The one in the middle got water only. This one" — he bent to stretch a stalk to its full height — "this one was given LSD. The one on STP has always been the shortest. The one on water was the tallest until a month or so ago. Then the one on acid took the lead."

Whether the LSD-nutured plant would bear fruit or not, Luce and the staff researchers were convinced that the psychedelic movement and its offshoots would continue to alert local physicians to the plight of the hippies in their areas. He, Jim Sternfield and other volunteers also began advising doctors in Berkeley who were thinking of founding a free clinic near Telegraph Avenue to care for the street people there. Delores Craton organized a number of volunteers from the Medical and Psychiatric sections who started making house calls in the country. And other volunteers under the direction of Ruth Fleshman, a nurse from the University of California, began work on a *Hip Health Home Handbook* to help those they had interviewed on the communes.

All this took money, of course. 409 and 558 Clayton Street still drew heavily on the Clinic budget, and although enough funds had been raised in October to underwrite their operation until the end of the summer, both facilities were now in need of more financial support. This problem had been anticipated before the November reopening, but the continual immigration of homeless adolescents to the Haight-Ashbury and the inauguration of new projects was causing a budgetary depletion that no one could have expected. The Clinic business manager now had his work cut out for him.

In spite of this current situation, Jerry Read had not been idle since the fall. He and the volunteers had already raised over one thousand dollars in private donations and had arranged for three fund-raising benefits, including a night of entertainment at a rock club called the Matrix and a Valentine's Day dance-concert at the California Hall. The third benefit was hosted for them by Chet Helms and the Family Dog, who sponsored a Spring Medicine Show on May twenty-eighth and ninth at the Avalon Ballroom with music provided by Santana, A. B. Skhy, and other third- and fourth-generation San Francisco bands. Two thousand dollars was netted at the Spring Medicine Show, stimulating Read's grandiose visions about presenting a huge benefit at the Palace of Fine Arts Festival on Labor Day.

Further difficulties would ultimately result in the Place of Fine Arts benefit becoming a major disaster. But before they did, Read turned his attention toward the free outdoor dance concerts he had always wanted to produce. The Golden Gate Park Panhandle had been declared off limits to rock musicians because of the opposition of local property owners long before this time, but the Recreation and Park Commission was still willing to let groups play on Speedway Meadows in the heart of the park. Read organized two weekend-afternoon performances in early July on the former site of the Summer Solstice Festival, the largest of which featured Big Brother and the Holding Company and attracted twelve thousand fans. These were followed by two additional dance concerts in the city hall plaza, where volunteers from 409 and 558 Clayton Street sold soft drinks and passed the donation can.

These proceeds were barely enough to cover expenses, but profit was not Read's primary objective. The Haight had grown more crowded with the coming of summer, and although not so many young people flocked to the area as did a year earlier, tension was mounting and tempers were continually flaring in the behavioral sink. The Clinic organizers hoped to decrease pressure in the district by providing free music which might draw young people off the streets. They therefore sanctioned Read's productions as a form of community therapy.

The need for such therapy was then documented by a second study of drug practices in the Haight-Ashbury conducted in June by Dr. Meyers, Dr. Smith and Frederick Shick. Shick distributed four hundred and sixty-two questionnaires in and around the Medical Section at the start of the summer and once again collated his findings on a computer. He then used the figures to draw several comparisons between this second survey and the one taken eight months earlier.

Shick found that whereas the respondents to his first questionnaire were almost evenly divided according to sex, only twenty-nine percent of the new sample were female while seventy-one percent were male. The median age of these respondents was twenty-one and a half years, almost a year more than those surveyed during the previous September and October. Only twenty percent had fathers in professional fields, as compared with the twenty-seven percent seen in 1967. Only thirty percent had gained some college experience. In addition, less than fourteen percent were from the Bay Area, while over forty-four percent were raised in large cities and only four percent came from rural areas.

The survey also revealed a consistent rise in every area of chemical experimentation and abuse. Well over ninety percent of the respondents had used alcohol and/or marijuana, for example, while eighty-nine percent were personally familiar with adulterated or pure hallucinogens. Over fifty-two percent had taken barbiturates and other downers; twenty-nine percent had tried opiates, although only a small percentage of these appeared to be addicted to heroin. By contrast, seventy-two percent had experimented with oral amphetamines — a rise of three percent from the previous survey. Approximately thirty-five percent had sampled these drugs in their intravenous form. And whereas only ten percent of the 1967 respondents were counted as intravenous abusers, a full fifty percent of the more recent sample could be considered habitual abusers of speed.

Aside from the obvious increase in chemical consumption indicated by these figures, the Clinic organizers realized that the new population had changed dramatically since the Summer of Love. For one thing, fewer females were either coming to the Haight or appearing on the street. Those who were arriving and/or remaining in the area seemed to be older, less educated and more often from deprived urban backgrounds than ever before. The new community had never been reestablished in the district, as Dr. Smith might have wished. Randy summed up the reasons why. "Like I tell you," he said, "this place is becoming a dope-fiend Bowery, full of junkies and freaks. It's too rough out here for girls, for candyass hippies and for kids."

These population changes explained the tensions which the organizers hoped to lessen through their dance concerts, but the city was also responsible for perpetuating the behavioral sink. No public funds had yet been used to improve conditions in the Haight-Ashbury, and Mayor Alioto, who tried closing Haight Street to automobile traffic for two days shortly after the altercation there in February, had long since abandoned his effort. He now appeared to be adopting what one Neighborhood Council member called a "domestic Vietnam policy" in the Haight. "This area had become Alioto's political albatross," she claimed. "He either has to call in more troops and level the Haight-Ashbury or stand back and let the natives slaughter themselves."

Dr. Norman Sissman, who had to spend over six hours one evening persuading the police from Park Station to transport a dangerously psychotic patient to Mission Emergency, thought that the mayor might follow the second tactic in the future. Other organizers at the Medical Section leaned toward the first alternative, but most agreed that San Francisco's public officials, like leaders in other cities, seemed unable to come to terms with alienated youth. They were hardly surprised in mid-July when the Haight was ripped by three nights of rioting which conclusively demonstrated that the district needed far more therapy than the Clinic could ever provide.

The Siege of the Haight-Ashbury

The siege of the Haight-Ashbury began around six P.M. on Tuesday, July sixteenth, when two undercover narcotics agents arrested a pair of Oakland men for selling speed at the corner of Haight and Clayton streets. The dealers began screaming that they were being unduly hassled and called upon the street people in their vicinity to help them fight off the narcs. A large, angry crowd soon collected and began pelting the police with sticks and rocks. Patrolmen from Park Station and members of the Tactical Squad then arrived, imposed a curfew, and began sweeping the street.

Peggy Sankot immediately called Don Reddick and asked if she should close 558 Clayton Street. Reddick advised her to open the door to injured young people, but after eighteen patients were admitted for broken bones and scalp lacerations, the police blocked the front steps. The staff then started leaving the facility, only to be caught in the Tactical Squad's sweep. Twenty-seven people were subsequently arrested, including an *Examiner* reporter and a volunteer.

Although the Clinic bondsman eventually bailed this young man out of jail, other innocent bystanders could not be helped. Three volunteers were chased off the front steps with riot clubs later in the evening, and the police also cornered the wife of a member of the Medical Committee for Human Rights. This nurse and frequent worker at the Medical Section was stopped while she was attempting to pick up her husband during the curfew. The police lectured her about trying to aid unruly adolescents and then beat her in the back of her legs until they were black and blue.

At 409 House, Lyle Grosjean and several seminarians were showing films and serving coffee in an effort to entice young people off the street. Roger Smith was standing in the walkway leading to his basement office around ten that evening when he saw a paddy wagon pull up at the intersection of Clayton and Oak to block access to the Panhandle. Two patrolmen alighted from the van and began rounding up a dozen people whom one of Father Grosjean's volunteers was urging not to retaliate. Father Grosjean then appeared and yelled at his assistant to come inside before he too was arrested.

The boy ran toward 409 Clayton Street and rushed inside, the police at his heels. When they reached the front door, Father Grosjean asked them not to precipitate a disturbance by entering the building and pointed at the sign advising "This Is a House of Peace." Disregarding both this notice and the clerical collar the minister was wearing, the patrolmen kicked him to the ground and worked him over with their fists. Father Grosjean rose from a pool of blood, shook himself off, and requested his assailants' badge numbers. The police floored him a second time, shouting, "You aren't going to get anything but this, you bearded son of a bitch."

One of the seminarians threw himself upon Father Grosjean at this point and the patrolmen decided to call it quits. But as soon as they had driven away from the blocked intersection, a Tactical Squad member appeared, started screaming obscenities, and stormed up the steps. Father Grosjean retreated to his office and subsequently filed a complaint with the Police Department, as did Roger Smith. Neither was acted upon. Both mentioned that the first major violent incident at the Episcopal Peace Center had been started not by young people but by the police.

All was quiet the day after these events, so Peggy Sankot, Judy St. Onge, Jackie and other staff members distributed leaflets urging nonviolence through the district. But around eight o'clock that evening, a dozen street people climbed onto the roof of a store adjacent to the Medical Section and hurled a Molotov cocktail into the street. Other street people hauled a large construction trash box into the intersection of Haight and Clayton and set it ablaze. An unmarked police car drove up; its occupants tried to arrest a girl and were swarmed over by the crowd. One hundred men from Park Station then appeared, and the Tactical Squad was called in once again.

Although arrests were soon made throughout the area, the center of action continued to be Haight and Clayton streets. A tug-of-war gradually developed there, with the police lugging the trash box onto the sidewalk and the young people pulling it back into the street. The Tactical Squad, meanwhile, was moving up and down the block busting heads. Fifty-seven patients, one of whom had been stranded with her baby in a nearby doorway, were treated for scalp lacerations at the Clinic. This girl's arm was fractured and her buttocks were bloody because the police had swatted her as she ran from them up the street.

After she was treated, Dr. Smith and Don Reddick decided to see what was happening outside. They had barely descended from 558 Clayton when ten Tactical Squad members rushed up the front steps of a nearby building and smashed in the door. A few minutes later, sixteen street people emerged from the residence, one of whom was beaten to the pavement. Dr. Smith then walked up, introduced himself as a physician, and told the police that the boy they were working over should be examined for a possible concussion. One of the Tactical Squad members pushed Dr. Smith with his riot stick and yelled to get out of the way. Reddick intervened and asked for the officer's badge number. He was shown the riot stick and told, "I'll use this on you too if you don't get inside."

While the administrative director was filing yet another useless complaint with the Police Department, a huge truck rambled up and carted the trash box away. Further violence followed, but by eleven o'clock the police managed to clear Haight Street. Few lights were left burning there by this point, save for those in the Medical Section. The street was quiet until the Tactical Squad finished a mopping-up operation and assembled on the corner below.

Then the stillness was suddenly broken by a scratchy sound. Dr. Andrew Weil turned to the front window from a patient whose scalp he was stitching and saw thirty officers lined up with their helmets over their hearts and riot sticks at their sides. The scratchy sound, he realized, came from a portable sound system on which a well-worn record was being played. "I knew it was 'The Star-Spangled Banner,'" he recalled later, "But 'Deutchland, Deutchland Uber Alles' kept running through my mind."

Aftermath

Dr. Weil was not the only one to hear echoes of Nazi Germany on Haight Street that evening. Although the siege of the district ended the next night, when Mayor Alioto announced that "we're not going to listen to any crybabies complaining about police brutality," the brutality decimated the Clinic. Some volunteers were so terrified by the recent events that they refused to reenter the Haight, while others who had tried to bridge the straight and hip worlds by working at 409 and 558 Clayton Street finally realized the precariousness of their position. "The worst thing about the riots," Carter Mehl said, "was that we couldn't identify with either side."

Particularly vulnerable to this realization were those older doctors who had risked their professional reputations by coming to the Haight-Ashbury. Dr. Breithaupt, who was under pressure from his family for spending so much time at the Clinic, decided that the Haight was hopeless and helped establish a drug-abuse center in Santa Clara County. Dr. Norman Sissman and his wife Hallie apparently realized they had learned all they could from the district and chose to stay in the drug-abuse field at Stanford. Dr. Bertram Meyer, who wanted to do more for Negro patients, devoted his future to the Black Man's Free Clinic in the Fillmore. And Dr. Meyers formally disaffiliated himself from the staff.

Also terminating their service were many young volunteers and staff members. Peggy Sankot and Judy St. Onge started making plans to leave the district long before the Medical Section was closed in the coming fall. Furthermore, only two of the former patients Miss Sankot had mothered remained with the Clinic after the riots. One was Randy, who enjoyed the action and had nowhere else to go. The other was Jackie, who considered rejoining her parents until she discovered that she would soon be a parent too.

Jackie's pregnancy was confirmed one week after the riots and two days after she broke up with her current boyfriend. She placed a long-distance call to her mother three hours later, but the mother seemed less concerned about her daughter's safety than her sex life. This naturally alienated Jackie, so although she discussed having a therapeutic abortion which would allow her to return home, she decided to have the baby and to stay in San Francisco at least temporarily. She therefore moved to a small apartment on Willard Street near the University of California and came to Haight Street only to shop, to see Dr. Dernburg, and to work at the Medical Section.

This was not the case with Alan. Alan had made considerable progress in therapy by this time, but he was more disturbed by the violence than Jackie was and therefore decided to migrate to the Wheeler Ranch to "clear out my head." Dr. Dernburg was saddened by his departure, particularly because Alan was still prone to asthma and other respiratory disorders. But he realized that his patient would not improve physically or psychologically as long as he remained in the Haight-Ashbury. Feeling the same about most of the young residents, he considered severing his ties with the Clinic and finally left the Haight after speed abuse peaked there during the frantic fall.

Dr. Dernburg quit the Haight-Ashbury, but before leaving he made a prediction which was seconded by many staff members at the Clinic:

Two years' experience in this district has convinced me that the hippie modality which surfaced at the be-in has been fully absorbed by American society, although the hippies have not been assimilated themselves. Individuals as unlikely as Charles Manson exhibit certain of its features, as do young people from every socioeconomic class.

Equally important, society is continuing to spawn the modality and reinforce psychological plateauing among the young. Families in almost every technologically sophisticated nation are fragmenting under the stress of divorce, dislocation and rapid change. The structure of our country is giving away to the cultural diffuseness once common only to California and is thereby encouraging adolescents to create their own institutions. Deprived of home life and family involvement, children are being forced to form alternative families with their peers.

Because of these and other factors, I feel that we are witnessing in this country the evolution of a vast youth subculture with poorly defined boundaries. Smaller and more specific subcultures will continue to exist within it, many of them based on a particular psychoactive chemical, as in the Haight. But the members of these different groups will have much in common. Multiple drug use and abuse is the coming pattern in the United States. Drugs are one lowest common denominator for our young people. Another is the new community's life-style.

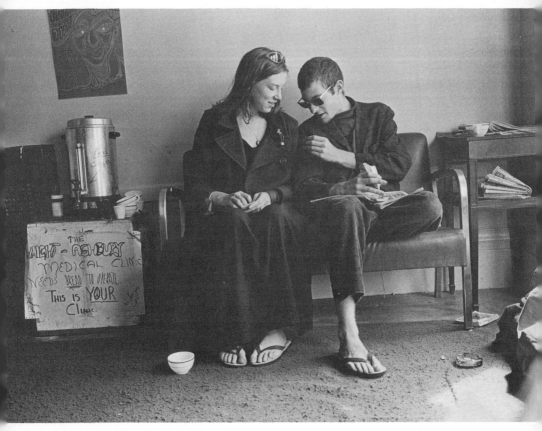

558 Clayton Street: marking time.
(Elaine Mayes)

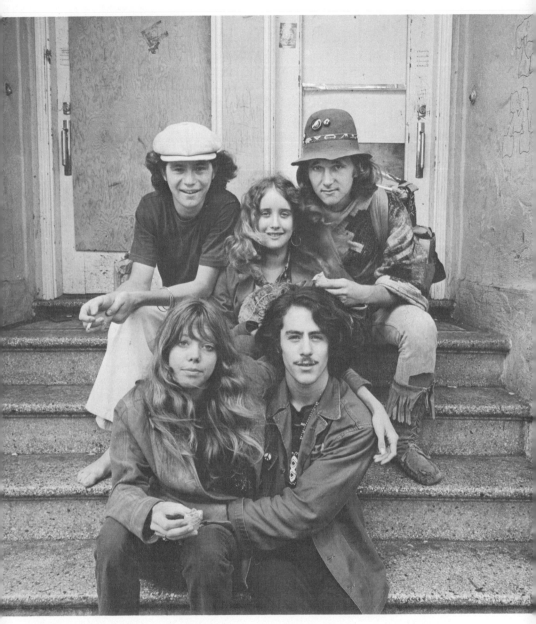

Haight Street: Shari, Bunny, Stephanie, Michael and Sean — "There's nothing wrong with having fun."
(Elaine Mayes)

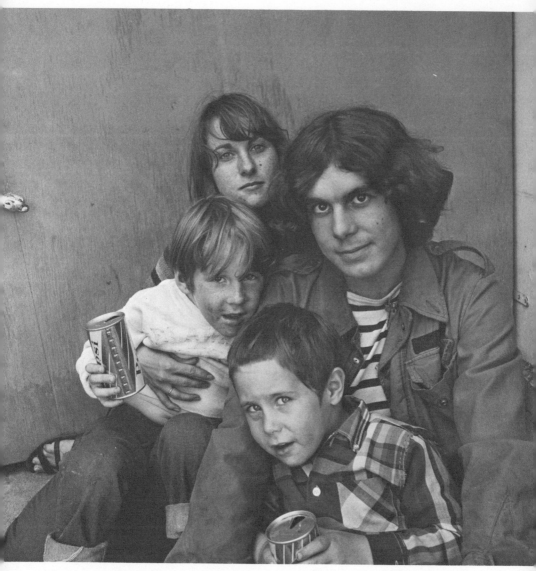

Clayton Street: Libra, Leo, Taurus and Gemini — "Love is all you need . . . all you need is love."
(Elaine Mayes)

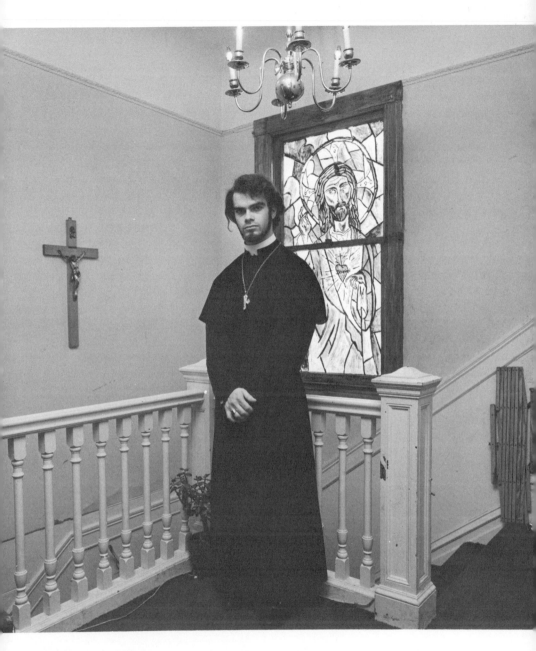

Frederick Street: "The Holy Father, Reverend Laurence, archbishop of Haight-Ashbury, deacon of the Devil's Church, alias Bishop James Pike, Bishop Fulton Sheen, Pope Pius — Who cares about my name?"
(Elaine Mayes)

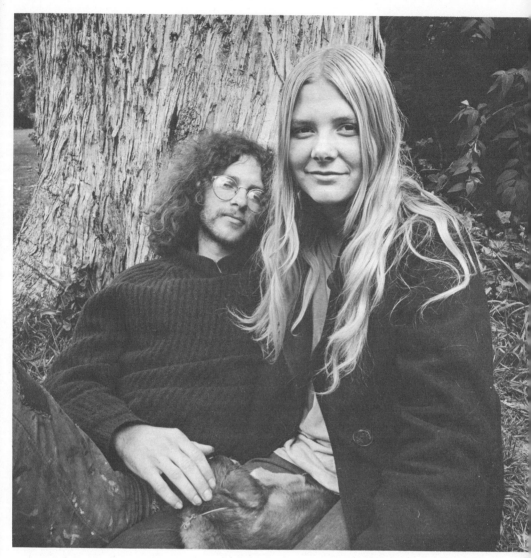

The Panhandle: Steve and Sue — "Life can be good if you let things happen to you."
(Elaine Mayes)

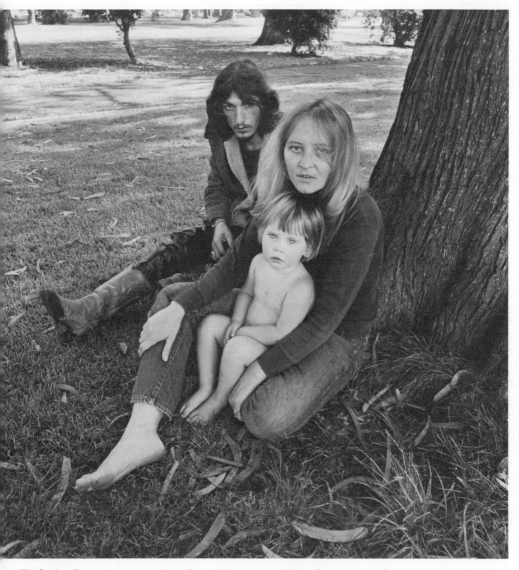

The Panhandle: Jerry, Asia and Tarin Djia — "You may not like us, but we're people, too."
(Elaine Mayes)

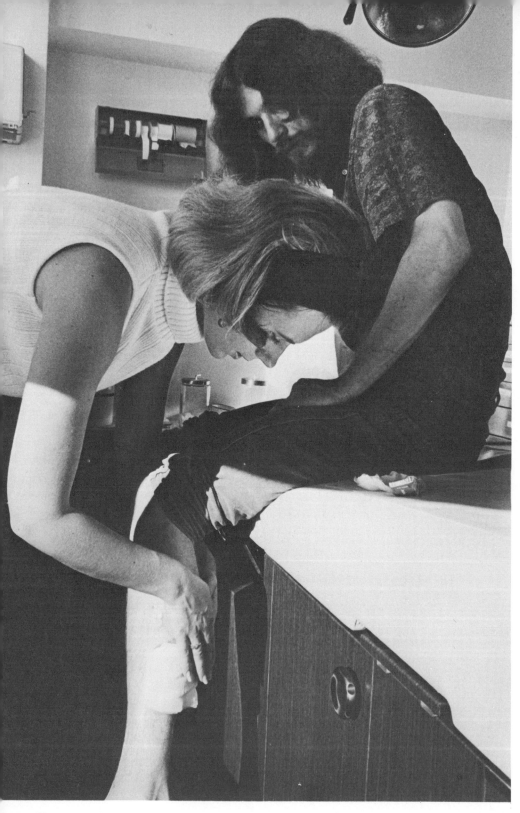

558 Clayton Street: another riot . . . more care.
(Jim Marshall)

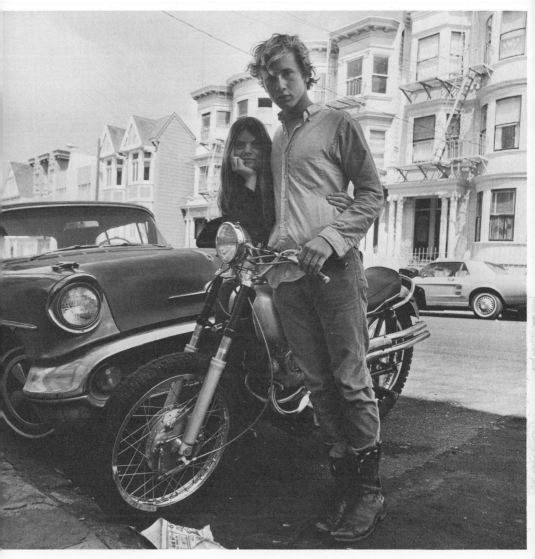

Clayton Street: Cookie and Jack — "We're getting out, to Berkeley, maybe. It's great being free and riding around. But there's nothing here but rip-offs and garbage cans." (Elaine Mayes)

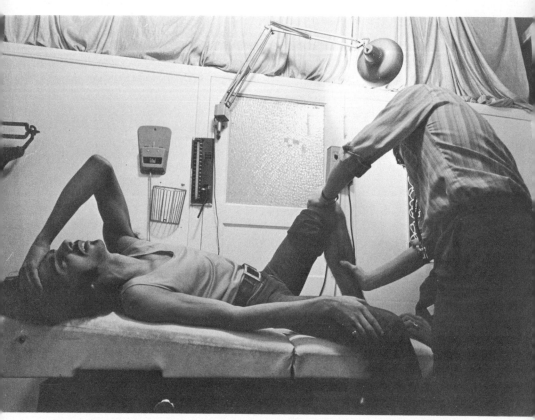

558 Clayton Street: only pain remains.
(Michael Alexander)

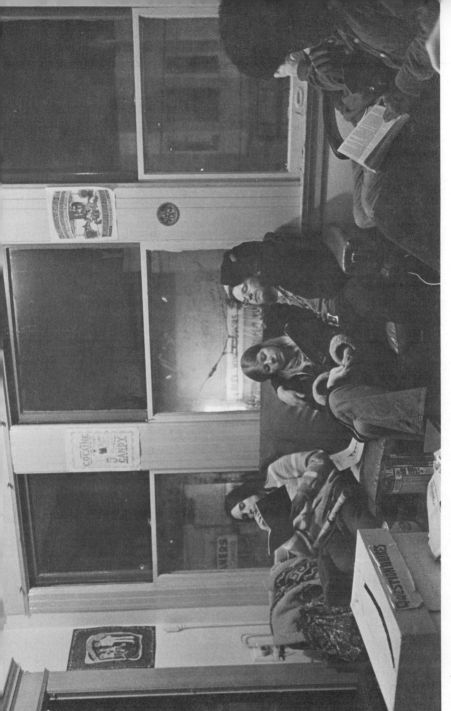

558 Clayton Street: night life in the waiting room.
(Michael Alexander)

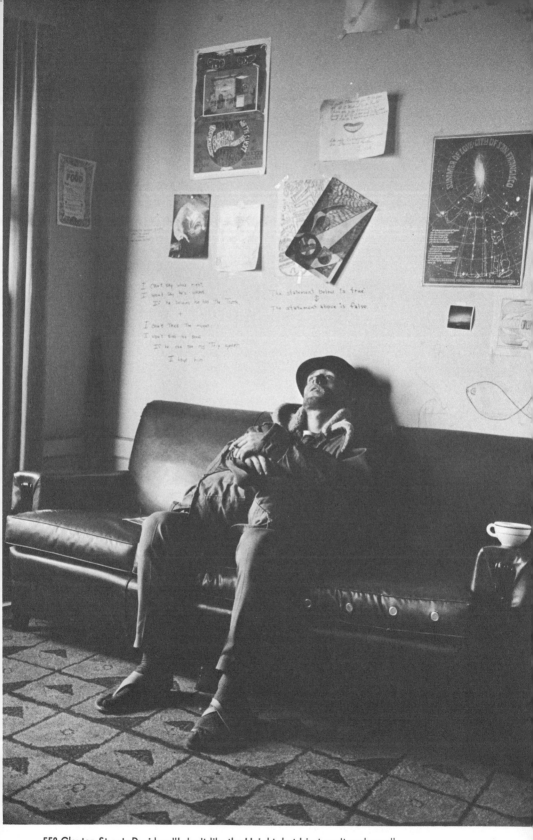

558 Clayton Street: David — "I don't like the Haight, but I just can't go home."
(Elaine Mayes)

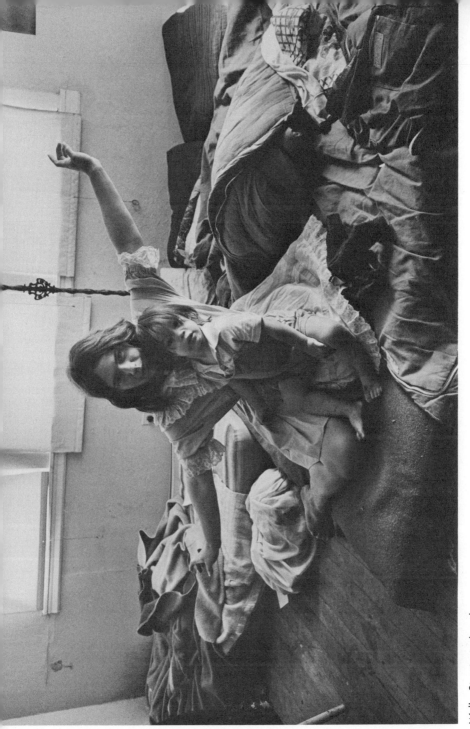

Waller Street: crash pad.
(Elaine Mayes)

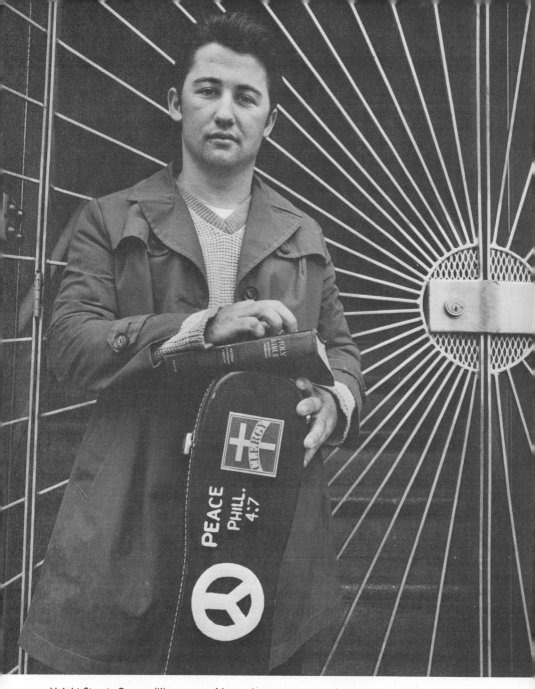

Haight Street: Gary — "I'm a man of love. Jesus is my strength; I don't need dope like they do. I just make music for Christ. . . . That's my thing."
(Elaine Mayes)

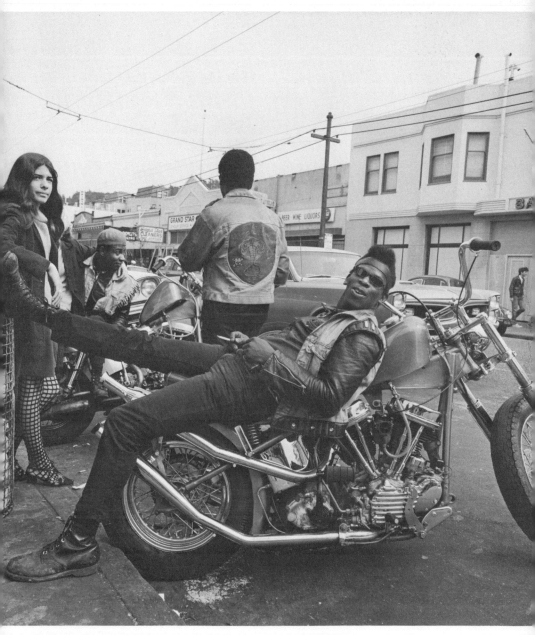

Haight Street: "You can take my picture, but I won't give you my name."
(Elaine Mayes)

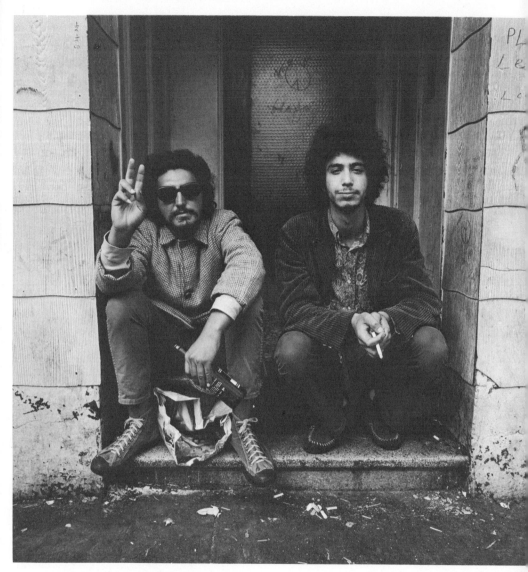

Haight Street: Art and Eddy — "Right on."
(Elaine Mayes)

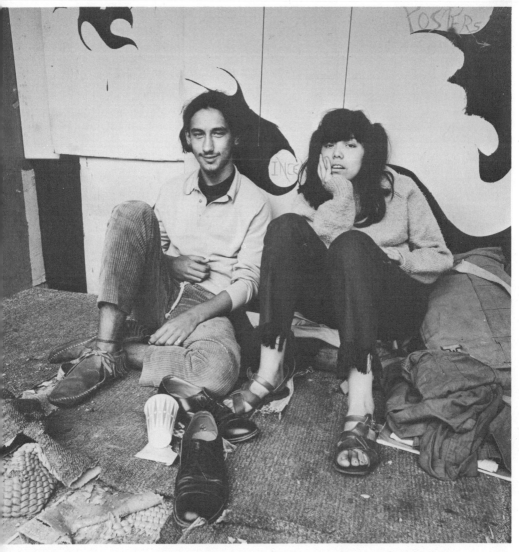

Haight Street: Adam and Hiawatha — "Self is the root of all evil . . . on high with the wind; people are twins."
(Elaine Mayes)

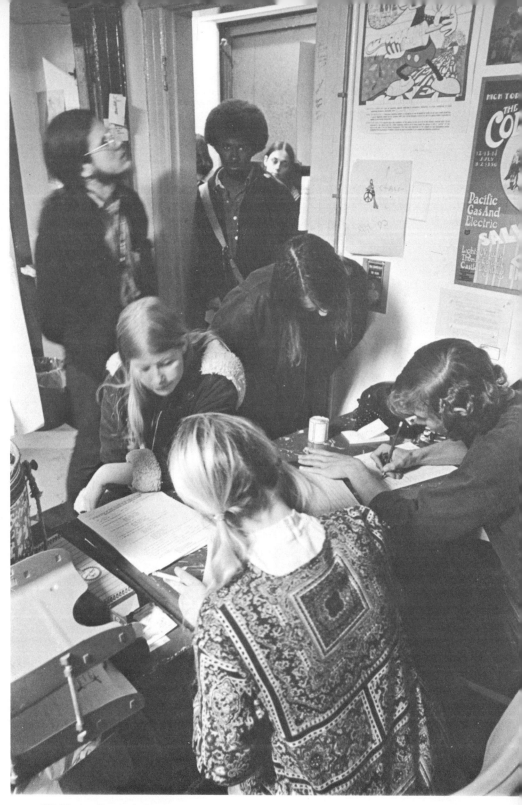

558 Clayton Street: signing in.
(Michael Alexander)

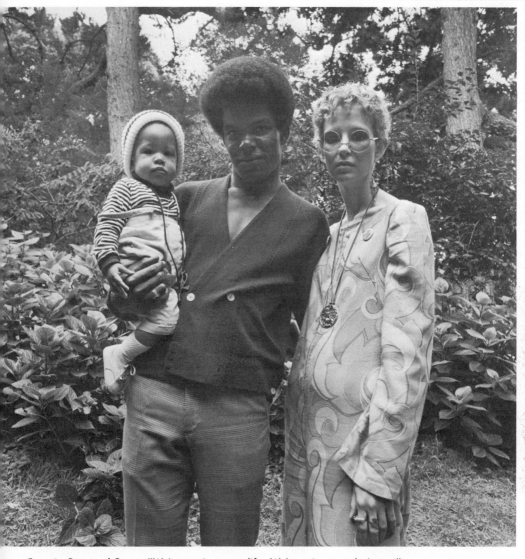

Georgie, Peter and Gay — "We're starting a new life. We're going to make it, too."
(Elaine Mayes)

Part V

Epitaph

The river's tent is broken: the last fingers of leaf
Clutch and sink into the wet bank. The wind
Crosses the brown land, unheard. The nymphs are departed.

T. S. Eliot, ''The Wasteland''

He had the heart, the eye of an eagle.
His hands were quick and his mind as well.
Now he just quivers and clings to his needle.
He's on the wrong road, the long road to Hell.

Genesis, ''The Long Road''

Humane treatment may raise up one in
whom the divine image has long been
obscured. It is with the unfortunate above
all that humane conduct is necessary.

Fëdor Dostoevski, **The House of the Dead**

That Was the Year That Was

Dr. Dernburg's belief that drugs and the new community's living pattern were now national common denominators was amply borne out during 1969. 1969 was "the year of the commune" according to *Newsweek*, which put Janis Joplin on its cover and reported that thousands of young people who followed her were settling in urban and rural communes. It was the year when more than five hundred new group living units sprung up in northern California and a dozen veterans of the new community formulated plans for an Earth People's Park in the Southwest on one hundred and fifty thousand acres inhabited by peyote-using Indians. It was the year in which over three hundred thousand people gathered for three days of peace and music near Woodstock, New York, and a slightly smaller number ripped apart the Altamont Speedway in San Francisco's East Bay.

1969 was the year President Nixon declared drug abuse the country's number-one educational problem and launched Operation Intercept to cut off the flow of marijuana across the Mexican border and thereby curtail consumption of the killer weed. It was the year when California's superintendent of public instruction proposed a Project Turnoff involving unannounced searches of student lockers by school officials and plainclothes policemen. It was the year in which the San Francisco Sound became one of the city's ten largest industries and Dr. James Stubblebine of the Public Health Department established what he referred to as crash pads (actually calm centers) to detoxify adolescents in local high schools.

It was the year ecology began to rival the Vietnam war, which had previously eclipsed civil rights, as the most urgent national issue. It was the year in which liberal politicians started speaking out against the dangers of urban congestion and applied the behavioral-sink concept to our major cities. It was the year when America noticed her dwindling natural resources. It was the year in which she forgot the Haight-Ashbury. And it was the year when the Haight became a biracial ghetto instead of a white teen-age slum.

This change was a long time coming, but few older residents of the district were caught napping when it finally arrived. Most of the straight merchants who had not quit Haight Street after the riots there the previous summer vacated their stores during 1969, while many Neighborhood Council members who saw their dreams of a model integrated community go up in smoke and tear gas seemed to take the fate of the Haight-Ashbury in stride. "We should have known what was going to happen," a fifty-five-year-old woman said. "We thought we could postpone the Haight's evolving into a ghetto in 1960, but the new community and the publicity it generated pushed our timetable ahead by at least ten years."

Although such acceptance was widespread in the district, a few residents protested that the deterioration was as yet limited to the Flatlands and set out to save the slope of Mt. Sutro. Some homeowners turned to Mayor Alioto for help, but others decided to form a Haight-Ashbury Neighborhood Development Corporation to stimulate private renewal efforts, raise property values, and apply for one hundred million dollars of federal aid. These leaders of the old community predicted publicly that Haight Street could be transformed into a tree-lined boulevard. Yet they admitted privately that the Haight would have trouble securing outside assistance in spite — or because — of its international fame.

Those who made it famous now had little invested in the area. Most of the hippies who lingered through 1968 left the Haight-Ashbury as 1969 began, as did the last of the H.I.P. shop owners. And as the year advanced, several elements of the new population that had survived the negative filter of police repression started to abandon the Haight as well. The Hell's Angels rarely roared down the street on the motorcycles during January of 1969, for example. They still shopped there for chemicals, but only the Gypsy Jokers and other lesser bikers continued to occupy the area.

Many hoodies had also had their fill of the Haight-Ashbury. The more sensible drug distributors began vacating their crystal palaces after the Ann Jiminez orgy, leaving only the lower-echelon dealers, the second-rate street commandos and the psychotic street people behind. Those who stayed to squabble over the speed marketplace had to spend as much time defending their positions in the subcultural hierarchy as they did selling amphetamines. Some organized themselves into groups like the Methedrine Marauders and escalated their ripoffs and cops-and-robbers games. Others were so hard pressed for status that they turned to ritualized murder to prove they were capable of gangland-style revenge.

The young Negroes of the Haight, who gathered daily in front of the liquor stores on Haight Street or sat by the curb in their flashy cars, profited most from this intracultural genocide. These blacks had maintained their own subculture since the early 1960's, when the district housed only a small bohemian colony. They had lived alongside the beats and hippies, exploited the adolescents during the summer of 1967, and endured after love left the area. Now they were growing numerically and emerging as a major force in the Flatlands.

One reason for the blacks' prominence was the absence of many former members of the new population. Another was the fact that few young whites were taking their places in the area. Grizzled winos were still coming to the district, along with heroin addicts and other habitual and/or multiple drug abusers whom Randy recognized from New York and elsewhere. A handful of servicemen also stopped by occasionally, but the only whites interested in the Haight were homeless San Francisco State students, high schoolers sampling from the Haight-Street smorgasbord and lower-income runaways who were so desperate for shelter and so dependent on chemicals that they still came to the district in spite or because of its well-advertised poverty, sickness and crime.

Some of these new arrivals were used to ghetto conditions and had lived on the periphery of black subcultures. But most found the Haight-Ashbury worse than their experiences or their expectations. The health of the district had suffered heavily after the Clinic's closing in the fall of 1968, and the departure of the last merchants had left Haight Street looking worse than a skid row. Other than a half-dozen liquor dispensaries, markets and well-lit storefronts, the street was a solid sheet of plywood from Masonic to Stanyan. "The place is burned out," one supervisor told his television audience. "It reminds me of Berlin after the Second World War."

The same description fit many of the young residents. Most of those who had been abusing hallucinogens since the summer of 1967 were now extremely disoriented, while Randy and his companions were physically and psychologically wasted from shooting speed. Their jaundiced faces, sunken eyes and emaciated bodies were only superficial indications of their interior disfigurement. Some were still hyperactive and euphoric, but others seemed to stay depressed. These young people had aged approximately one year for every two months of their high-dose amphetamine consumption. They now needed more insulative drugs to shield themselves from their environment.

So did the alcoholics, older abusers and young Negroes. Most had always preferred depressants to stimulants, even though some took speed because of its availability. Now many were increasing their intake of alcohol, marijuana, barbiturates and opiates to smother their anxiety and depression. Their numerical superiority, combined with certain developments in the amphetamine-based subculture, had a profound influence on drug-taking practices in the district. The change in chemical tastes, along with the continued apathy of San Francisco's political and health leaders, helped the Haight become a ghetto in 1969.

The transition was gradual, but although speed remained popular in the district for several months, sedating agents soon began to set its drug tone. Thus, while 1969 may have meant many things to other regions of the country, it was the year of the downers in the Haight-Ashbury. Young people arriving in the area were now exposed as often to traditional ghetto compounds as they were to stimulants and hallucinogens. It was downers which the volunteers faced after January thirteenth, 1969, when the front door to 558 Clayton Street was opened once again.

Another Try

The organizers had anticipated the downer problem the previous December, when Dr. Herbert Freudenberger of New York warned them that the Haight would become a depressant-dominated Harlem within the coming year. But they had no way of telling when the change in drug-taking would happen. They also had little idea of the nature and the needs of their new patients. And although they described the Medical Section as part of a multiservice center at their press conference on January seventh, 1970, the services it could offer were painfully few.

For the first time in the Clinic's history, this situation related less to financial difficulties than to a shortage of manpower. The organizers had raised enough money from Norman Stone and other contributors to guarantee a budget of eight thousand dollars for their combined operations for several months. They had also managed to restock 558 Clayton Street with medications, but few staff members were available to administer them. Most of the medical staff had gone on to new projects: Dr. Dernburg was involved with Hospitality House, a social center for street people in the Tenderloin district, and was also active at a residential treatment facility called Walden House near the University of California; Dr. Meyers was seeing patients in his office, helping out at Walden House, and donating what was left of his spare time to Reality House, an in-patient detoxification center for heroin addicts in the Fillmore.

The only two doctors regularly on hand at the Medical Section were Dr. Alan Matzger, who became assistant medical director after the Palace of Fine Arts benefit, and Dr. Richard Gleason, who would soon leave on the S.S. *Hope*, a floating hospital, for Vietnam. Other physicians were too frightened or depressed by the Haight-Ashbury to work there, and Don

Reddick, Dr. Nesbitt, Professor Loomis and Dr. Smith were the only organizers from the summer of 1967 who wanted to give the district another try.

The clerical and paramedical staff was also depleted. Carter Mehl was willing to resume operations at 558 Clayton Street in his new title of supervisor. So was Delores Craton, the new operations manager, Renée Sargent, assistant operations manager, Jackie, now seven months pregnant, and several others who had remained in the Haight after the Clinic closed. The staff members received two hundred dollars a month for their efforts and served at the Medical Section from six to ten P.M. on weekdays in keeping with Don Reddick's revised schedule. But they had fewer volunteers to work with than when the facility started in the Summer of Love.

This shortage did not prove to be a serious handicap at first, for only seventy-five patients came to the Clinic on the evening of January thirteenth, one-half the number that arrived the previous November and one-quarter the number present six months earlier on the seventh of June. A few had familiar faces, such as a pair of monks from the Krishna Consciousness Temple who once begged on the corner of Haight and Clayton with Alan and a half-dozen hippies living near the Medical Center who crowded around Jackie and admired her swelling abdomen. Two ex-Diggers also sought treatment, as did Randy and twelve others who were strung out on speed. But one-half of the patients lived outside the Haight-Ashbury, while many of those who gave addresses in the district had never been seen at the Medical Section before.

Among them were four older alcoholics, one of whom had to be taken to San Francisco General Hospital after he passed out in the front hall. Clifford, the American Indian, came by looking for a new friend now that Peggy Sankot was gone. He was followed by two young people stoned on barbiturates, a heroin addict who asked for detoxification, a fourteen-year-old amphetamine abuser from the posh Pacific Heights district and a seventeen-year-old male prostitute from the Tenderloin. A busload of hippies drove in from a commune in Marin County, as did two dozen others who knew Delores Craton and Carter Mehl. Six long-haired young people arrived from the Western Addition and said that they had been using the Black Man's Free Clinic, which was temporarily closed. Three of Dr. Bertram Meyer's black patients also sought treatment, one of them from the Flatlands and two from the Fillmore.

All had common complaints, but their health was uncommonly poor. Most would not use public facilities unless they were unconscious, and many had not seen a doctor since 558 Clayton Street was closed. The Clinic physicians saw twenty traumatic injuries, twelve cases of chronic bronchitis, one case of pneumonia, four of dysentery, twelve urinary and/or genital tract infections and six cases of periodontal disease on the evening of January thirteenth. They referred nine females for pregnancy tests, birth control pills or abortion counseling, helped two epileptics, and found nine cases of serum hepatitis and twelve of VD.

By ten o'clock that evening, it was clear that the condition of these patients was worse, and their medical needs greater, than ever before. At least fourteen had toxic psychoses and one female speed freak who arrived topless was covered with abscesses and open sores. Another was so malnourished that he could not walk. A nineteen-year-old girl brought in a baby who had not eaten in over a week. One young man who had dropped eighteen tabs of street acid was taken to Mt. Zion Hospital. A twenty-three-year-old woman had to be hospitalized after she slashed her wrists in an attempted suicide.

The hopelessness of these patients was contagious. Many of the doctors were gratified by the long-awaited presence of black people at the Clinic, but they still felt disheartened by the fact that so many of the patients they treated seemed so devoid of life and so eager to die. Dr. Matzger described his reaction to the evening of January thirteenth as "one of disbelief, even horror. I was glad I had a sense of humor and a surgical background. In my specialty, you learn what you can do and how to avoid breaking down completely when you can't do anything more."

Dr. Matzger was tempted to leave the Haight after the reopening, but he called a meeting instead and instituted new procedures for the staff. He and the other physicians first decided to augment their shuttle service to San Francisco General with more comprehensive referral services to the University of California, St. Mary's, Mt. Zion and other hospitals the patients were willing to use. They then began offering thorough examinations and treatment for gonorrhea at the Medical Section because their patients would not keep their appointments at the city's Venereal Disease Clinic. They contracted with six local pharmacies for cut-rate prescriptions for those patients who could not afford medication. They arranged for some young mothers to be helped by Federal Aid to Families with Dependent Children. And they made yet another plea for volunteers through the *Chronicle* and *Examiner,* the underground press and a local FM rock station, KSAN.

Over two dozen doctors responded to this publicity. Included were four physicians from Letterman Hospital in the San Francisco Presidio, two of whom were en route to Vietnam. Interns and residents from other facilities offered their facilities, as did Dr. Marcus Conant, chief of the Dermatology Clinic at the Medical Center, who brought his students to 558 Clayton

Street every Thursday evening. Dr. David Berman, a doctor with the United States Public Health Service who once worked at the Open Door Clinic in Seattle, became involved in the Clinic. The Medical Committee for Human Rights, of which Dr. Berman was a member, also continued to furnish aid.

Another important addition to the roster was a thirty-nine-year-old anesthesiologist named George "Skip" Gay. Dr. Gay came to San Francisco in 1967 by way of St. Louis and the University of Chicago Medical School. He volunteered at the Medical Section during the Summer of Love but had to discontinue his activities until he established a local practice. He had accomplished this by January of 1969, so he could devote his free time to the Clinic. Dr. Gay saw community medicine as "a way of gaining personal contact with my patients — everyone I deal with is asleep when I practice anesthesiology. I always found it ironical that most of my patients were anesthetized in the Haight-Ashbury, too."

Several others became staff members during this period. Gene Dobson, a withdrawn young man from Michigan who was on probation for having refused induction into the army, signed on as a night watchman and janitor. With him came Jeannie Kubicki, a twenty-one-year-old former patient at the Psychiatric Section, who was put in charge of referrals. Four young people who had recently quit Vista and the Peace Corps in disgust over the Nixon-Agnew administration also began serving at 558 Clayton Street. And John Luce, who was taking premed courses, counseling patients, and preparing a pamphlet on speed abuse for the Amphetamine Research Project, became the Clinic's first historian and director of public affairs.

Finally, the facility acquired its third and most competent business manager. Bill Essen was a nineteen-year-old ex-student from Cleveland, Ohio, who moved to the city in January and worked for two months as a computer programmer until he volunteered at the Medical Section and met Carter Mehl. Mehl realized Essen's abilities and his dissatisfaction with the social irrelevancy of his position. He encouraged him to drop out of computers and into the Clinic. Essen did and gradually replaced Mehl as the leader of the Clinic family.

As a result of this recruitment, 558 Clayton Street had the youngest staff in its history. The people who now worked there resembled the early flower children in their nonviolence and therefore had little to identify with in the Haight other than humanity. They were virtually alone in the district, cut off from hip and straight worlds and still at odds with the city and its medical establishment. Yet they were committed to the Clinic and determined to carry on Peggy Sankot's tradition of intensive personal care.

The staff members also had several advantages over their predecessors.

They were aided by the shorter working schedule, by the lessened press of patients and by the fact that the procedures the organizers had initiated were now a matter of routine. Furthermore, they had few adverse hallucinogenic drug reactions to treat in the calm center and could call on their counterparts at the Annex to detoxify speed abusers. Because of these several factors, their efforts improved the operations at the Medical Section and greatly enhanced those at 409 Clayton Street a block away.

409 House was similarly blessed because it no longer had to carry the extra burden of medical treatment it did during the fall. This allowed for an expansion in the Publications Section, which soon housed not only the Clinic's educational service, speakers' bureau and film library, but also several research projects as well. The Commune Research Project that evolved out of the rural visits of the previous summer had to be suspended after the 1969 reopening because of staff limitations and because the winter weather precluded visits to many communes. But the staff was able to create a liaison with the Haight-Ashbury Research Project, a long-term study of young residents of the district which was conducted by the chief of psychiatry at Mt. Zion Hospital and a young psychologist, Dr. Stephen Pittel.

A third program was the Marijuana Research Project that was being conducted by Dr. Smith and Carter Mehl. Both men had seen few bad trips from marijuana in their experience in the Haight-Ashbury and were therefore surprised to find a much higher incidence of adverse reactions in San Francisco's population at large than they expected. Mehl and Dr. Smith learned that over ten percent of the approximately two hundred people they interviewed in a special sample had experienced acute anxiety, nausea, and perceptual distortions from smoking and especially from eating marijuana. These cases did not show up clinically because most young marijuana users reacted to their overdosage as if they were drunk — they feared being ridiculed by their peers if they became panicky, avoided public health treatment, and preferred to medicate themselves at home and sleep off their symptoms. This was particularly true of those younger adolescents who had problems with such high tetrahydrocannabinol preparations as the Supergrass available in the Haight, which was alleged to come from Vietnam.

At the same time, Mehl and Dr. Smith found that marijuana had precipitated acute psychoses in several patients throughout the city and confirmed their suspicion that adverse reactions of all sorts were most common in those who were turning on with marijuana for the first time. Their research was facilitated by a recent survey taken by the Langley-Porter Neuropsychiatric Institute which indicated that over seventy-five thousand San Franciscans, many of them adults, were now experimenting with grass.

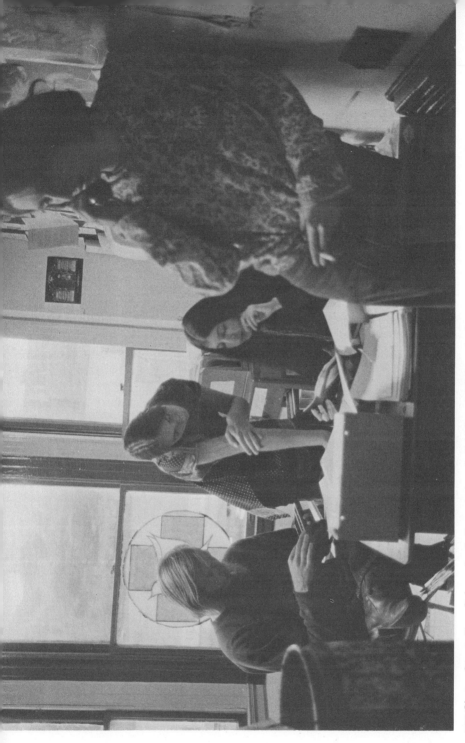

558 Clayton Street: Gene Dobson, Renée Sargent, Jeannie Kubicki and Bill Essen in the reception area.
(Elaine Mayes)

One such person, a disc jockey on a local classical music station, called the Clinic one evening after he became anxious while smoking marijuana during his radio show. Another, a stockbroker in his early forties who was a heavy drinker, apparently triggered a mild psychosis after he ate a pound of brownies spiked with marijuana. The stockbroker then picked up two hitchhiking hippies who delivered him to the Medical Section. Over four hundred straight persons like him sought treatment for drug problems during 1969. Although most were terrified by the Haight-Ashbury, the Clinic was one of the few medical institutions in San Francisco where they knew they would be neither arrested nor condemned.

This was the case in over thirty other cities which had their own free facilities by January, so Mehl, Dr. Smith, Alice deSwarte, a teacher of emotionally handicapped young people who had been his girl friend since the founding of the Clinic, Jim Sternfield, and three other criminology students who were helping organize the Berkeley Free Clinic began to formalize plans for a National Free Clinics Council. After contacting the Open Door Clinic in Seattle, Dr. Joseph Brenner's clinic in Cambridge and several other centers, they recognized the need for an organization which could circulate information, advise other drug-abuse centers, and provide for group malpractice insurance and funding.

Since political lobbying was a stated purpose of the organization, Dr. Smith proposed a National Free Clinics Conference at the Medical Center in 1970 and informed President Nixon and Robert Finch, then secretary of Health, Education and Welfare, of his plans. The President had paid considerable attention to private efforts to meet drug and adolescent health problems during his campaign, so the National Free Clinics Council hoped for a reaction from him or his adviser. Three detailed letters were sent to Washington during 1969. None received a reply.

Dr. Smith tried to remedy this unresponsiveness through the Drug Abuse Information Project, and also offered consultation to private treatment facilities and to the three hundred educational projects that were active in California by 1969. Concurrently, he, Dr. Meyers, Dr. Fort and others continued to fight for legislative change. Yet little was accomplished during 1969, for Governor Reagan and the legislature reemphasized punishment as a technique for controlling chemical consumption and rejected any attempt at education or therapy.

The governor vetoed one bill to lower the penalty for possession of marijuana to a misdemeanor and another which would have allowed hospitals to encourage addicts to seek treatment and rehabilitation by removing the requirement that they had to be reported to the police. The legislature, meanwhile, allowed the use of methadone in research projects but still limited its availability for treating heroin addiction. It also refused to remove marijuana from the pharmacologically unwarranted narcotics category. Over fifty thousand young people were therefore arrested for possession of this compound in California during 1969.

The only redeeming note in the legislative session that year was the defeat of a statute favored by Governor Reagan which would have made being under the influence of any psychoactive chemical a misdemeanor except under a doctor's care. In addition to tying up the courts for centuries, this desperate measure would have empowered the police to make mass arrests at places like the Clinic and thereby undermine their efficacy. The physicians were naturally relieved when this bill was defeated. But they interpreted it as yet another indication that government was still unwilling to take positive action in the drug-abuse field.

Once again, they answered this inaction with programs of their own. Among them were the efforts of Professor Loomis and twenty-five volunteer counselors and psychiatrists on the second floor of 409 Clayton Street, who were now seeing more than forty regular or short-term patients a day. Professor Loomis and others donated nine hundred patient hours a month at the Psychiatric Section, making it one of the most productive out-patient facilities in San Francisco. Their efforts were closely coordinated with those of Father Grosjean, Roger Smith and Gail Sadalla, who were conducting interviews in the back of the basement downstairs.

With Roger Smith involved in research, Father Frykman was now in complete command of the Drug Treatment Program. He shared his responsibilities with a staff of ten, including Bill Bathurst, an Amherst graduate and marine corps veteran who once worked in a therapeutic community for addicts in England, Bob Cronback, and John Hatch, who began volunteering at 558 Clayton Street after serving with the special forces in Vietnam. Their primary task was the training of physicians, school leaders and others who hoped to get young people off drugs and out of their self-destructive life-style.

Most of these counselors worked in the front of the basement, which also housed Father Frykman's office, a room for detoxification and a receiving area into which patients were funneled from other areas of the Clinic. This space was necessarily crowded, but the staff tried to make visitors feel at home by minimizing history-taking and other mechanical procedures. They offered a variety of services to those patients who responded positively. Some were detoxified under the supervision of physicians from the Medical Section or were referred to Mendocino, the Youth Drug Unit, Reality

House, Walden House and other facilities. Others were encouraged to participate in informal rap sessions or to join the nightly encounter groups run by the staff.

The Drug Treatment Program drew heavily from Synanon, the Esalen Institute and the Youth Drug Unit in designing these meetings, but it rejected the savage in-fighting so common to Synanon and prevented the groups from degenerating into the often grotesque acting-out ceremonies at Esalen. Father Frykman wanted his patients to realize, yet not act upon, their hostile feelings. He believed that many were too confused to profit from an intense emotional bombardment and therefore turned the encounters into a more gentle and supportive form of group therapy.

Although several hundred patients were reached by such methods, the core of the Drug Treatment Program was a therapeutic community. Its center was a group house at 1495 and 1497 Page Street that was divided into two flats. One of these housed several staff members and served as an auxiliary detoxification area; the other was occupied by from six to twelve patients who stayed an average of one month apiece and supported themselves by odd jobs. Drugs were not allowed at the group house, whose members were required to participate in the encounter sessions and were encouraged to undergo individual therapy.

Father Frykman originally conceived of his community as a loosely structured family in which people could be helped, but not steered, through their difficulties. He also hoped to provide treatment away from institutional facilities and within his patients' environment in keeping with the concept of community medicine. He started with eight young people, five of whom were amphetamine abusers. All swore off chemicals during their stay in the community, while three remained to help their comrades.

Yet there were problems with the program from its inception. Four of its initial eight members went back on drugs after they left the group house, as did so many veterans of the Mendocino Family. Many who followed were unable to outgrow their dependence on chemicals and refused to admit that they and not society were the source of their immediate problems, a habit which was reinforced by several of the volunteers. Bill Bathurst felt that "all of us benefited in one way or another from the residential program." But as Dr. Dernburg predicted, those who benefited most did so because they became members of the staff.

Furthermore, although Father Frykman maintained an excellent rapport with the patients, most of them required much more supervision than he intended. They related to him as a parent and needed much more nurturance and direction than he or the Clinic could provide. They also disobeyed constantly, giving Father Frykman little choice but discipline, which illu-

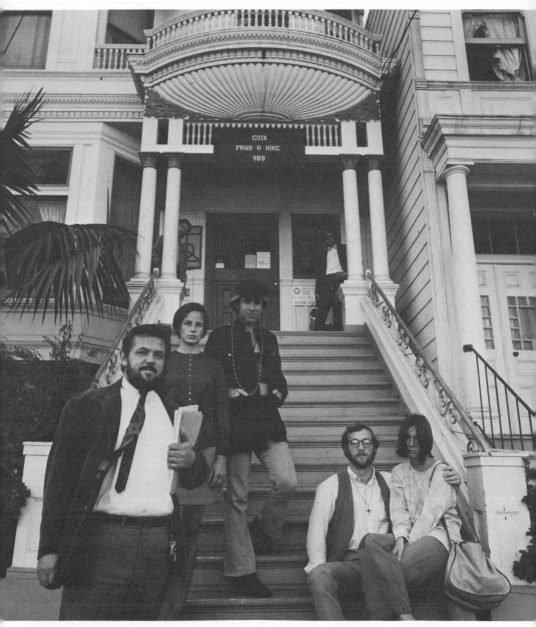

409 Clayton Street: Father John Frykman, Ramsey Raymond, Bill Bathurst, John Hatch and Dianne Gueldin of the Drug Treatment Program.
(Elaine Mayes)

minated the fact that he and the Clinic had still not found the midpoint between authority and acceptance which is crucial to successful therapy.

Finally, the program was so plagued by financial limitations and by the nature of the new population that it could not reach all of the Haight-Ashbury. The young blacks remained wary of white counselors; the hoodies were not amenable to treatment; and so many patients suckered the staff out of time and money that it had to be educated about the intransigence of psychopaths. Father Frykman was willing to be a father to people like Randy, but not on a full-time basis. Father Frykman needed professional help, particularly when the street people began using barbiturates instead of amphetamines.

Sedation and the Relief of Anxiety

Barbiturates are classified pharmocologically as nonselective central nervous system depressants because they can depress all excitable areas of the nervous system. Dr. Meyers further notes that they should be considered sedative-hypnotic-general anesthetics because graded doses of the compounds produce the same four stages of depression seen with alcohol. True barbiturates are derivatives of barbituric acid, a condensation of malonic acid and urea that was prepared by a German chemist in 1864. The first hypnotic barbiturate, barbitol or diethylbarbituric acid, was introduced into medicine in 1903 under the trade name Veronal. The second, phenobarbital, was introduced as Luminol in 1912. Over twenty-five hundred barbiturates were subsequently synthesized, fifty of which are in wide use today.

Barbiturates may be divided into four general types on the basis of their duration of action. They include long-acting compounds, with a duration of six hours or more; intermediate-acting, with a duration of from three to six hours; short-acting, with a duration of less than three hours; and ultrashort-acting, with a duration of several minutes. The most widely employed long-acting barbiturate is phenobarbital, while the most common intermediate-acting is probably amobarbital sodium (Amytal). Examples of short-acting barbiturates are pentobarbital sodium (Nembutal) and secobarbital sodium (Seconal). The ultrashort-acting ones include sodium thiopental Pentothal). Amobarbital is also mixed with secobarbital in Tuinal; a combination of amobarbital and dexedrine sulfate is marketed as Dexamyl; and a phenobarbital-methamphetamine mixture is sold under the trade name Desbutal.

Closely related to these true barbiturates are several sedative-hypnotic-general anesthetics which have been misrepresented as tranquilizers by certain pharmaceutical companies. Among them are the intermediate-acting glutethimide, or Doriden, and the short-acting meprobamate (Equanil or Miltown), chlordiazepoxide (Librium), diazepam (Valium) and chloral hydrate, the active ingredient in the "Mickey Finn." These compounds differ from true tranquilizers like Thorazine in that they produce four stages of central nervous system depression, including disinhibition. They also cause physical addiction, psychological dependence, anticonvulsant action and voluntary muscle relaxation in high doses and with continuous administration. True tranquilizers do not cause anesthesia, are convulsant in their action, inhibit impulses, are not habituating or addicting and possess atropinelike peripheral effects. They are used in treating psychotic patients, while barbiturates and barbituratelike drugs should be employed to suppress anxiety.

The peripheral effects of barbiturates and their equivalents are comparable to those of other sedative-hypnotic-general anesthetics. The effects vary with dosage and are likely to include a decrease in respiration and heart rate, a relaxation of the smooth muscle of the gastrointestinal tract and a reduction in urine flow. The central effects of these compounds stem from a progressive depression which may be initially experienced as disinhibition and euphoria. The compounds possess few of the analgesic properties of alcohol but do provide some relief from pain by also causing a drowsiness and sedation that may culminate in sleep. This differs from true physiological sleep in that most of the drugs, with the exception of chloral hydrate, reduce the time spent in the rapid eye movement or dreaming phase.

Although reduction in REM sleep may be psychologically harmful, the short- or intermediate-acting barbiturates and barbituratelike compounds are often prescribed in single one hundred or two hundred milligram doses to induce sleep on a temporary basis or as part of the treatment of chronic insomnia. Long-acting preparations are also used in fifteen to thirty-five milligram doses three or four times daily to provide sedation and relief from stress and either situational or neurotic anxiety, or to diminish the excitement generated by amphetamines and other agents while maintaining, and actually strengthening, their mood-elevating effects.

Barbiturates and their equivalents are also of great value in controlling the acute convulsions that occur in tetanus and grand mal epilepsy. Preparations with rapid onset and relatively short duration of action are usually given intravenously for these purposes, as they are to combat the convulsions caused by cocaine, strychnine and other local anesthetics and poisons. In addition, intravenous injections of ultrashort-acting agents like Pentothal are employed to provide anesthesia prior to surgery.

These drugs have comparatively few undesirable aftereffects, a fact which explains their wide use in medicine. Yet barbiturates and barbituratelike compounds can be harmful. The drowsiness they produce may lead to serious accidents. They can impair coordination and performance while deluding users, as amphetamines do, into thinking their abilities are increased. They often cause dizziness, a hangover and a feeling of lingering lassitude. And many users become dependent on sedatives and sleeping pills and develop a tolerance which forces them to increase their dosages and results in severe physical symptoms when the drugs are withdrawn. As with amphetamines, the distinction between therapeutic use and abuse of these chemicals is frequently blurred.

One reason is that many people take sleeping pills to induce an intoxication comparable to that of alcohol. The oral ingestion of a one-hundred-milligram dose of short-acting barbiturates usually causes sleep if the drugs are used in an appropriate setting with that purpose in mind. But if sleep is neither achieved nor intended, people may show signs of euphoria and confusion resembling those of alcohol intoxication. The disinhibition characteristic of this acute toxicity usually leads to sluggishness, slurring of speech, increased emotional lability and nystagmus, an involuntary oscillation of the eyeballs. Excessive irritability and moroseness are also common, as are hostility and paranoia.

In larger doses, these drugs produce a state of deep anesthesia which is followed by respiratory and circulatory depression. Such overdosage is particularly frequent in those whose toxic confusion leads them to forget the extent of their dosage, in those who consume barbiturates with alcohol and thereby intensify their effects, and in those who use the chemicals singly and in combination to commit suicide. Acute barbiturate toxicity and overdosage have become major problems in most urban centers and reached an incidence of over ten thousand cases in New York City from 1963 to 1969. About one-half of these attempted suicide; twenty percent of them succeeded. Barbiturates and their equivalents in combination with alcohol have also figured in the deaths of Marilyn Monroe, Judy Garland, Alan Ladd and a host of celebrities and movie stars.

Adverse reactions are usually treated in intensive care units, as are those to alcohol. Patients should be urged to keep moving and talking if they are conscious and may be induced to vomit, although this increases the risk of their gagging or suffocating on regurgitated fluids. If coma has occurred, they require supportive treatment to maintain an air passage and to continue breathing so that their lungs do not fill up with fluid. Respiration may be assisted mechanically, while electrocardiographic monitoring is necessary. The patient's blood pressure should also be monitored, and blood, plasma and glucose may be administered if shock occurs. Secondary lung infections can develop in cases of depressed breathing, so antibiotics may be necessary to prevent pneumonia, along with diuretics to increase urine flow.

An equally grave problem is chronic barbiturate toxicity, which resembles alcoholism. Its symptoms consist of extensive neurological damage, greatly impaired coordination and emotional lability, skin rashes and malnutrition. Patients who are taking barbiturates intravenously may also experience cellulitis, immense abscesses of the subcutical fossae and an inflammatory reaction that follows the infiltration of the drugs under the skin. Treatment is comparable to that for chronic alcoholism and includes the administration of glucose, proteins, thiamine and other vitamins. It also usually requires extensive aftercare and treatment for withdrawal.

Because of the pharmacological similarities between true barbiturates and drugs like Miltown, the term general depressant withdrawal syndrome is applied to all. A typical course of withdrawal from short-acting compounds is much more serious than that from opiates like heroin. It usually begins with extreme anxiety about the time of the next scheduled dose. Cramps and nausea, which may leave patients too weak to walk, follow. These symptoms increase within twenty-four to forty-eight hours of abstinence, at which point convulsions of the intensity of grand mal epilepsy may occur.

Some patients who have seizures may then show improvement, but more than half of those reported proceed to a psychotic reaction that mimics the delirium tremens of withdrawal from alcohol or the paranoid-schizophrenic reaction associated with amphetamines. Anxiety mounts during this period, while frightening dreams may be followed by insomnia. Visual hallucinations, disorientation of time and space, and agitation may then lead to exhaustion and cardiovascular collapse. The treatment of depressant withdrawal is based on the twin principles of hospitalizing patients and never attempting abrupt withdrawal. Patients traditionally have been given regular doses of a short-acting barbiturate to maintain a continuous state of mild intoxication which is gradually tapered off after seven to eight days.

Improvements on this technique suggested by Clinic researchers may be necessary in the future, for acute and chronic barbiturate toxicity has increased dramatically at all levels of our society. Many of these compounds are classified as dangerous drugs, the illicit manufacture, sale and/or possession of which is prohibited by state and federal law. Yet they are widely available by ordinary medical prescriptions which can be refilled repeatedly or obtained from more than one physician. Dr. Joel Fort notes that over one million pounds of barbiturates and so-called tranquilizers were dispensed by prescription alone during 1969, a year in which hundreds of thousands of

Americans were estimated to be misusing and abusing the chemicals. This distribution is sufficient to provide every person in the country with at least one one-hundred-milligram sleeping pill a day.

Most of these people are housewives, businessmen and other adults — the same kind who abuse pharmaceutical amphetamines. But barbiturate abuse is also common in the underground, where the drugs are obtained from legitimate or forged prescriptions, from drugstore or warehouse robberies or by way of Mexico, where they are ordered in huge quantities from American pharmaceutical companies. The compounds are known by a number of slang terms on the black market. Included are Amytal (blues, blue devils, blue dolls), phenobarbital (phennies), glutethimide (goofers), Librium (sleepies, tranks), chloral hydrate (coral), Tuinal (double trouble, rainbows), Nembutal (nembies, yellows, yellow bullets, yellow jackets, yellow dolls), and Seconal (seggies, reds, red devils, red bullets, red dolls). The abuse of these underground drugs far exceeds that of narcotics today.

Valley of the Dolls

Reds containing one hundred milligrams of Seconal cost a quarter in the Haight-Ashbury, where barbiturates and barbituratelike compounds were taken in every possible way. Some bikers and sidewalk commandos swallowed the drugs by the half-dozen to obtain a euphoric high and to demonstrate their *machismo*. Others medicated themselves with oral doses of barbs and speed comparable to the drugs used by their counterparts in straight society. Many high school students who shopped at the smorgasbord went on weekend sprees in the Haight and then dropped reds, blues, or yellows during the week before class.

The members of the new population often dissolved barbiturates in water and injected the mixture directly into their veins. They obtained only a slight orgasmic rush when compared to that of speed or heroin, but they did manage to sedate themselves. They became stuporous after shooting up and would stumble up and down Haight Street glowering at everyone. A few of the more notorious barb freaks took as much as three thousand milligrams of Seconal in several doses a day. Two Valium addicts were seen at the Medical Section, as were four alcoholics who injected barbiturates to sedate themselves during alcohol withdrawal. One fifty-eight-year-old abuser told the physicians that he had "started with Veronal in the good old days."

Dr. Smith also observed a ten-year-old barbiturate abuser who was first seen at 558 Clayton Street when he came in to be detoxified. He was the son of a local real estate salesman and apparently acquired his habit from taking his mother's sleeping pills. The patient was frequently stoned for weeks at a time, yet his parents never noticed his condition. At first he never took a high enough dose to develop more than a slight dependence. But his parents left him alone for three weeks while they attended a sales convention, at which point he increased his intake, became addicted, and was sent to the Medical Center to begin withdrawal.

Although this patient had a single drug dependence, many of those seen at the Clinic had substituted barbiturates for or mixed them with other compounds as early as 1968. Several young people said that they took Seconal with LSD, the peace pill or STP to decrease the latters' peripheral effects. One patient, a nineteen-year-old male, came to the Medical Section for treatment of an abscess after missing his vein while injecting an STP-LSD-Nembutal combination. "I wanted a smoother trip," he said. "Shooting acid makes the world look pretty, and barbs are great for getting down."

More common during the early months of 1969 was the practice of using barbiturates or their equivalents in place of or in addition to heroin. Well over three hundred opiate addicts were living in the Haight-Ashbury at this point, and many switched to barbs after they found the local heroin to be high in price and low in potency when compared to that in other areas. Prolonged high-dose barbiturate consumption helped these addicts withdraw from narcotics, but they then had to be eased off barbs.

A case in point was one twenty-eight-year-old woman who arrived at the Clinic in the early stages of withdrawal after shooting approximately fifteen hundred milligrams of Seconal daily for several weeks. She had begun using heroin at the age of seventeen in New York City and was hospitalized there on two occasions. The patient moved to the Haight in late 1968 "because New York was too much of a hassle." After finding that the West Coast heroin was "overcut and too damned expensive," she turned to barbiturates as substitutes until she sought treatment to avoid the possibility of convulsions during withdrawal.

Over three dozen such patients were seen during January and February of 1969, but they were a minority when compared with those who were using barbiturates in place of amphetamines. Barbs had been essential to the speed subculture since its beginning, and many young people used a combination of the two drugs to achieve a heightened mood elevation or employed the depressant to counteract the stimulative effects of amphetamines. As the subculture grew, its members began to fear the comedown from high-dose speed consumption as badly as barbiturate addicts feared withdrawal. One girl told Roger Smith that "it was so rough I kept going on a run when I was physically goddamn incapable of it, just because I was so righteously afraid to crash. I couldn't face the fucking comedown and I would do a couple more hits of crank until I could find something to ground myself. Things kept getting worse, and I needed more and more barbs."

Another common use of the drugs documented earlier by Smith was to bolster courage. Randy acknowledged this in explaining that "barbs are what make you really mean and nasty, specially if you want to be. It's the combination of the two. Once you've got enough goofers so you're ready to kill some cat, you have to shoot up the crank so you get the energy to do it. Barbs really tear your head apart. They overpower the speed and the speed gets you where you're paranoid and when you're coming down it's real fear. But everybody out here is looking for a mellow downer. I don't know a speed freak alive who doesn't use barbs."

Although Randy began his search for a mellow downer as early as the fall of 1968, the rest of the amphetamine-based subculture did not catch up to him until January and February of 1969. Some young people turned to opiates to achieve sedation and Terminal Euphoria at that point, but barbs were more immediately popular than heroin because they were cheaper in price and because they lacked a Negro identification. They therefore became drugs of choice within the district as its young residents tried to escape their environment and overcome their despair.

But escape was impossible, and those street people who used barbiturates developed almost as many psychological and physical symptoms as they did with speed. They also increased their criminal activity, both because their tolerance required a greater financial investment and because of the toxic effects of the compounds. Their greater violence in turn made the barb freaks outcasts until the rest of their companions joined them in becoming addicts. The amphetamine subculture thus became in part a barbiturate subculture whose members streamed into the Clinic for aid.

One example was an eighteen-year-old girl who injected amphetamines for six months during 1968 until she was on the verge of psychosis. Her physical problems also increased, so she started shooting reds. The patient missed the orgasmic action of speed but obtained a comparable euphoria and felt relieved as her paranoia abated. She then became addicted and was raped by three dealers when she could not pay for their products. She arrived at 558 Clayton Street with a fresh scar running down her right cheek and a two-inch-diameter abscess bulging from her left arm.

This patient asked for detoxification and withdrawal on a permanent basis, but little could be done for her. She and her contemporaries needed their drugs for medicinal purposes; one went so far as to write "Give me Librium or give me meth" on the waiting-room wall. These young people could be treated for their abscesses and other complaints at the Medical

Section, yet because neither it nor 409 House were appropriate settings for detoxification, many emergencies had to be taken to Mission Emergency Hospital.

The Clinic physicians regretted this procedure, for they had little faith in the drug-abuse medicine practiced by the Public Health Department. Their feeling stemmed in part from their experience with a volunteer at 558 Clayton who was taken to San Francisco General after making a suicide attempt with five thousands milligrams of Seconal. The girl had been shooting barbs for several weeks, but her physician failed to determine the tolerance she had developed and instead treated her acute intoxication as an isolated episode. After giving her a cursory examination and a lecture on her moral degradation, he released the girl from the hospital. She began convulsing the next day because his treatment sent her into withdrawal.

The patient eventually recovered after Dr. Fred Shick, who was now taking his internship in San Francisco, stayed up all night assisting her. But Dr. Smith and others were so upset by her case that they made every attempt to place patients for several weeks in private facilities and at the Mendocino State Hospital. This approach proved to be successful, and several returned from Mendocino to start counseling at the Psychiatric Section. Father Frykman managed to assimilate seven of them into his family.

By February, the Clinic was being visited by more than ten barbiturate abusers a day. Having so many patients forced the staff to rely more on General Hospital, but they employed a technique worked out during 1968 by Dr. Smith, a psychiatric resident and an intern to facilitate withdrawal. This treatment method was inspired by the substitution of the long-acting narcotic, methadone, in treating withdrawal from heroin and other opiates. The doctors started by taking detailed patient histories. Then, instead of using the traditional regular doses of short-acting barbiturates with their patients, they began giving them phenobarbital over a short period to achieve a stabilized and less dangerous intoxication. They then gradually lowered the phenobarbital dosage while using methadone with those addicts who were simultaneously undergoing heroin withdrawal.

The physicians found that this substitution technique shortened the withdrawal period, lessened the suffering of their patients, did not increase the incidence of seizures, and proved successful in most cases. An example was a forty-year-old white male who was formerly taking twenty-five hundred milligrams of Nembutal and Seconal with varying doses of heroin and codeine each day. He was withdrawn from opiates and barbiturates in six days. He then joined Synanon, where he overcame his addiction while a resident there.

The doctors also had their share of failures. One was a thirty-year-old barbiturate and heroin addict who was initially given methadone and phenobarbital. Her dosage was reduced after the fourth day of treatment, but she left the ward that afternoon and returned to her abuse pattern. She died from a barb overdose within ten days.

In addition to this patient, hundreds of people in the Haight-Ashbury remained addicted to barbiturates. Over one hundred and eighty eventually came to the Clinic, but although the facility helped some of them, it probably had its greatest impact outside the immediate area. Drs. Smith, Gay and Matzger and Father Frykman spoke often at local grammar and high schools during this period and were instrumental in educating teachers about the drugs that were beginning to appear in their classrooms. And in the doctors' absence, young people in the Haight who abused barbs became even more desperate.

"Rip-offs are quite the fashion now that reds are big," one young man told Roger Smith. "People who used to pride themselves on dealing would rather go and rip these days. Like Shotgun Mike, who is just about the best rip-off artist around. He comes in, sticks a gun in your head, and says, 'O.K., motherfucker, give me your bread or I'm gonna kill you.' He either has a pistol or a sawed-off shotgun, and he will usually put a shot in the wall on one side of your head, so you better do what he says."

Smith believed that this increase in burns and rip-offs tended to accelerate the tempo of ritualized gang warfare in the Haight-Ashbury. Thus, he was hardly surprised when, a week after the nine bikers were convicted of raping and murdering Ann Jiminez, three young people were found in an apartment on Page Street with their hands tied and bullet holes in the backs of their heads. The police identified this as a revenge-type killing and seconded Smith's prediction about increased violence. A week later, it was the Clinic's turn.

Early Monday morning, February sixteenth, three young blacks pried open the front door of the Medical Section and surprised Gene Dobson. They bound and blindfolded him and threatened to hit him with a hammer unless he opened the safe and the pharmacy. Dobson swore that he did not know the combination, so his assailants broke into the pharmacy, only to learn that narcotics and dangerous drugs were not kept on the premises. They then stuffed Dobson in a broom closet and walked off with two typewriters and three-hundred-dollars worth of medical supplies.

409 Clayton Street also experienced a rash of violence during February. One of Professor Loomis's students was almost killed by a Seconal addict, and the receiving area of the Drug Treatment Program was frequently invaded by young people stoned on barbs. Although two of these invaders improved considerably in the therapeutic community, others were difficult

to manage because of their surliness and paranoia. Guns were drawn on several occasions at the group house, and a knife fight was started by the son of a southern California pharmacist who was using Nembutal and speed.

Shortly after the knife fight, two volunteer nurses were assaulted by a barb freak, while three Gypsy Jokers stabbed a black resident after he walked down Haight Street with a white girl. His death was followed by a ritualistic knife slaying involving a street dealer who was once associated with Superspade. A twenty-four-year-old white man used a hunting rifle three days later to kill a seventeen-year-old black boy. In all, seventeen murders, fifty-eight rapes, two hundred and nine cases of assault and almost fifteen hundred burglaries were reported in the Haight during the first two months of 1969. "The street population is the smallest we've had since 1964," a police lieutenant said, "but we've seen a steady increase in murder and violent crime."

Not reported to the lieutenant were at least a dozen murders of informers and other victims of gangster-style revenge which were disguised as overdoses to confuse the authorities. Roger Smith learned of one case in which an infamous burn artist was injected with ten thousand micrograms of acid and left to die in the Mission district. He was also told of a runaway who refused to ball seven motorcycle riders and was then injected with eight thousand milligrams of Seconal.

A third case was related by an interviewee at the Amphetamine Research Project:

My sister was going with a biker who's on trial for trying to murder her ex-old man. They fed him full of one hundred reds and ditched him in a cemetery out in south San Francisco for three days. And he was still alive — he testified. They did it because he took them for dope, money and for guns. He ripped them off for four pistols, which were, you know, hot pistols — but good ones.

And there's definitely going to be more violence. There's a lower type of society — there's less money — and more competition for it. A lot of people here now can't go to the Tenderloin or North Beach because they don't know many people; not so much the cooks or big distributors — they're known everywhere — but your street dealers and sidewalk commandos. They have only one place where they can be, and that's here. I'm convinced they're running out of places to hide.

Another Exodus

Roger Smith needed no convincing about the fate of the Haight-Ashbury. He had interviewed over two hundred amphetamine and barbiturate abusers by this time and knew that violence would continue to increase in the district. Three tape recorders had been stolen from the Amphetamine Research Project during February, prompting Smith and Gail Sadalla to erect wire screens and install a series of locks to protect the basement. In March, they made plans to move out of 409 Clayton Street. In May, they finally joined Dr. Meyers in his offices at the Medical Section.

Several other staff members preceded Smith and Miss Sadalla out of the Haight. The first was Jackie, who gave birth to a seven-pound boy on March tenth at the University of California Medical Center. Over two dozen former and current staff members were outside the delivery room that evening to wish her good fortune and to say good-bye. For Jackie had decided to raise her son, whom she named Siddharta, outside the city. They and three volunteers from the Medical Section were safely nestled in a large farmhouse in Mendocino County by the middle of May.

Jackie's departure served as a signal to the rest of the staff. Shortly after she left San Francisco, Carter Mehl, who was tired of working with difficult patients, announced that he would soon return to Ohio State to finish his studies and to create a commune on his parents' land. Judy St. Onge, who had been working at a local halfway house since leaving the Clinic, decided with four other ex-staff members to join him. Bill Essen stayed on as business manager and also assumed Mehl's administrative duties. He shared them with Renée Sargent and Delores Craton until Miss Craton decided she was losing her influence at the Clinic and also chose to leave town.

Gene Dobson and Jeannie Kubicki then moved up the staff ladder, as a half-dozen young people whom Essen recruited from Cleveland and elsewhere filled clerical and paramedical positions. But there staff members were even younger than their predecessors, so the physicians took a stronger parental role. Several doctors began giving the employees extra living allowances out of their own pockets; Dr. Smith and Alice deSwarte held staff dinners and meetings at his new house near the University of California; and in June the Clinic leased two flats at 120 and 122 Del Mar Street to protect and perpetuate the 558 Clayton Street family.

Although most of the staff members remained in the district that summer, several took time out with Dr. Smith and Ruth Fleshman to revisit the urban and rural communes. They were assisted by a young medical student and his wife, who traveled extensively through the western United States dispensing health information and checking on former members of the new community and the staff. In northern California, the researchers found Jackie and her companions living peacefully, planting a vegetable and marijuana garden, and planning to enroll in a nearby state college in the fall. They also encountered Alan, who was still bothered by respiratory problems but seemed healthy and happy to be alive. Alan had emerged as a respected guru in his living group. The same was true of Allen Cohen, former editor of the *Haight-Ashbury Oracle,* who was now raising chickens and educating young people about natural child-rearing on a twenty-acre farm.

Delores Craton organized several medical visits to these and other establishments before she left the Clinic. The doctors found the sanitary and health conditions of most of the communes unchanged from the previous summer. They observed many more infants and learned that the rural residents still suffered problems with hepatitis and venereal disease. The physicians gave what medications they could to the hippies and also treated a number of fractures. But because they lacked the necessary financial resources, no thorough delivery of medical services could be made.

One thing which was accomplished during the summer was an expansion of the Commune Research Project under the leadership of Dr. Smith and Jim Sternfield. They began by collecting information about the size, location and living conditions of the many residences that had been visited. Dr. Smith then met with Dr. Bennett Berger, a sociologist from the University of California at Davis who had launched his own NIMH-funded research project. A cooperative agreement was reached, after which Dr. Berger applied to the National Institute of Mental Health for a five-thousand-dollar grant that would provide small salaries for Gene Dobson and Jeannie Kubicki to assist him on a study of child socialization in hippie communes.

Another research project was initiated in the early summer by Dr. Alan Matzger. The Clinic had given up with the city at this point, but the continual pressure of the *Chronicle* and the constant improvement in its own services had resulted in the facility being accepted, albeit reluctantly, by the Public Health Department. The Medical and Psychiatric sections drew support from Dr. Francis Curry, who would succeed Dr. Ellis Sox as public health director after Dr. Sox's wife died under mysterious circumstances. Dr. Curry gave no money to the Clinic, but his cooperation allowed the organizers to finally apply for federal aid.

One possible source was the National Institute of Mental Health, which had recently allocated over one million dollars to four areas in the city. One such area was in the jurisdiction of the Westside Mental Health Center, a consortium of facilities located in the section of San Francisco which included the Fillmore and the Haight-Ashbury. Because a portion of the Westside budget was earmarked for drug-abuse treatment, Dr. Matzger assumed that 409 and 558 Clayton Street would qualify for part of the grant. But the original director of the Westside consortium wanted the money for competing projects and insisted in spite of evidence to the contrary that drugs were not a problem in his area.

A second consortium was the proposed Northeast Mental Health Center, to be under the direction of Dr. Arthur Carfagni. The Clinic did not fit geographically into the area to be covered by this consortium, which included North Beach and the Tenderloin, but Dr. Carfagni believed that it would qualify for assistance because it had served so many former and present residents of the section and had been so neglected in the past. He also felt that its chances would be enhanced if Father Frykman expanded the Drug Treatment Program into the Tenderloin and North Beach, both of which were beginning to rival the Haight and the Fillmore in the severity of their drug problems. Father Frykman took his advice and started to look for donated space within the two districts during the summer. Meanwhile, Dr. Matzger continued to negotiate with both the Westside and the Northeast Mental Health centers for funds.

At the same time, he was urged by Dr. David Berman of the United States Public Health Service to apply to that organization for a forty-thousand-dollar grant through which he might determine the health needs of the Haight-Ashbury, design a program to meet them, and then reapply for further finances to implement his plan. Dr. Matzger wrote up a grant proposal, adding a provision that would give Renée Sargent and two other staff members paid positions. He was awarded the grant in October and thereby became the Clinic's first full-time physician. This timing proved to be crucial, for the search for mellow downers brought many young people in the Haight to opiates by the early fall.

Death without Permanence — Life without Pain

The natural alkaloids of opium, their semisynthetic derivatives and the synthetic opiate analogs, or opioids, are classified pharmacologically as central nervous system modifiers because they manifest both depressant and excitory effects on the nervous system. These compounds differ from sedative-hypnotic-general anesthetics in that they do not cause nonspecific depression in low doses. They are categorized as narcotics because they can induce sleep and as narcotic analgesics because they are employed primarily for the relief of pain.

Morphine, codeine and some twenty other alkaloids occur naturally in the seed pods of the opium poppy, *Papaver somniferum,* which is indigenous to Asia Minor. The alkaloids are extracted from a gum which is exuded from the plants and collected by a laborious manual process. They are then either used directly, modified to produce such semisynthetic derivatives as dihydroxomorphone (Dilaudid) and dihydroxohydroxycodeinone (Percodan) or converted by a simple and illegal process into heroin, which is approximately twice as potent as morphine in its central effects and is known chemically as diacetylmorphine. These drugs are pharmacologically similar to such synthetic analogs as phenylpiperdone or meperidine (Demerol), phenyhelptylamine or methadone (Dolophine) and propoxyphene (Darvon).

Although the latter compounds are of recent origin, the use of opium alkaloids predates recorded history and is mentioned by the Sumerians as early as 4000 B.C. The word "opium" is derived from the Greek name for juice, and the opium plant was employed medicinally and recreationally by both the Greeks and the Romans. It was also used to treat dysentery in China, where it was taken orally and by sniffing or was smoked in the small bowls of pipes which are heated by a flame that vaporizes the crude opium and allows it to be inhaled.

Western scientists began studying the opium poppy in the eighteenth century, when a German pharmacist isolated the plant's most potent alkaloid and named it after Morpheus, the Greek god of dreams. Other alkaloids were soon discovered, and they, rather than crude opium, spread throughout the medical world. A search for new synthetics was then initiated, while the importation of Chinese labor during the nineteenth century and the introduction of the hypodermic needle increased the rate of traditional forms of opiate addiction and caused the beginning of an intravenous pattern of abuse in Europe and the United States. Morphine, codeine, and other opiates and opioids were employed in a wide variety on nonprescription medications which hundreds of thousands of people used and abused in this country prior to the First World War.

At that point, the drugs were made subject to the restrictions of the Harrison Narcotics Act, a punitive piece of legislation which has severely limited medical efforts to treat addiction until this day. Persons using morphine and other compounds are now subjected to a complicated prescription procedure, while states like California have imposed two- to ten-year sentences for first occurrences of possession of illegal narcotics and life imprisonment for further offenses.

The natural alkaloids and their equivalents have marked peripheral actions, the most immediately noticeable of which is a constriction of the pupils to pinpoint size. The drugs suppress coughing, cause a warm, flushed skin because of their dilating effect on surface blood vessels, and depress respiration and the heart rate in high doses. They also depress the secretion of gastric acid and liver bile, decrease urine flow, and reduce the propulsive contractions of the intestines, thereby exerting a constipating effect that explains their role in the treatment of dysentery.

More pronounced is the opiates' mixed stimulative and depressant effect on the central nervous system. Their essential central effect is to relieve pain not by blocking impulse transmission in the nervous system but by altering the perception of and the psychological reaction to pain. This analgesia occurs before and often without sleep when the chemicals are administered in small or moderate doses; that is, in amounts from five to ten milligrams. Pain is relieved regardless of its origin and intensity, while euphoria is frequently achieved.

Dr. Meyers explains that such euphoria is not a universal reaction. Morphine will often produce a subjectively unpleasant reaction which is often accompanied by nausea and mental confusion in people unfamiliar with the drug and not in pain. But if pain is present and euphoria is desired, morphine may cause it while inducing complete sedation and relief of anxiety in even the most potentially distressing situation. Persons using the compound under these circumstances are often aware of the source of their pain, yet they gain a supreme indifference to suffering.

The indifference stems in part from the fact that narcotics, more than any other drugs, can suppress those instinctual drives that usually motivate people to assuage hunger, seek sexual gratification, and respond to provocation with anger. They thus produce a state of drive satiation and a feeling of nurturance which is comparable to that enjoyed by fortunate children in early infancy. These compounds do not induce the sense of protoplasmic consciousness associated with hallucinogens, the general depression of barbiturates, the general stimulation of amphetamines or the delirium of such parasympatholytic agents as atropine. But if taken intravenously, they bring about an orgasmic rush that is as powerful than that of amphetamines. This feeling is followed by a toxic numbness and insulation which one addict has described as "death without permanence — life without pain."

Although the intensity of the intravenous state is unfamiliar to most people, many have experienced the numbing effects of morphine and other opiates used in medicine. These agents are often administered orally, subcutaneously or intramuscularly in five-milligram doses with a duration of action of approximately four hours to soothe the agony of intestinal spasms, terminal illness and surgery. They are also employed to control extreme anxiety in certain cases, to suppress coughing, and to treat severe diarrhea. Paregoric, or tincture of opium, is usually prescribed in the latter situation, while codeine, which is much less potent than morphine, is used in such over-the-counter cough preparations as Robitussin A-C and Romilar. These medications are relatively safe, but some patients do experience nausea, restlessness, confusion, constipation and recurrent depression from their continuous administration.

The greatest danger from prolonged use or abuse of the opiates is the psychological dependence and physical addiction that occur because the drugs alter the body's chemistry in such a way that normal metabolic functioning becomes impossible if they are withdrawn. Patients frequently become dependent on morphine in hospital settings or abuse Darvon and other prescription preparations. So do doctors and nurses. Their most common drug choice is usually meperidine, or Demerol, which is erroneously assumed to be less addicting than morphine.

Two hundred thousand Americans were estimated to be addicted to legal and illegal narcotics in 1969. Although some were health professionals and could obtain narcotics through hospitals or pharmacies, the great majority used heroin that was smuggled into the country from Mexico or the Middle and Far East by professional criminals or brought in by servicemen returning from Southeast Asia. Then, as now, experimental narcotics use usually begins by smoking opium, sniffing or snorting heroin, or taking heroin and other compounds orally. Users may proceed from this point to skin popping, in which they inject the drugs under the skin. The next step is intravenous injection, or mainlining, which is alleged to be desirable both because of the attendant rush and because of the self-feeding implications of the needle. Most users are known as junkies at this point in their addiction. Others consider themselves chippers or occasional users and insist, perhaps euphemistically, that they can regulate their consumption through self-control.

Such occasional use is complicated by the fact that tolerance to the effects of narcotics develops more rapidly and to a much greater extent than tolerance to other drugs. Although it is possible to obtain analgesia and sedation from doses in the therapeutic range for indefinite periods with intermittent use, persons given repeated and progressively larger doses over a six to eight week period are soon able to tolerate many multiples of the original dose and may consume as much as three thousand milligrams of morphine or heroin in several doses a day. In the process they develop a cross-tolerance to other narcotics.

This tolerance is a comparatively minor problem to physicians and wealthy users who have access to a steady supply of pharmacologically consistent drugs. But to other addicts the acquisition of opiates becomes an extremely expensive procedure. A kilogram of morphine costing three hundred and fifty dollars in Vietnam or Turkey is worth more than two hundred and fifty thousand dollars after it is converted into heroin, passed through upper-level distributors, and sold on the street in fifteen cent (fifteen dollar) and quarter (twenty-five dollar) balloons or glassine bags containing from three to four hundred milligrams of white or brown powder. The thirty to forty milligrams of heroin (which is also called "H," "horse," "Harry," "junk," "shit," "stuff," "skag," and "smack") in these containers is generally mixed with procaine, quinine or milk sugar. Because of its low (three to five) percent composition, many addicts develop such a tolerance to street smack that they are soon shooting from three to fifteen quarter bags a day.

Some people manage to limit themselves to nickel and dime bags used for sniffing or skin popping, while others attempt to curb their tolerance by taking barbiturates, amphetamines and/or alcohol. But most become trapped in an addictive pattern which leads them to depend on opiate dealers, who are called connections and/or pushers, as they might depend on a doctor for medical care. The addicts develop hustling skills to pay for their medication and engage in such criminal practices as petty theft, forgery, prostitution, burglary and/or dealing. Assuming that each of the two hundred thousand narcotics addicts in the United States had a one-hundred-dollar-a-day habit, the total cost to society from their thefts, robberies and related offenses exceeded six billion dollars in 1969.

This figure included relatively few crimes of violence, for opiate addicts are characteristically unassaultive, especially while stoned. Unlike amphetamines, barbiturates and alcohol, narcotics per se seem to inhibit aggression; it is the need for them, rather than their pharmacological action, that motivates criminality. The drugs also have few debilitating effects on the mind and body, so that addicts should be able to live as long as nonaddicts. The fact that they do not is related less to the chronic action of narcotics than to their illegality and to the dangers which accompany their abusers' life-style.

These dangers are comparable to, although more intense than, those associated with all underground drugs. Narcotics addicts run a regular risk of being poisoned if they have untrustworthy connections. They stand a good chance of being beaten up or arrested by the police or being burned by competitors when they try to cop, or acquire chemicals. They are subject to malnutrition because they rarely eat while intoxicated. They often overlook their physical condition because of the analgesia they experience from opiates. They are exposed to the high disease rates of their environment and are particularly prone to such problems as abscesses, septicemia, tetanus, bacterial infections and serum hepatitis from unclean needles. And they may die from acute opiate toxicity following overdosage. Overdosage difficulties are sometimes related to impurities in street heroin but are caused most often by uncommonly pure preparations which impose too great a demand on the user's constantly fluctuating tolerance. People who take large doses of the drugs may fall into a drowsy state of shallow and irregular breathing that is called being on the nod. Others who have intentionally or unintentionally overdosed may become close to nodding out or losing consciousness. Still others become comatose and barely alive.

If patients have not yet reached the coma stage, they should be asked questions which require their attention, and may have to be reminded to keep breathing because the depressant action of narcotics prevents involuntary respiration beyond a certain dosage. In cases of coma, patients need respiratory support and transfusions. Their air passages must be cleared, and they may also require antibiotics to prevent pneumonia and the sequelae of pulmonary congestion.

One advantage opiates have over barbiturates in terms of treatment is that their effects may be counteracted with nalorphine (Nalline) and other narcotic antagonists. These compounds exert a narcotic action by themselves but immediately terminate the effects of other narcotic analgesics in the body. They are administered to intoxicated patients to treat overdosage and to mothers who have been given narcotics prior to and during delivery. This latter procedure prevents the possibility of respiratory depression in newborn babies.

Nalorphine is also employed to determine the presence of opiates in suspected addicts in some states either as a prelude to incarceration or as a test to determine suitability for probation and parole. In the Nalline test, an injection of the antagonist is given and the pupillary response is monitored; the pupils will dilate if the person being examined has used opiates within the last twenty-four hours. The same conclusion can be reached by a urine analysis, but the police generally prefer the former procedure. They thereby intoxify persons who are not using narcotics and plunge others who are addicted into an immediate and life-threatening withdrawal.

The character and severity of these withdrawal symptoms depends upon several factors, including the kind and amount of opiates taken, the interval between doses, the duration of usage, the tolerance developed and the health and personality of the patient involved. In cases of morphine or heroin addiction, withdrawal symptoms usually occur six or more hours after the final dose and persist for forty-eight hours or longer, while the duration is shorter and more intense in the case of short-acting meperidine and longer and less intense in the case of methadone. Although withdrawal can be quite severe with older, imprisoned addicts, Dr. George Gay compares the withdrawal of younger addicts from low-quality heroin in settings like the Haight-Ashbury to a bad case of the flu.

The first withdrawal symptoms are anxiety and hyperexcitability shortly before the time of the next scheduled dose. Excessive yawning, sweating, tearfulness and rhinorrhea, or nasal discharge, begin at this point and may lead to a restless sleep known as the yen from which patients awake even more anxious than before. Their pupils then dilate widely; the hair on their skin stands up in a gooseflesh pattern and the skin becomes cold, resembling that of a plucked turkey. This condition accounts for the term "cold turkey," applied to any form of abrupt and/or nonmedically assisted withdrawal.

Contractions may pass over the walls of the stomach a few hours after the onset of cold turkey, causing an explosive vomiting. Abdominal pain also increases as the intestines contract and the previously constipated bowels are voided. Weakness becomes prominent, the heart rate is elevated, and marked chilliness, alternating with skin flushes and sweating, may occur. So may the muscle spasms and kicking motions which are the basis of the expression "kicking the habit." Convulsions and delirium tremens, however, do not occur.

As these conditions persist, patients usually become emaciated and dehydrated because they cannot eat or drink during withdrawal. They may improve, but they remain weak and often suffer from lingering diarrhea. These and other symptoms will disappear if narcotics are administered, so physicians often use methadone, a long-acting and orally active synthetic, to ease the pain and remission rate of withdrawal.

Methadone is a potent analgesic that was developed in Germany as a substitute for morphine and is often prescribed for terminal cancer cases and for patients who have recently undergone surgery. It provides few of the euphoric effects of morphine and heroin and serves to blockade their actions so that persons taking methadone cannot obtain concurrent highs from, and lose their hunger for, other narcotics. Methadone is administered during withdrawal in doses appropriate to the patient's tolerance. The dosage is then reduced and the patient is withdrawn from methadone over a longer period.

Although this technique minimizes the distress during withdrawal, treatment with methadone is limited to hospital settings and cannot be employed on an out-patient basis. A few addicts may acquire methadone on the black market, but most can only obtain sedatives and antipsychotic tranquilizers to help them through withdrawal. The unavailability of methadone thus discourages addicts from seeking proper treatment and allows them to claim that the anticipation of physical suffering forces them to stay addicted and to avoid withdrawal.

A much more serious impediment is the psychological depression which follows abstinence from most toxic chemicals but is especially prominent in the case of opiate withdrawal. These drugs are such gratifying substances that many addicts talk about — and to — them as if they were people. They relate to the compounds as an infant might to its mother's breast or to another source of nurturance. When the symbolic breast is removed, the addicts manifest an infantile inability to tolerate frustration and usually sink into depressions that resemble bereavement after the loss of a loved one.

The extent of such depressions and the interpersonal voids most addicts attempt to fill with narcotics presents a severe problem to voluntary psychotherapy. Most confirmed addicts are extremely dependent people with limited ego functions and psychopathic tendencies who rarely seek help and are difficult to reach even if they do so. Thus, although intensive verbal methods have proven to be useful with young, experimental opiate abusers, they are no more effective with older narcotics addicts than they are with alcohol addicts.

Involuntary treatment practiced in such institutions as the federal narcotics hospitals at Lexington, Kentucky, and Fort Worth, Texas, prior to

1961 has been even less effective. In fact, it was rightfully regarded as a pointless bureaucratic exercise by most opiate addicts. Illegal drugs were sold by enterprising guards at these facilities, as they are today in most prisons, while long-term confinement and crude psychiatric intervention was followed by a ninety percent rate of relapse when inmates returned to the streets — and to heroin. The cost to the public for their so-called treatment was in excess of one thousand dollars a year per patient. This is less than the total accrued by an addict with a one-hundred-dollar-a-day habit, but the disregard for the importance of motivation in therapy implicit in the hospital approach is hardly to be desired.

Motivation does play heavily in a third treatment modality involving the administration of nalorphine and other narcotic antagonists to postwithdrawal patients on a regular basis to discourage readdiction. Unlike Antabuse and other compounds employed for a similar purpose in treating alcoholism, Nalline and comparable antagonists merely blockade the effects of opiates in the body and do not cause a violent physical reaction, although they may precipitate withdrawal. Clinical experience with highly motivated addicts who ask for antagonist therapy has been extremely encouraging, especially because the use of medications may serve as an introduction to rehabilitative therapy.

The most traditionally successful method of rehabilitation involves placing addicts in authoritarian environments that seem to provide the external structuring they require. Synanon, the Mendocino Family and other groups of this sort attempt to replace the addicts' dependence on drugs with an allegiance to a nurturing and protective organization which ultimately alleviates many of their difficulties by abrogating their individuality. Like Alcoholics Anonymous, these therapeutic communities succeed only when addicts stay within the family structures or create similar structures for others whom they may reciprocally "save." Furthermore, the leaders of such programs sometimes play upon the paranoid and antisocial tendencies of the members of the therapeutic communities. They can keep their followers only by perpetuating a constant, albeit nonviolent, war against society.

A modality which attempts to overcome this problem is the British System. It is based on the fact that addicts can function for prolonged periods without disability if they receive regular doses of opiates and on the operating premise that addiction is a sickness, not a crime. As originally conceived, this technique allowed British physicians who were convinced that complete withdrawal would endanger an addict's health to prescribe maintenance doses of his drug of choice. The program had the great advantage of making narcotics legally available and thereby making it unnecessary for addicts to steal in order to support their habits.

The British System also had disadvantages. Some doctors grossly over-prescribed heroin to addicts, who in turn sold their medication on the black market, and opiate addiction increased in Great Britain almost as dramatically as in the United States. This led the government to change the program in 1968 so that only specially designated clinics could prescribe drugs in uniform dosages. The British are continuing their medically oriented program and improving the clinics so addicts may obtain other health services. They are also exploring other avenues of rehabilitation.

The sixth and perhaps most promising approach to the problem of confirmed addiction in older people is the methadone maintenance program which was pioneered by Drs. Vincent Dole and Marie Nyswander in New York in 1964. They have found that establishing a tolerance to methadone on an in-patient basis and subsequently maintaining the tolerant state with a constant daily oral dose on an out-patient basis allows them to blockade the action of heroin and eliminate their patients' hunger for narcotics. The daily oral dose of methadone can be administered in fruit juice from which the narcotic cannot be reconstituted. It does not impair an addict's functioning and costs as little as ten cents a day.

The standard methadone procedure requires former addicts to report regularly for at least a year to a facility where their urine is checked to determine if they have remained clean of other narcotics and therefore suitable for continued admission to the methadone program. The patients are counseled during this period and are either helped to taper off from the synthetic or maintained on it for the rest of their lives. Drs. Dole and Nyswander have found that over eight-five percent of the patients they have treated since 1964 have remained heroin — and crime — free.

In spite of this unprecedented success, critics have argued that out-patient maintenance programs merely substitute addiction to one narcotic for another. Dr. John C. Kramer, former research director of the California Rehabilitation Center responds by noting that "this is inconsequential when one considers the alternatives — disease, death, degradation and prison — which affect most addicts in our society. The fact that methadone is dependency-inducing is irrelevant if one determines that long-term treatment is desirable. We insist on a similar use of antipsychotic drugs with hundreds of thousands of psychiatric patients and anticonvulsants with an equally large number of epileptics whose lives are significantly improved. Withholding methadone from an addict is tantamount to denying a diabetic his insulin."

Arguments against methadone also make little logistical sense, for although continuous supervision is vital to maintenance programs, the only problem in dispensing methadone relates to the security and scheduling of the drug. Paperwork and staff time are held to a minimum in programs like that of Drs. Dole and Nyswander. Hospitalization is also minimized, a fact of great significance because ward space is limited and hospital beds cost up to one hundred dollars a day. Although methadone programs may be only intermediate therapeutic steps, they offer practical advantages and an end to human suffering at a low personal and social cost.

These advantages were apparent in 1969, but California and many other states refused to allow out-patient methadone withdrawal and/or maintenance on a productive scale during that year. Local statutes even limited research on the drug, and the only methadone program in northern California was that first applied for in 1966 by Dr. Fort and subsequently supervised by Dr. Barry Ramer, his successor at the San Francisco Center for Special Problems. Dr. Ramer's program, which was launched in June of 1969, could provide for only thirty-five patients in a city whose addict population was estimated at between five and seven thousand. It had only a slight impact in the Haight-Ashbury, where heroin abuse became epidemic as early as July.

The Smack Scene

Narcotics were not new to the Haight. Dr. Frederick Shick's survey revealed a substantial amount of opium smoking and heroin experimentation during 1967 and 1968, while the Medical Section saw a half-dozen patients using opiates each week through the early months of 1969. But narcotics consumption was confined to a minority in the district so long as its subcultures limited themselves to amphetamines and hallucinogens. This pattern was disturbed during 1969, when the influx of older addicts, the emergence of the black subculture and the speed freaks' dissatisfaction with amphetamines and barbiturates led almost inexorably to the establishment of a smack scene.

This scene was strikingly silent in comparison to those which preceded it, for heroin exerted a dampening effect both on its users and on the Haight-Ashbury. Yet although precipitous violence decreased in the district, petty theft, prostitution, dealing and burglary continued to rise. Paranoia also increased because the members of the heroin subculture lived in constant fear of one another and the law. They maintained a certain fragile fellowship, but only by putting abusers of all other toxic chemicals down.

This snobbery was specious at best, for the addicts in the Haight were ridiculed by those who remained loyal to speed or acid and were considered garbage junkies by other abusers who had access to more potent narcotics elsewhere. Most of the smack sold on Haight Street was brought in by black and white dealers who purchased their products either from Vietnam or from professional criminals who channeled them through Mexico. The local smack was notoriously high priced and low in quality, so that its abusers were even more desperate than their counterparts in other cities. Thus, although they were sometimes as pacific and unthreatening as the early hippies, their depression and isolation was much more intense. "It's quiet, almost dead, with everyone out here on the nod," Dr. Matzger said during August. "But as in all ghettos, you can feel the people screaming inside."

The screams became more audible during September, when President Nixon's Operation Intercept partially cut off the flow of marijuana into the Haight-Ashbury. The diminished supply prompted several local dealers to begin marketing a concoction called Angel Dust which was alleged to contain synthetic marijuana but turned out to be mint leaves or oregano sprayed with phencyclidine. It also forced those new arrivals who did not enjoy alcohol or barbiturates to find their sedation in heroin. As their opiate experimentation increased, several Clinic patients complained that they would never have used junk if they could have obtained marijuana. One volunteer who was concerned over the plight of her companions entered All Saints' Episcopal Church and prayed for a fresh shipment of grass.

Although the federal policy contributed to the growth of the narcotics subculture, Randy offered another explanation for its birth. "The real reason is the Haight's so full of freaky people," he said. "Everybody's been strung out on something or other since I got here. You've got these big superpros coming and these little kids who think they're so tough. Smack is expensive. It's trouble to cop and hard as hell to come off. I still shoot speed and barbs too to keep my habit down, but I tell you, heroin is the greatest. Man, when it comes to shit, I can't get enough."

Randy obtained sufficient heroin to build up a seven-bag daily habit by the first of October, when Dr. Matzger received his United States Public Health Service grant and began working full time at the Medical Section. The facility was then treating only twelve addicts a week, but during the second week of October, a supply of unusually potent smack arrived from the East Coast and sent nineteen overdosed persons between sixteen and eighteen years of age to San Francisco General, three of whom were dead on arrival. By the third week in October, the Clinic was seeing more than fifteen patients with opiate problems a day.

These patients came to 558 Clayton Street for a variety of reasons. Some were adolescents who were either acutely toxic from narcotics or eager to be cleaned up before they became completely addicted. Others were older addicts who had either been busted or beaten up once too often or were trying to come to terms with themselves before committing suicide. Many had attempted cold turkey and were suffering from insomnia, cramps, jitteriness, nasal congestion and diarrhea. Most merely sought help when they ran out of drugs, money and the energy necessary to sustain their life-style.

The patients hoped to be given tranquilizers and sedatives which would ease their agony, tide them through the weekend, and/or lower their tolerance and thereby reduce the cost of their habits. They abused the Clinic as much as they did the chemicals but were impressed by the treatment they received. Thus, if their pain increased after their first visit to the facility, they were less hesitant the next time to ask for complete withdrawal.

Methadone could not be used at the Medical Section, but Dr. Matzger and the other physicians managed to detoxify over thirty patients and sent fifty more to private institutions where they could start withdrawal. No fatalities occurred during October, although operations ground to a halt on several evenings as the staff prevented seventeen patients from nodding out. Word of their work then spread through the Haight-Ashbury, and dozens of people who had previously avoided treatment began to seek aid. "It was as if the floodgates were suddenly opened," Dr. Matzger said, "and the junkies realized there was a safe alternative to their private hell."

Twenty addicts were arriving daily at 409 and 558 Clayton by the end of October, including many blacks who had never visited the Clinic before. The situation eventually became so acute that Dr. Matzger asked Dr. Gay to help out at the Medical Section from two to five in the afternoon. Dr. Gay responded by setting up an emergency out-patient Heroin Detoxification Program in a section of the old calm center. He first established a screening procedure whereby patients were initially seen at the Drug Treatment Program. He then began to use several drugs, including Darvon for analgesia, chloral hydrate for sleeplessness and Valium for nervousness, to facilitate their withdrawal.

Dr. Gay tried not to dispense sedatives with a high abuse potential that might be resold in the underground. He also urged an extensive follow-up with his patients, even if they only wanted pills so they could reduce their habits. And he learned to look out for the junkie shuck employed by those psychopaths who said they felt guilty but had little interest in abstinence. Dr. Gay spent extra time with young people who were sincere about kicking their habits and placed dozens in the Drug Treatment Program, the Psychiatric Section, the Mendocino Family, Walden House and other facilities. Although he was too busy at the time to keep track of all his patients, he completed a study of one hundred and sixty-five of them in December which allowed him to gauge his success so far.

Dr. Gay found that forty-six of these patients were female and one hun-

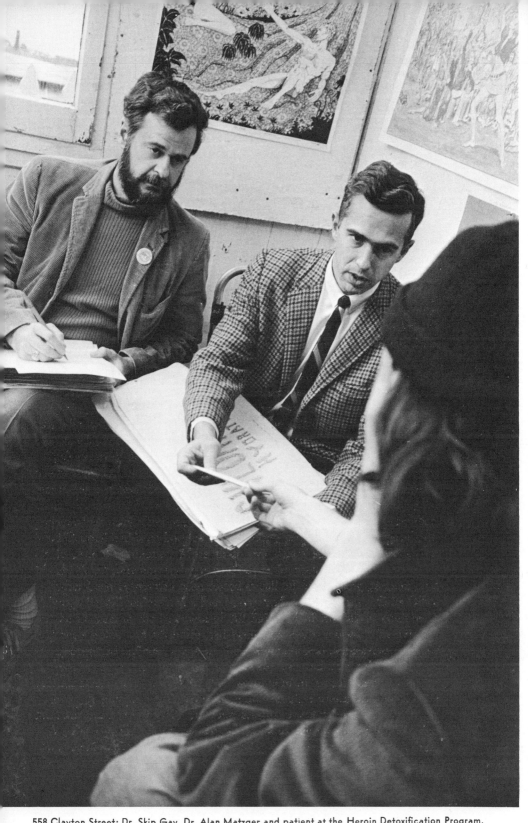

558 Clayton Street: Dr. Skip Gay, Dr. Alan Matzger and patient at the Heroin Detoxification Program.

(Elaine Mayes)

dred and nineteen were male. They ranged from seventeen to fifty years of age, with a median age of approximately twenty-four years. Although most of the thirty-two patients who were older than thirty were long-term black and white addicts, the younger ones were largely late arrivals or veterans from as far back as the Summer of Love. Thirty-eight of the patients had habits of from one year to one month. One hundred and twenty-seven had been hooked for over a year. One hundred and eighteen were spending less than one hundred dollars a day for their habits. Forty-seven had habits of over one hundred dollars. Fifty-four of the one hundred and sixty-five patients were married. Only thirty-two had regular jobs.

Furthermore, only thirty-two of these came from the Haight-Ashbury: eighty-one lived in the Tenderloin, North Beach, Mission, Western Addition and Fillmore districts, while fifty-two were from out of town. Sixty-five had no previous withdrawal history. Twenty-one had tried withdrawal on at least five occasions, while seventy-nine had attempted withdrawal from one to five times. Fifty-eight had tried cold turkey; seventeen had received medical attention; nineteen had medicated themselves with street drugs; thirty-eight had either been in the Dole-Nyswander program or had used black-market methadone.

Almost all of these patients could be considered habitual and multiple abusers of other drugs. Forty were or had been heavily involved in alcohol, and ninety-two used marijuana regularly, although not necessarily as a stepping-stone to heroin. Sixty-four took hallucinogens, one of whom shot LSD and smack together to experience what he called "psychedelic dreams." Barbiturates were used by fifty-four of the patients; four also took cocaine. Sixty-nine had been or were speed abusers, and many had followed a sequential course from alcohol to marijuana to hallucinogens to amphetamines to barbiturates and to heroin.

Finally, the patients gave many reasons for coming to the Clinic. Seventy-one made only one visit for medication or to determine whether or not they would be arrested there. Thirty-one came on two occasions; forty-two came on three, four or five occasions; twenty-one came more than five times. Eighteen of the one hundred and sixty-five stayed clean for one month or more following their last visit. Seven reduced their habits to the chipping point. Nine were known to have resumed their addiction, while one hundred and thirty-one either disappeared or were referred to other programs. Almost all of those who did want further treatment asked for methadone.

In summing up his results, Dr. Gay concluded that only ten percent of the patients had remained clean after participating in the Heroin Detoxification Program but that a much larger number could be helped in the future if methadone was available at the Clinic. He also predicted that his case load would increase in 1970, which Dr. Smith and Dr. David Bentel, his associate on the Drug Abuse Information Project, referred to as "the year of the middle-class junkie." Dr. Gay therefore joined the fight to liberalize the state statutes governing methadone withdrawal and maintenance and called upon the Drug Treatment Program to become more active in battling the heroin-based life-style.

This urging was unnecessary, for Father Frykman and his staff were swamped with opiate addicts after October too. The receiving area at 409 Clayton was frequently full of addicts who required extensive emotional support, especially if they were undergoing or about to attempt withdrawal. Approximately seven overdosed patients were treated weekly at the Annex, none of whom died. The informal rap sessions and encounter groups also ran long after midnight on many occasions as the Drug Treatment Program became a center for insomniacs of every conceivable personality, background and age.

This diversity among the patients was so pronounced that Father Frykman said, "The only typical thing about junkies is that they're not typical at all." Among the patients he counseled were an eight-year-old Mexican boy whose five brothers and sisters dealt heroin, a seventy-three-year-old black longshoreman who had abused narcotics all his adult life, two army corporals who became addicted in Southeast Asia, a sixty-year-old antique store owner with a one-hundred-dollar-a-day habit and the eighteen-year-old daughter of a prominent local businessman. She started with LSD in 1967, was wired on speed at her high-school graduation, began shooting one hundred dollars worth of smack a day and came to the Clinic when "I realized I would either have to kick horse or sell my body in the Tenderloin."

This girl and over a dozen other addicts joined Father Frykman's therapeutic community. Five of them made considerable progress because they helped one another stay off drugs and subsequently became members of the staff. Jobs were found for two others outside the Haight-Ashbury, while one twenty-two-year-old went home to his parents. But another family member was jailed after he left the group house, and four who remained in the Haight returned to heroin.

These results were unimpressive but Father Frykman and his co-workers decided to expand, rather than improve, their existing program. In December, they qualified for inclusion in the Northeast Mental Health Center by opening one office in the Tenderloin Y.M.C.A. and another in the International Hotel at 848 Kearny Street between North Beach and Chinatown. These offices were staffed with counselors and therapeutic community graduates. They detracted from work done in the Haight but offered help to Tenderloin residents and Chinese adolescents as well.

Although the financing for this expansion was supposed to come from Dr. Carfagni's budget, the National Institute of Mental Health grant which the Clinic was counting on was held up, apparently because of the Vietnam war. This forced Father Frykman to raise private funds. He was assisted by Roger Smith, who had finished his report for the Amphetamine Research Project, moved out of Dr. Meyer's office, and begun organizing a drug-abuse program for the town of Pittsburg in the San Francisco East Bay. Smith and Father Frykman obtained two gifts of stock worth eleven thousand dollars during December and secured a second grant of twelve thousand dollars from the Luke Hancock Foundation. Meanwhile, Dr. Smith applied for twenty-five thousand dollars from the Merrill Trust. His application was shepherded by Mrs. Inez Folger, a Clinic volunteer and member of the Folger coffee family.

These several sources guaranteed operations in North Beach, the Tenderloin and the Haight-Ashbury, but Father Frykman remained pessimistic as "the year of the middle-class junkie" approached. "Heroin is almost an unsolvable problem," he said. "The present treatment modalities make it impossible to keep people off junk. The best we can hope for in many cases is to achieve an equilibrium in which patients are stabilized at occasional use of narcotics, not cured. Methadone is probably the best answer. But until we can use it, we can still reach people who have never been reached before."

End of the Road

Ed was one person who achieved equilibrium through the Drug Treatment Program. He was a tall, gangly man who had been part of many scenes yet never belonged to one. Ed was not particularly intelligent, but he was psychologically sophisticated because of his exposure to several kinds of therapy. He smoked four or five packs of cigarettes daily and spoke and moved ponderously, as if his entire body were draped with an oppressive gloom.

Ed made the most of his somberness and self-pity and appeared to be burdened by a conscience which some people assumed was crippling and others dismissed as a sham. As a Clinic veteran, he joined Father Frykman's therapeutic community in November of 1969 and clung to the program long after his stay at the group house. He spent most of December in the basement at 409 Clayton Street alongside Randy and the other addicts. He also participated in the rap sessions and encounter groups and claimed to be improved by his involvement. Yet Ed remained detached, waiting for some external agent to soothe his spirits and motivate him.

This was a habitual pattern, for Ed had apparently lived with anxiety and depression almost from the day he was born. He was raised in the Richmond district of San Francisco, the son of a building contractor who left the family to marry his secretary when his son was one year old. Ed lived with his mother after his father's departure. He remembered her as an emotionally inconsistent castrater who drank a great deal. "She was crazy; one minute she cut me down, the next she was spoiling me," he told John Luce. "I never knew where she was at. It was like being in a tug-of-war."

Ed stayed with his mother until he was six, when she married a service-station owner and decided to put her son up for adoption. He was taken in by his paternal grandparents, who begrudgingly moved to the city from their home in rural Oregon to care for him. Ed's grandfather lived off his pension and mediated between his wife and grandson. "I really loved that cat," Ed said, "but my grandmother was like my mother: up and down. She used to tell me I was the reason my father left. There were fights when my grandfather got drunk and bitching about money all the time."

Ed did well in school to please his grandparents and because he welcomed a diversion from his home. He also spent much of his youth in the hospital for allergies, gastrointestinal problems and an undiagnosed blood condition. "They never did find out what was wrong, but I was always hurting. These doctors would come in with their fucking charts and ask questions, one after another. And they were always putting spikes in my arm."

These hospital visits continued until Ed was fourteen, when his grandfather died and many of his symptoms abated. He then moved with his grandmother to a small apartment in the Mission district and entered public high school. Ed also started drinking.

I drank on the weekends — sometimes during the week, too. I really dug school until adolescence, but all these feelings started coming out of me. I had these weird thoughts in my head, like I'd see myself with some woman and — I really couldn't handle it all. I was anxious — there was something missing in me, some part that everybody else had.

I used to do all these destructive things; I'd get loaded and swipe cars. I didn't need the money too much, but I dug boosting — I always felt better afterwards, like I'd just let go of myself a little, gotten rid of some of the shit inside. I really had hot pants, too. All I wanted to do was fuck. But I felt embarrassed. I just didn't think I could handle myself around chicks, that's all.

So I made it through high school and started city college, going just to see if I still had a brain. But I couldn't concentrate, even after six months in the marines. I got out but I didn't know where I was going — I didn't give a shit, you know? So I went back to school. Some of it I really picked up on, like the dramatics; I was a real funnyman, a clown. I got lots of attention for a change. But things got worse with my grandmother, so — I was about nineteen — I got married to this Catholic girl. A pretty intelligent chick, but she was naïve. She had a lot of ideals that are pretty blown now.

We lived in the Mission with her working while I tried to finish school. Then we had a kid, so I quit college and sorted mail at the post office for a while. That was the most stable time. I liked my kid, but I started running; I had a few chicks to go when my wife laid it on. Sometimes I'd go off on my own, just walking around trying to get it together. I remember it was about a year after I got married that I started reading, about the time my kid came. I did Kerouac and Ginsberg and all those guys. I really got romantic. Like I had tried the JD [juvenile delinquent] trip but this was new to me, going on the road and all. I'd go to the beach and write poetry with a bottle of wine.

I used to go to North Beach too, one of the weekend beatniks there. But the scene was all over and the Haight was beginning. This was like 1966 and 1965. My wife and I were going through these changes. We had another kid — she wouldn't use pills or a diaphragm. So I started living with this chick out here and still seeing my wife, fucking her, making promises, paying for the kids 'cause I still had my job. She wouldn't come to the Haight, but I dug it. I moved in with some good people, these three girls from back East. They really turned my head around.

It was the hippie bit, right on. I wasn't really one of them, I guess, like I didn't go in for all this Hare Kriskna shit, but our place felt like a home. My chick turned me on to grass, which was a good thing! It got me off the booze. Then I took some acid. Beautiful: good stuff, you could still get it then. Man, I remember my first trip — I didn't ever want to come down.

Then I had a real bummer. It was around the start of the big summer; I was back with my old lady off and on but still shacking with the chick here and things got rough one night. I was already behind acid and she said, "Here, try this." It was STP. And that did it. I started flashing on my wife and my kids and here I was in the Haight-Ashbury fucking this chick all the time. I knew what a shitty father I'd been but I couldn't help it. I wanted to kill my-self — I thought I'd really blown my mind.

They took me to the Clinic, but it was full of people and I started getting more freaky. Then some shrink talked to me and he put me straight. Anyway, I started seeing him a few times and my old lady says, "Either you come back with me or we get a divorce." Now that's a big thing for a Catholic, so I tried to put our thing back together. I turned her on to grass, but she had a bad trip and kept saying something bad was going to happen. She really blew it — we were so close.

After that my wife split and, man, I was nowhere. I started going with this other chick who really dug pills. We were into bennies and we shot crank a couple of times, but I was still pretty down and I couldn't get off the way she could. Finally she got strung out and it was so bad out here with all the freaks that I moved back to the Mission, near where I used to live. Then this cat turned me on to codeine and barbs. We shot smack too, but I cooled it for a few weeks. Then I got so anxious without an old lady. I told myself, aw fuck, it's easy to stop — you did it before. So I started again and moved out here after the speed thing died down.

Smack is the best, make no mistake. It keeps your head straight. First I can feel my stomach growl like I'm real hungry, then I taste it and I can feel the rush. Like, blam, my body turns liquid and I'm really relaxed. My head isn't working; I'm just sort of stowed away. I get this feeling that everything's taken care of — no one can touch me.

The rush is the best part. After that you're just fixed. You don't have any hassles, but it's nothing positive — it's like a neutral feeling, normal. You can work on heroin real well though. I can really do these physical things if I want to. But I like to lie back and get into dreams. Everything's sweet and warm, like I'm floating in a bathtub. My body's here but my head is somewhere else.

That goes only for the good stuff. The shit on the street now, it's so full of talcum powder you only get a little rush and you're back where you started in a couple of hours. It's a bad scene. But I've got a good connection, a white cat who cops in the Fillmore. I just won't mess with spades myself; you're going to get burned. Most guys I know feel the same. We stay together. None of the rapping you get with the speeders. In fact, we don't talk too much. We shoot together now and then but it's not like the hippie days. The only ritual now is deciding who's going first.

The worst thing is the hassle. I OD'd [overdosed] once out here too, fixing up in a car, not even a full bag but it was such righteous stuff I damned near died. The next thing I knew I could feel myself sliding down the seat, like I was in a roller coaster. These two guys I was with were in the Safeway trying to rip off a carton of cigarettes. They wanted to take me to General but I made it over to the Clinic instead. Renée and Bill Essen were there and they talked with me; it must have been four hours. The next day I was really scared but I still needed to get stoned.

I was driving a cab then — I'd stage a robbery, like someone had ripped me off, then keep the bread. Me and this guy were into burglary too — we'd get into places where I knew the people were away — no strong arm, just boosting stuff. Then my partner got busted and my connection split and I couldn't get any decent smack. I tried to kick on barbs and grass until I saw Skip Gay for detox.

Skip I like. He doesn't do what most doctors do — they get you when you're hurting and lay down this rap when all you are doing is screaming for tranks. He cleaned me up and said he could get me into all kinds of programs: Mendocino, Synanon, the whole bit. But they treat you rough at Synanon, and I wasn't sure about Mendocino. So I went into Frykman's program: one, one and a half months. He has a way of getting involved that I like. You don't feel trapped.

The group house was good for me. I had my only jacket ripped off but the place helped me get together — it was like my old hippie house. Now, I don't know what's going to happen. I don't dig the Haight, but I've got a pretty good place to live I don't want to give up yet. My roommate, he's O.K.; we can tolerate each other and we don't fight. He was a speed freak who got into smack and went through Drug Treatment. We try and keep each other straight. I'm still chipping, but I think I'm over the hump. There's still a lot of shit inside me, but I'm seeing Stu Loomis and I think my attitude is a whole lot better. I keep telling myself, "You're not such a bad guy after all!"

The biggest problem is keeping myself up, finding something to do. I get into these moods and I can't stand anyone around me; I just want to get away. But I can't go anywhere else, you know? A lot of the people here feel like that; it's the hanging out. Like some days I'll just sit at Drug Treatment for hours, maybe stoned, not just because I like it here, but because I haven't got anyplace to go.

What I really want is to get onto the staff or go on methadone. But I want to be clean before I ask for a place. It's hard staying off the stuff — I haven't had an old lady in so long. But I can help here; I've worked on a couple OD's with Bill and I'm pretty good working with the kids. They talk a lot about how they can handle heroin, like this cat from New York in earlier. But I know better. Junkies are losers, man, pure and simple. Smack is the best ride there is, but for me it's the end of the road.

Altamont

Ed was not the only person whose ride was over in December. Indeed, some of the beats he once emulated had also reached the end of the road by 1969. Dr. Francis Rigney, the psychiatrist who studied fifty-one bohemians in North Beach ten years earlier, found that two of his original subjects were now in mental institutions, while seven were alcoholics, fourteen had gone straight, thirteen had remained bohemian, two were dead and thirteen were unaccounted for. Neil Cassady had been buried in 1968. Jack Kerouac died from excessive liver damage in a suburban home near St. Petersburg, Florida, in 1969.

Norman Mailer was still alive and preaching philosophic psychopathy. So was Ken Kesey, who had to roust over three dozen camp followers before he could begin growing crops on his Oregon farm. But Dr. Timothy Leary, whose southern California commune had recently witnessed a drowning, was now facing a long sentence on two counts of possession of marijuana. Although the High Priest had achieved martyrdom, he was finally prevented from urging young people to do their thing.

Thousands of followers who had taken Dr. Leary's advice were already in hospitals or behind bars. Among them was Randy, who was held in San Francisco General during November for treatment of a chronic toxic psychosis, or brain syndrome. Randy had been taking heroin, intravenous speed, alcohol, marijuana, codeine, cocaine, diet pills and barbiturates interchangeably before his stay in the hospital. He spent several weeks there recovering from hepatitis, withdrawing from smack and barbs, and stocking up on the vitamins and proteins so alien to his system. He then escaped and returned to the Haight-Ashbury, where he resumed his multiple addiction and was arrested for possession of marijuana for a second time.

Randy could now be sent to San Quentin for twenty years. But Dr. Arthur Carfagni, who knew Dr. Zoom intimately, managed to have him committed instead to a state hospital for the criminally insane — where he might have to stay even longer. In early December, Randy wrote to Father Frykman, who had recommended that he compose his autobiography while an inmate, and asked him to check on a companion who was also in jail. His last words to Father Frykman were: "I'm glad you still have an interest in me. At least I'm not alone in this world."

A week later, the Clinic learned of the fate of another former patient. This was Charlie Manson, who was arrested with Susan Atkins, Patricia Krenwinkel, Linda Kasabian and three other members of his infamous family. Charlie was ultimately charged with the monstrous murder of actress Sharon Tate and six innocent bystanders in a home once occupied by Doris Day's son, Terry Melcher, near Beverly Hills. Included in the list of his alleged victims was Abigail Folger, whose mother had just raised twenty-five thousand dollars from the Merrill Trust for the Clinic and its Drug Treatment Program.

John Luce obtained a three-thousand-dollar donation from *Life* magazine in exchange for a report of the Clinic's experiences with Charlie, but many media used Manson only as an example of how morally bankrupt the psychedelic movement of which he was supposedly a part had become. Roger Smith, Dr. Dernburg, Dr. Smith and Alan Rose, who had returned to San Francisco, explained to the press that Charlie was not a typical hippie and tried to prevent a public backlash against all commune dwellers. Dr. Smith received several threats from members of the underground in return for his efforts. And his defense of the psychedelic movement was lost in the publicity which followed the weekend of December sixth and seventh, when the Altamont rock concert was held.

This event looked like another Woodstock in the making in November

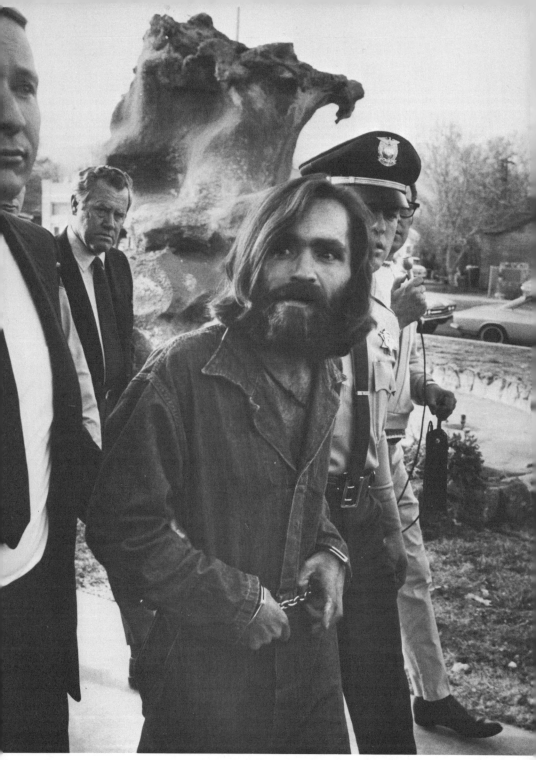

Charlie Manson.
(Vernon Merritt, **Life** magazine (c) Time Inc.)

after the Rolling Stones agreed to give a free concert comparable to the be-in in northern California and were joined by most of the prominent San Francisco bands. But Owsley, the Grateful Dead, Chet Helms, Emmett Grogan, several Diggers and the other producers were deprived of their location for the affair twenty-four hours before it was to be held. Instead of canceling their plans and being upstaged by the promotors at Woodstock, they agreed to give the concert at the Altamont Speedway, an arid and previously unheard-of racetrack in the East Bay.

The site they settled on was near a freeway and surrounded by ranches whose owners were never warned about what to expect that weekend. Sanitary, food and medical facilities were neglected, just as they were in the new community. The sound system was barely audible; the stage was too close to the audience and located in an area ultimately packed with people and paramedical personnel. Furthermore, the local police refused to impose permit restrictions or patrol the concert. The Rolling Stones' manager therefore offered the Hell's Angels five-hundred-dollars-worth of beer to protect his musicians from their fans.

The Angels were not on duty until Saturday morning, so Altamont was relatively peaceful the night before. Dozens of tents lined the speedway that evening, as young people played catch with Frisbees under arc lights used by the technicians setting up the stage. Meanwhile, the roads from San Francisco were crowded with hippies, hoodies, bikers, high school students and others of every age and description. Over five thousand were settled in sleeping bags by midnight, when the dealers started to arrive.

Hundreds of other drug salesmen set up shop the next morning, as the hills were swept by an army of young people trampling over the fences and private property which stood between them and the speedway. Every popular toxic chemical was waiting for them there. One group from Berkeley dispensed over five thousand tablets of adulterated acid during the morning. Speed and smack were available, and at least two cases of Seconal were passed out at the front of the stage. A Clinic volunteer saw a girl hand out STP and the peace pill to the audience. He moved away from the bandstand around noon, when, in lieu of other leadership, the Hell's Angels assumed control.

The Angels busied themselves at first by popping pills and downing the alcohol which the Rolling Stones' manager allotted them. They then proceeded to earn their keep by repulsing dozens of screaming groupies who were throwing themselves against the stage. A member of the Jefferson Airplane incurred the Angels' wrath a minute later, when he tried to prevent them from ganging up on a black man. Several onlookers then

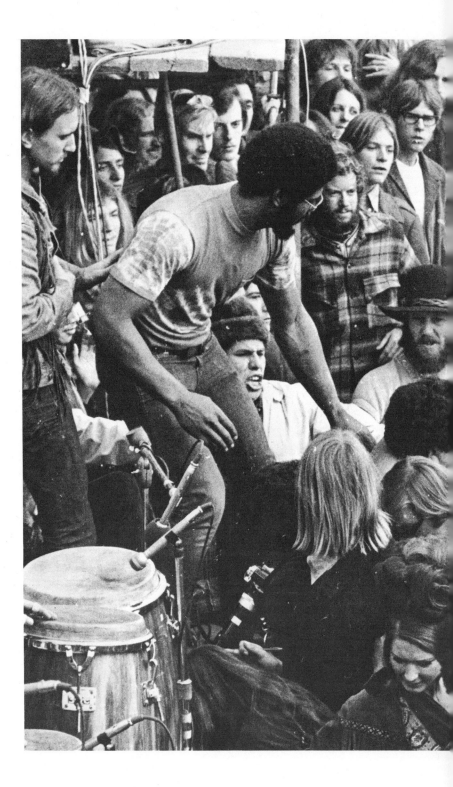

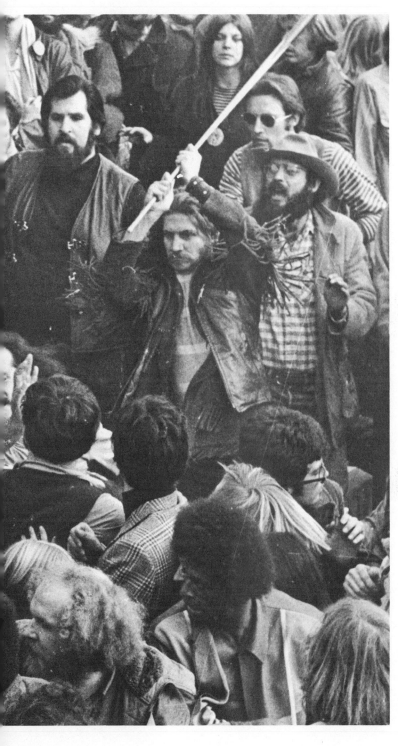

Altamont.
(Bill Owens)

bumped into an Angel's motorcycle. At that point, the outlaws grabbed weighted pool cues and went hunting in the crowd for heads to bust.

No precise records were kept on the Angels' victims. Nor were statistics available on the number of adverse drug reactions experienced that afternoon. Yet the fifty physicians and paramedical workers from the Haight-Ashbury and Berkeley free clinics who manned the first aid station treated so many bad trips that they ran out of Thorazine after half an hour. The volunteers tried to talk down young people using contaminated LSD but their efforts were hopeless because of the paranoia in the crowd. They also attempted to remove some psychiatric patients from the concert environment but were unable to secure the helicopter they were promised. One doctor who detoxified over forty young people said, "We're seeing the Summer of Love all over again."

A member of the Medical Committee for Human Rights who once worked at the Clinic treated over seventy cut feet, scalp lacerations and broken facial bones during the afternoon. He also assisted a female musician whose skull was fractured by a beer bottle and helped seven young people who had overdosed on heroin and/or barbs. "This place reminds me of the Haight during the 1968 riots," the physician said. "It's so violent you'd think somebody turned loose the Tactical Squad."

The violence increased after dusk settled on the speedway and a dry wind spread the noxious odor of hundreds of cooking fires. Many young people huddled together on the slopes of Altamont then began to wash down mescaline and psilocybin with wine. The music was turned off for an hour. Dozens of fights started as the audience waited nervously for the Rolling Stones to finally perform.

The Stones, who had been lounging backstage, strolled to the microphones and started singing a song entitled "Sympathy for the Devil." But they were interrupted by a disturbance in the front of the crowd. An eighteen-year-old Negro named Meredith Hunter apparently pulled a revolver on a Hell's Angel. Hunter had no chance to use it, for the biker stabbed him repeatedly in the back as a dozen others swarmed over the young man. The Stones threatened to stop their performance at this point. But instead of trying to restore order, they played through the incident and ended their set with "Street Fighting Man."

Meanwhile, Hunter was carried to the first aid station and dumped in front of the doctor in charge. The physician knew that his patient needed an immediate operation to repair ruptured blood vessels. But there was no way to get Hunter through the crowd and to a hospital. The doctor cupped his head in his hands and watched Hunter die.

Three other deaths followed in short order. Two twenty-two-year-old men from Berkeley were killed around midnight when a sedan plowed into them and several other young people sitting around a campfire. Next was a thirty-year-old hoodie who succumbed of asphyxiation due to drowning after he slid into an irrigation canal.

The crowd of three hundred thousand deserted Altamont by Sunday, leaving twenty tons of uncollected garbage behind. Then began a flurry of charges and countercharges as law suits were filed by neighboring ranchers against the speedway owner and by the parents of Meredith Hunter against the Rolling Stones. The local Board of Supervisors also threatened legal action, while Bill Graham told the press that the only good thing that could come out of Altamont was the end of all large rock festivals. He blamed the producers for holding the event, the police for not stopping it and the audience for its lack of self-control.

Ralph Gleason then commented on the episode in his *Chronicle* column. He compared Altamont to a religious gathering of a movement that first surfaced in San Francisco and was subsequently misrepresented by the media, exploited by commercial interests, and perverted by violent psychotics and psychopaths. He claimed that Hunter's death was due in part to a preoccupation with Now-ness on the part of many young people. And he concluded his piece with an appropriate — and long overdue — epitaph.

In the beginning, the word was tribalism in contrast to the individuality which was assumed to have led to the exploitive society being rejected. But paralleling the tribalism was the do-your-thing ethic which said that the responsibility inherent in tribalism was to be ignored. And that seems to me to touch upon the lesson of the Altamont disaster, for it was a disaster even though the incidence of death and violence was not disproportionate to twelve hours in a city of three hundred thousand.

It was a disaster because the clear irresponsibility of so many of those in charge produced the situation which caused the murder. The whole role the Hell's Angels played (was it only a dozen years ago that Allen Ginsburg called them 'saintly motocyclists' in "Howl," confusing beards for beatification?) implied the moral disaster that the Haight Street dream ended with . . . What started as a dream on Haight Street in 1965 may well have ended in Meredith Hunter's blood in front of the bandstand on December sixth when the Rolling Stones sang "Sympathy for the Devil" as Hunter died.

Today

The Haight Street dream did die with Meredith Hunter for many people at the Clinic. John Luce, for one, looked on Altamont as an indication of the degree to which drug-taking had progressed throughout the youth subculture. Like Ralph Gleason, he interpreted the concert as a final demonstration of the irresponsibility and social impracticality inherent in the eupsychic ethic. He traced the tragedy back to Norman Mailer, Allen Ginsberg, Ken Kesey and other bohemian writers who apotheosized mass disinhibition and psychological primitivism before the new community began.

The specter of Hell's Angels swinging pool cues also convinced Dr. Smith once and for all of the danger of allowing everyone to do his thing. He had once overlooked the psychopathology of the Haight in an attempt to defend and nurture the psychedelic movement and spread its ideals into straight society. But events like Altamont helped him see that, for all its idealism, the new community contained the seeds of its own destruction in its refusal to accept social and individual controls and its acceptance of unbridled experimentation. Experience in treating speed, barbs and narcotics made Dr. Smith more conservative in his political thinking and more professional in his approach towards drug problems.

Because of this, he began spending more time and exercising more authority at the Clinic. So did Bill Essen and others who returned to business as usual two days after Altamont was held. By the end of December, a study revealed that close to twenty-five thousand patients had been seen during 1969 at 409 and 558 Clayton Street, over two-thirds of them for one or more times. An even larger number was anticipated as Altamont faded into memory and "the year of the middle-class junkie" began.

1970 started badly for the Clinic, as Don Reddick suffered a heart attack from overwork and had to resign from his position as administrative director. But although no one could be found to replace Reddick, January was a period of growth for every part of the multiservice agency. Especially busy was the Medical Section, where the staff members treated a steady stream of from fifty to one hundred patients a day. More and more of these patients lived outside the district, for the Haight-Ashbury and Berkeley free clinics were now firmly established as the major local medical facilities for street people and other alienated white youth. But a few older residents of the Haight also sought treatment, as did several hundred young blacks from surrounding areas.

Although these patients had standard complaints, the Clinic witnessed a continued increase in both hepatitis and VD. Hepatitis had assumed epidemic proportions a year earlier, and a state survey indicated that over twenty thousand cases were reported in California during 1969. Gonorrhea officially reached the ninety-thousand mark during the same period, while one physician put the probable real estimate at five hundred thousand cases, half of them occurring in young people under twenty-five. San Francisco trailed only Atlanta, the location of the United States Public Health Service's Communicable Disease Center, in per capita gonorrheal infections during 1970. Over ten cases were seen daily at 558 Clayton. Syphilis, an extremely contagious venereal disease which is caused by the organism *Treponema pallidum,* was found in two patients for the first time.

The appearance of syphilis did not cause panic at the Medical Section, but Dr. Matzger was sufficiently alarmed to take additional steps in the daily battle against VD. He first dispatched a half-dozen volunteers to seek out patients on the streets outside the Clinic as their predecessors did during the Summer of Love. He then began working with the Communicable Disease Center in Atlanta and the University of California Medical Center to determine the incidence of gonorrhea in female patients suspected of having the disease.

At the same time, Dr. Matzger launched the Clinic's first attempt at manufacturing medication with the University of California School of Pharmacy, which prepared an inexpensive, nonprescription lotion in place of Kwell for the crabs. Patients were charged a nominal fee for the lotion and were also afforded pregnancy tests on the premises at slightly less than cost. Dr. Matzger reported these developments to the United States Public Health Service as part of his research project. They were also announced at the first National Free Clinics Conference, which attracted over eight hundred representatives of the rapidly expanding free clinic movement to the Medical Center during the last week in January. Among them were Dr. Herbert Freudenberger, who had recently opened a private drug-abuse facility on New York's lower East Side.

The conference was followed by the inauguration of a Dental Section at 558 Clayton in February. This service, the first of its type in America, obviated the necessity of sending patients to sympathetic dentists, to the University of California Dental Clinic and to the Oral Surgery Unit at General Hospital. It was initiated by Dr. Ira "Ike" Handelsman, a thirty-year-old dentist from San Francisco who objected to fee-for-service treatment because it complicated the patient-doctor relationship and prevented the poor from receiving proper care. Dr. Handelsman conceived of the Dental Section during the summer of 1969, when he applied for a five-thousand-dollar grant to study the relationship between chronic drug abuse and periodontal disease at the Clinic. Yet it took him over six months to implement his plan.

His main obstacle was the San Francisco Dental Society, which was opposed to any form of free service to indigents beyond its own charity program. The Dental Society threatened to forbid its members from participating in the project until Dr. Handelsman obtained the endorsement of the University of Pacific Dental School for his efforts. He then began recruiting faculty and students to assist him, contacted his fellow professionals for funds and equipment, and secured three donated dental chairs.

The chairs were installed in the rear of the Medical Section in the space once occupied by the calm center and laboratory. The latter was then moved into another office, while Dr. Handelsman stored his supplies and anesthetics nearby. The anesthetics had to be moved into the pharmacy after three patients tried to carry off a tank of nitrous oxide, but no further management problems were encountered. By February first, when Dr. Handelsman received his research grant from the United States Public Health Service, he and twenty assistants were treating more than two dozen patients a day.

The Dental Section was involved with the Heroin Detoxification Program both because of their physical proximity and because of the patients they shared. Dr. Gay had refined many of his techniques by this time and was gaining a reputation throughout the city for his work with addiction. Although he made his major progress with young whites new to the Haight-Ashbury, he was also accepted by the older junkies on the street. One such person, a forty-year-old ex-addict recently released from prison, became Dr. Gay's assistant at the Detoxification Program. They were dealing with three hundred patients, half of whom had never before used the Clinic, by the end of February.

Dr. Gay's success contrasted with Father Frykman's difficulties, so March meant reevaluation for the Drug Treatment Program. Father Frykman was forced to close his group house during this period because several junkies disrupted his communal family. He also had problems in the Kearny Street office, which was picketed by a racist Chinese youth group, the Red

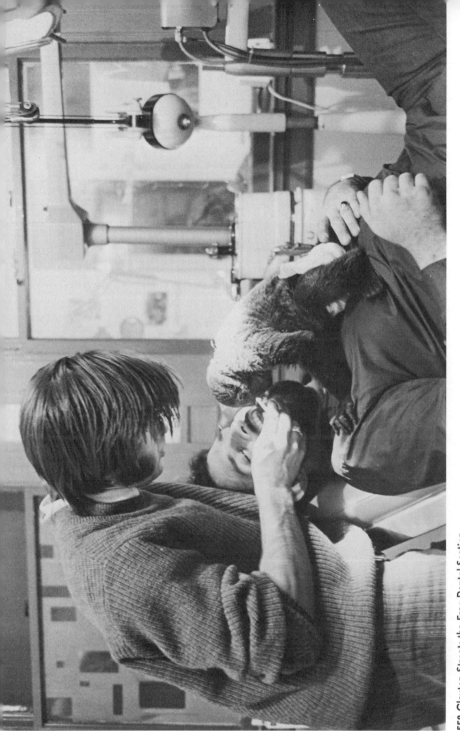

558 Clayton Street: the Free Dental Section.
(Michael Alexander)

Guards. And the continued exclusion of the Drug Treatment Program from Westside and Northeast Mental Health Center funds prevented him from taking Ed and other candidates onto the staff.

The program's complete collapse was forestalled by two large donations to the Clinic. The first was a twenty-five thousand dollar grant from the Readers' Digest Foundation, for which Dr. Smith was serving as a drug-abuse consultant. This was followed by a gift of twenty-five thousand dollars from Princess Raineri de San Faustino of San Francisco and the Bothin Helping Fund, arranged by Mrs. Inez Folger. The money allowed Father Frykman to start looking for a new North Beach office and to formulate plans for a halfway house in the Haight where he might create a more structured therapeutic community. With opiates becoming more of a problem, he decided to pattern his future efforts after the professional medical model of the Heroin Detoxification Program.

Professionalism was demanded more than usual in late March, when the Clinic had hundreds of unfamiliar patients to deal with. Two factors accounted for the sudden influx: a strike at San Francisco General and the closing of the Black Man's Free Clinic in the Fillmore. The first was led by interns and residents fed up with intolerable working conditions and insufficient patient services at General Hospital. The second came after a group of Black Panthers and other Negro militants objected to sharing their facility with whites and ordered Dr. Bertram Meyer, who created the clinic and then served as its medical director, to resign.

After Dr. Meyer left, the clinic fell apart as the black radicals attempted to do their own thing. Few Negro doctors were willing to work at their facility, and no one could equal Dr. Meyer's investment of time and money in the project. The Black Man's Free Clinic was therefore closed, while many of its former patients began coming to the Haight-Ashbury for aid.

April was a cruel month in the Haight, beginning with a bombing of Park Police Station and ending with the demise of the Peugeot station wagon that had served the Clinic for almost three years. May was also brutal: Al Rinker closed his Switchboard at the start of the month, and Dr. Arthur Carfagni failed to allocate a promised portion of his Northeast Mental Health Center budget to pay Dr. Gay's salary. But the Clinic rallied once again. Bill Bathurst and several other staff members from the Drug Treatment Program joined Dr. Gay at 409 Clayton Street; Ed, who finally swore off heroin under Dr. Gay's supervision, was given a full-time position which he handled capably; and plans were formulated for moving the project onto the first floor of 409 House because Father Grosjean and his Episcopal Peace Center were running out of money. Meanwhile, Dr. Smith, Dr. Fort, Dr. Eugene Schoenfeld and a dozen other physicians and addicts filed a class action suit against the state for the right of private facilities to use methadone in treating narcotics addiction. And John Luce and Bill Essen began planning a benefit with Bill Graham of Fillmore West to raise funds.

These developments boosted the staff's spirits, but they were only a drop in the bucket so far as Dr. Alan Matzger was concerned. He had completed his study of the Haight and its young residents by this point and was convinced that both needed more help than the multiservice agency as presently constituted could ever provide. Dr. Matzger felt that the district was beyond the self-improvement advocated by the Neighborhood Development Corporation. He also believed that its real residents required more comprehensive medical maintenance in addition to crisis intervention. These thoughts were the basis of the master plan for community health services which he forwarded to the United States Public Health Service in late May.

Dr. Matzger's plan called for a one million dollar annual grant, approximately one-half of which would go towards salaries for a full-time medical and paramedical staff. The remaining funds would be used to support the activities of several sections that might either be housed separately or in a location like the still vacant Safeway Supermarket on Haight Street. Included would be the Medical, Psychiatric and Publications sections, the Drug Detoxification and Treatment programs and a new Outreach Project, which would utilize street workers and mobile health vans. Other future efforts might include a Prenatal Section operated in conjunction with the University of California, a Family Planning Agency and a Rehabilitation Center through which the Clinic could consolidate its many counseling programs and help drug abusers reenter society.

Dr. Matzger's plan was acceptable to the Neighborhood Council and other community organizations, but he believed that it would be approved and not funded by the government. He also felt that the Clinic would be turned down for philosophic reasons by the Nixon-Agnew administration. Because his research grant had run out by this time he decided to combine his activities as chief of the Medical Section with a surgically oriented general practice for poor patients in the Mission district after the end of May.

Although Dr. Matzger's comprehensive health plan was not funded during the summer, Ruth Fleshman of the Clinic and the University of California secured in June a twenty-five-thousand-dollar grant from the National Institutes of Health for commune health education. A Commune Health Section was subsequently established in the Clinic, providing a vehicle for research and the giving of inoculations, prenatal care and family planning and childbirth information. Miss Fleshman and the staff encountered opposition from some gurus and witch doctors who resented their influence, but they succeeded in bringing preventive medicine and treatment to hundreds of young people and children in both urban and rural communes.

June also saw the formalization of a Free Clinic Consultation Section administered by Alice deSwarte. Thirty letters were arriving weekly during this period from individuals interested in starting facilities like those in the Haight-Ashbury, and staff members from the Medical and Psychiatric sections were advising residents in Isla Vista and Santa Barbara who had decided to establish a center for street people after spring disturbances near the University of California campus there. Particularly active in this effort were Dr. David Berman, Bob Cronbach and others who were supervising the Drug Treatment Program.

Drug Treatment needed their assistance, for it was all but disbanded by the end of the month, when Father Frykman left to assume the position of drug abuse counselor to the school department in Carmel. Dr. Berman and Cronbach took over as co-administrators, but their effectiveness was limited by the Clinic's lack of a residential treatment program for heroin addicts. In July, Dr. Berman and his girl friend were beaten up and arrested by Tactical Squad members after they witnessed the policemen harassing a black woman. Dr. Berman cut back on his Clinic involvement to raise defense funds, as Professor Leonard Wolf had done two years earlier. He then moved to Isla Vista to head its free clinic. Bob Cronbach also left, and Pat Bebout, a longtime staff member, fell heir to the Drug Treatment Program's offices in the Haight and the Tenderloin.

Meanwhile, the Clinic found a good friend in the person of Willis Duff, vice-president and general manager of the FM rock station KSAN. Duff first learned of the facility's work with heroin addicts in New York, where he heard Dr. Smith lecture. He then volunteered to assist John Luce and Bill Essen with the benefit they were organizing with Bill Graham. The result was a three-week period of educational announcements about the heroin epidemic and the Clinic over KSAN and two dozen other radio and television stations. This educational effort, which Duff coordinated, culminated in an antiheroin H Week between August tenth and fifteenth. On the latter date, Alice deSwarte and Dr. Smith were married.

H Week included two late-night benefit film screenings and an evening at Fillmore West with Creedence Clearwater Revival, the Bay Area's most popular band. Duff obtained Creedence for the evening of August eleventh and worked out arrangements for their appearance with Bill Graham. His help, along with that of other H Week contributors, generated a great deal of publicity for the Clinic, prompted the organizers to plan future benefits, and raised ten thousand dollars for the Heroin Detoxification Program.

This money was crucial, for Dr. Gay's program had treated one thousand patients in its first ten months of operation and was now seeing approximately fifty addicts, many of them new to the Haight-Ashbury, each day. Over half of these people were blacks who had little respect for the Clinic and its philosophy of nonviolence. One of them held a doctor at knife point on August twentieth until he opened the pharmacy. This attempted theft was averted by a prompt response from the police at Park Station, but two nights later another black addict with a lacerated tendon started breaking medical equipment when he was told there was no surgeon in residence to treat him. After being asked to leave the Clinic by Bill Essen and other staff members, he pulled a gun and waited to waylay them outside.

Park Station was notified and two patrolmen arrived within ten minutes to subdue the assailant, thereby cementing a close working relationship with the Clinic which exists to this day. But Essen and the other staff members, whose flat on Del Mar Street was ripped off twice during the summer, rightfully decided that the Medical and Dental sections could not operate in the same building as Heroin Detoxification. They were close to collapsing from nervous exhaustion when the funds collected from H Week allowed Dr. Gay to relocate his program.

Dr. Gay had once hoped to take over Father Grosjean's space in 409 House, but this move was prevented by the Episcopal Peace Center's last minute securing of funds. Dr. Gay therefore started looking for housing elsewhere and in September leased a four-story building at 529 Clayton for four hundred dollars per month. He planned to offer detoxification and counseling in the new center, along with a residential thrapeutic community supervised by himself, Ed, other former addicts and several medical student volunteers.

Although this new facility was expected to ease pressure on the other Clinic sections, the Haight-Ashbury was still difficult, if not impossible to deal with in the fall. Most of the difficulty was caused by the continued deterioration of the district and by the increased size of its Negro population. Haight Street became even more dangerous and depressing during September, forcing Stuart Loomis and Carter Mehl, who had returned to San Francisco and assumed Trina Merriman's duties as administrator of the Psychiatric Section, to avoid walking there. Volunteer dentists also grew more frightened of the street, and the periodic brutality of black patients was too much for the paramedical staff to bear. Renée Sargent quit in

September, and Bill Essen, the Medical Section's mainstay for so many months, tendered his resignation, effective in January.

Bill and Renée's absence will be hard felt at the Clinic, but, at this writing, the future looks far from grim. Other qualified young people have offered to fill the vacant staff positions, and the various Clinic sections are operating with more efficiency and structure than ever before. The Medical Section sees about one hundred people daily, one-third of them black. Dr. Ira Handelsman of the Dental Section, working with an ever increasing patient load, will soon receive his second research grant from the National Institute of Mental Health.

Father Grosjean is also in business, as are the Psychiatric, Commune Health, Publications and Free Clinic Consultation sections and the Drug Treatment programs. An expanded Executive Committee meets monthly to oversee these projects. And the Clinic has finally found a new executive coordinator to replace Don Reddick, whose health and business have suffered since his heart attack in January, 1970. He is Clyde Gardner, a former director of a convalescent hospital whom the authors recently met during a national workshop on drug-abuse education in San Francisco.

Gardner's main task will be the utilization of the Clinic's talent and the allocation of its resources in the months to come. Some staff members want him to expand the Commune Health Section and establish a New Community Medical Clinic outside the Haight where patients would be charged one dollar a visit for medical and psychiatric services. Others seek a strengthening of the Drug Treatment Program and the Medical and Dental sections within the district and hope to turn these services over to a black staff. Still others see a combination of these approaches to realize Dr. Matzger's plan for comprehensive health care.

We hope for — but do not count on — city, state or federal help for these projects. Yet whether or not aid is given, we believe that our experiment in the Haight-Ashbury will continue to grow. The Clinic can go any number of ways in the future; it may even be assimilated into an established agency like the University of California Medical Center, where John Luce is now studying, if San Francisco's health care delivery system becomes more responsive to the needs of minorities. But we trust that the Clinic will never be co-opted, that it will continue to be an amalgam of individual efforts, an alternative to bureaucratic in action, a search for a better way. It looks like Terminal Euphoria has finally killed the Haight, which has been declared an "intense poverty pocket" by the Economic Opportunity Council. But the Clinic has fulfilled its destiny as a community based multiservice agency, and we believe that, one way or another, it will never close.

Where Do We Go from Here?

Time will test our prediction about the Clinic. But time is something our country cannot afford. Although heroin may eventually run its course in the Haight-Ashbury, it and the other psychoactive chemicals that have been introduced to the district are becoming increasingly available in every part of America. New toxic compounds are likely to appear in the future, as are new patterns of abuse, new life-styles and new adolescent health problems. If we are to profit from the history of the Haight and its Free Medical Clinic, we must do something about these difficulties now.

First and foremost, we must place the Haight-Ashbury in proper perspective and realize that ours has been, is now, and perhaps ever shall be a drug-dominated society. Almost every culture in human history has used toxic chemicals for relief and recreation, but ours relies on these substances most of all. Social scientists note that the pressures of modern life are intensifying as our traditional family structure disintegrates, our cities become more congested, and our environment evolves into a vast behavioral sink. In the future these factors will probably lead us to depend more and more on alcohol, marijuana, tranquilizers and other agents to alter our moods and mental states and to regulate internal and external stimuli.

The young are most vulnerable to such pressures because of their limited psychological armamentarium and their susceptibility to the influence of peers. It is therefore hardly surprising that the steady increase in drug use and abuse throughout the United States has been most obvious in those subcultures which have sprung up in areas like the Haight over the past decade. Young people there and elsewhere now appear to be melded together in one rapidly expanding youth subculture. This subculture is certain to change in the future. But no matter what form it takes, its members will never be unique in their chemical consumption. They will continue to be a reflection of the dominant culture that they have rejected — and that has rejected them. Although their specific choices may differ, the children of tomorrow will use and abuse drugs primarily because their parents and parent surrogates do today.

This fact can best be appreciated if we bear in mind that old and young alike take toxic chemicals predominantly for therapeutic purposes. Whether they seek to overcome affective numbness and to control their anger like Alan, to satisfy peer-group pressure and prove their independence like Jackie, to disguise their dysfunctioning and gain a sense of mastery over their emotions like Randy, to validate their delusions and manipulate others like Charlie and early leaders of the psychedelic movement, to escape their depressions and fill their emptiness like Ed, or to insulate themselves from anxiety and stress like so many parents, people use and abuse drugs not because they are criminals but because they are in pain.

Use and abuse are therefore medical and social, not legal problems. The Supreme Court has acknowledged this by declaring alcoholism an illness rather than a criminal action. Yet most Americans accept and endorse punitive legislation against dependency and addiction to other compounds, support political leaders like Ronald Reagan who adopt "get tough" policies toward abuse and allow the police to violate civil rights in attempting to control the traffic of illegal chemicals. We have progressed to the point where mentally ill patients are no longer straitjacketed and thrown into dungeons in this country. But we still do not recognize that abuse of all drugs, including alcohol, is a disease.

One reason for this blindness is that most people, even if they smoke cigarettes to settle their nerves or drink coffee to wake up in the morning, refuse to see their actions and those of other addicts as forms of self-medication. Another is that some people project their own unconscious appetites onto others whose weaknesses are more apparent — or less carefully concealed. Furthermore, as Dr. John C. Kramer states, "The major conceptual obstacle to accepting addiction or dependence as a disease is that it is usually self-initiated and self-sustained. Other diseases seem to be thrust upon their victims from the outside.

"Yet," Dr. Kramer continues, "there may be less willfulness in becoming drug dependent than it seems. Initially the motivating force may be curiosity or proving one's boldness or for social acceptance or as a protest against the conventions of the larger culture; foolish, perhaps, but not criminal. Once initiated, the drug use may also be self-perpetuating. Dependency-producing drugs are by definition strong reinforcers, and the desire to resume the drug effect can be powerful enough to carry the user beyond questioning the propriety or the legality of his actions."

Dr. Kramer's points have been conclusively demonstrated in the Haight-Ashbury. So has the fact that abuse beyond the experimental or social levels is almost invariably a symptom of underlying psychological problems. These difficulties may be insurmountable in certain habitual and multiple abuse cases. But they may be relatively simple to solve in adolescents who use toxic compounds to help them avoid or ameliorate the process of growing up. Dr. Ernest Dernburg believes that many young people today have a propensity toward psychological plateauing which is enhanced by society and by their subcultural involvement. If they are further alienated by adults, they may remain in the youth subculture for the rest of their lives.

The Haight should teach us to eschew such negative reinforcement. Yet our elected leaders still throw tantrums when their opinions are not respected and continue to use repressive tactics against rightful dissent. They also ridicule the younger generation, fail to hear and respond to grievances, and maintain a distance which exacerbates the feelings of rejection common to so many adolescents. In the process, they intensify the alienation and the self- and socially destructive behavior of young people. They allow self-acknowledged gurus to seize leadership in their absence. The Haight-Ashbury should remind us that adults give the young much to fight against but precious little to struggle for.

The Haight should also show us the failure of two ethical systems. The first, the eupsychic ethic, has led to mass irresponsibility, commercial exploitation and a collective acting-out pathology which culminated in the disaster at Altamont in December of 1969. Yet doing your thing has been no more than an historical response to social inaction. It and the tired "law and order" clichés of reactionary politicians represent the opposite ends of the present ethical spectrum. As such, they are probably destined for failure. But constructive progress can be accomplished if we work within the two extremes.

To facilitate this, we must amend our current drug policies to encourage medical research and treatment and to discourage the alienation and criminalization of the young. This requires us to rewrite state and federal statutes to meet scientific drug classifications and to make the penalties for violating such statutes consistent with the pharmacological properties of psychoactive agents and commensurate to the abusers' alleged crimes. Marijuana, for example, should not be categorized as a narcotic any longer. Its possession should not be regarded as a felony offense. And we should consider making standardized preparations of *Cannabis* legal to persons over twenty-one years of age.

At the same time, we should seriously consider curtailing or completely revising antipossession laws. Drs. Meyers and Fort favor this approach, noting that such statutes have never begun to achieve their ostensible purpose of limiting chemical consumption. Instead, they have distracted the police from their proper duties, given politicians a smoke-screen issue, and imposed a major burden on the taxpayer. They have also prevented some people from seeking or receiving treatment and attracted others to drugs because of their illegality.

The alternative is to uniformly enforce the existing legislation. Such fairness had never been traditional in our country, a fact that is not lost on the young. They know that there is no justification in penalizing adolescent users of black-market drugs while adults are allowed to stockpile barbiturates and amphetamines. One answer to this situation would be to require triplicate forms for sedative and stimulant prescriptions, as is done with narcotics, and to place strict production quotas on the domestic pharmaceutical companies which manufacture them.

Indeed, uniform enforcement of statutes governing the manufacture and sale of toxic substances is a necessity. Operation Intercept and the Federal Bureau of Narcotics's efforts against opiate importation ease unemployment but do little to counteract the foreign-based drug flow. They also fail to deal with the flood of toxic chemicals from domestic pharmaceutical companies. If we must continue to rely on legislation, let us at least spend the same amount of time and money policing the people responsible for filling our medicine chests with amphetamines and barbiturates as we do barbs dealers and underground manufacturers of speed.

In addition, let us require these people to clearly state the adverse effects of their products. Alcohol is as hazardous to health as tobacco. So are most pain-killers and diet and sleeping pills. The Food and Drug Administration should regulate the manufacture of these substances and others which are either medically useless or hazardous. Yet it has been emasculated by budgetary restrictions and undercut by politicians whose campaigns are financed in part by the drug industry.

The same industry should be condemned for the deleterious effects of its advertising. Drugs were a problem before Madison Avenue emerged as our Fifth Estate, but there is little doubt that the use of enticing advertisements and the exploitation of human weakness by pharmaceutical companies is largely responsible for engendering the climate of abuse in our country. The impact of advertising on fostering destructive attitudes should be curbed by legislators advised by pharmacologists and psychiatrists. So should the television industry, which helped create the Haight-Ashbury in the first place and may well be contributing to the passivity so common among the young.

Education is another answer. Along these lines, we should encourage the study of sex, hygiene, health, and drug use and abuse in the home and in grammer school, recognizing that young people will otherwise learn about them in places like the Haight. Whether these subjects are presented in the separate human ecology classes we are now designing or as part of a general curriculum, those who teach them should not attempt to isolate abusers or stamp out psychoactive agents but accept them as facts of life, as their students do. They should avoid using teaching machines, poorly produced films and other technological crutches which young people rightfully condemn — and which are no substitute for interpersonal relationships. They should realize that perhaps the best thing they can teach is discrimination in using drugs. They should present scientific fact rather then moral bias. They should let young people, when possible, do most of the teaching. And, most important, they should educate parents and professionals in the latest drug-abuse trends.

This is crucial, for few of the approximately two million young people who have passed through the Haight-Ashbury in the past ten years would have done so if they had sufficient reason to stay home. Most of these youths have suffered from parental rejection, insufficient nurturing and an inability to cope with our antiquated and rigid social institutions. They have viewed the Haight, its Free Clinic and other organizations as political alternatives to the status quo and as places to find substitute families. Our country desperately needs alternatives like the Clinic which give young people a sense of competency and involvement. It also needs a new or modified model of home life. Short of placing infants in urban kibbutzim, as Dr. Bruno Bettelheim has suggested, the ultimate answer to the drug-abuse epidemic in the United States would be a massive mental health program designed to shore up or selectively improve the crumbling structure of the American family.

Such suggestions do not exceed the scope of our national capabilities, but we doubt they will ever be acted upon; abuse is symptomatic of social, as well as personal ills. These ills run deep in America, yet many adults, including those whose children have run away to the Haight, refuse to admit to them. Wide-scale treatment is impossible in a country which annually allocates thirteen dollars per person for health and four hundred dollars for war.

Until this situation is reversed, until we regain our sense of national purpose, we cannot reach the young and reconstitute our society. Nor can we expect our older political and medical leaders to do the job. Men like Ronald Reagan have repeatedly refused to allocate funds for education and treatment and have thereby encouraged the growth of teen-age slums modeled after the Haight-Ashbury in at least a dozen major cities. The United States Public Health Service is restricted in its budget, while such local public health departments as San Francisco's have seemed more interested in their own longevity than that of their patients. The American Medical Association, which spends more money on the election of conservative candidates than on the distribution of health information, remains extremely resistant to purposeful change.

The Haight-Ashbury Free Medical Clinic and other facilities like it maintain a different approach to drug, health and social problems. They do not offer solutions to the problems, for at present there are none. Nor do they claim to be ideal organizations: their structures are extremely fragile, and their experience has most often been gained the hard way. Yet, as Dr. Philip Selznick writes, "The character and direction of new instruments of intervention have been born out of social crisis, set out piecemeal as circumstances have demanded; they have not come to us as part of a broad and conscious vision." The Clinic and the new community which inspired it were created in response to this lack of social vision. The new community is now dead. The Clinic is struggling for survival. And the vision is still lacking today.

Perhaps today's free clinics are clumsy models for the delivery of health services tomorrow. Yet they do offer a concept and an alternative applicable to other existing institutions. The clinics have gained a wide popularity by respecting the needs and the imperfect humanity of their patients. They have revitalized the doctor-patient relationship and shown its relevance in modern, computerized medicine. They have demonstrated the desirability and practicality of minimizing red tape in dealing with people. They have pioneered the use of paramedical volunteers and staff workers in a country faced with a severe shortage of doctors and professional personnel.

Finally, the free clinics have proven their ability to reach alienated economic, racial and philosophic minorities. They have advanced the goals of community medicine by seeking out patients in their own environment and by regarding the environment as an organism capable of being healed. They have provided an outlet for idealism and social frustration. And they have served as a conscience for the country. These are the true meanings of Love Needs Care.

Bibliography

Glossary

Appendices

Bibliography

The following articles, books and monographs have been used in the preparation of *Love Needs Care* and are recommended as references for our readers. Also listed are a number of journals, books and films associated with the Haight-Ashbury Free Medical Clinic and available through its Publications Section at 409 Clayton Street in San Francisco.

I. References and Suggested Reading

Adler, Nathan. "The Antinomian Psychotherapies." Presented at the 76th Annual Convention of the American Psychological Association, San Francisco, 1968.

Alexander, Franz. *Psychosomatic Medicine.* New York: W. W. Norton, 1950.

Alexander, Franz, and Selesnick, Sheldon. *The History of Psychiatry.* New York: Harper and Row, 1966.

Alighieri, Dante. *The Divine Comedy.* New York: Washington Square Press, 1968.

Arieti, Silvano. *The Intrapsychic Self.* New York: Basic Books, 1967.

Asimov, Isaac. *The Human Body.* Boston: Houghton Mifflin, 1963.

———. *The Human Brain.* Boston: Houghton Mifflin, 1964.

Becker, H. S. *Outsiders: Studies in the Sociology of Deviance.* New York: The Free Press, 1963: 150–185.

Bell, Daniel. "Charles Fourier: Prophet of Eupsychia." *The American Scholar* 38:1 (1963–64): 41–58.

Bettelheim, Bruno. *The Children of the Dream.* New York: Macmillan, 1961.

———. *The Empty Fortress.* New York: The Free Press, 1967.

Blacker, K. H. "Aggression and the Chronic Use of LSD." Appeared as "The Acid-heads." *American Journal of Psychiatry* 123:5 (1968): 97–107.

Blos, Peter. *On Adolescence.* New York: The Free Press, 1962.

Brainerd, Henry; Margen, Sheldon; and Chatton, Milton J. *Current Diagnosis and Treatment.* Los Altos, California: Lange Medical Publications, 1969.

Brenner, Charles. *An Elementary Textbook of Psychoanalysis.* New York: International Universities Press, 1955.

Brown, Norman O. *Life Against Death.* Middletown, Connecticut: Wesleyan University Press, 1959.

Camus, Albert. *The Plague.* New York: Random House, 1950.

Carey, James T. *The College Drug Scene.* Englewood Cliffs, New Jersey: Prentice Hall, 1968.

Castaneda, Carlos. *The Teachings of Don Juan.* Berkeley: University of California Press, 1968.

Cohen, S. "The Therapeutic Potential of LSD-25." *A Pharmacologic Approach to the Study of the Mind,* edited by Robert M. Featherstone and Alexander Simon, pp. 251–259. Springfield, Illinois: Thomas, 1959.

Columbia University Press. *The Columbia Encyclopedia.* New York: 1969.

Davies, Hunter. *The Beatles.* New York: Dell Books, 1968.

Davis, Fred, and Munoz, Laura. "Heads and Freaks: Patterns and Meanings of Drug Use Among Hippies." *Journal of Health and Social Behavior* 9:2 (1968): 156–164.

DeRopp, Robert S. *Drugs and the Mind.* New York: Grove Press, 1957.

Didion, Joan. *Slouching Towards Bethlehem.* New York: Farrar, Straus and Giroux, 1968.

Dole, V. P.; Nyswander, M. E.; and Warner, A. "Successful Treatment of 750 Criminal Addicts." *Journal of the American Medical Association* 206:12 (1968): 2708–2711.

Dole, V. P.; Robinson, J. W.; Orraca, J.; Launs, E.; Searcy, P.; and Caine, E. "Methadone Treatment of Randomly Selected Criminal Addicts." *New England Journal of Medicine* 41:5 (1969): 1372–1375.

Dole, V. P., and Warner, A. "Evaluation of Narcotic Treatment Programs." *American Journal of Public Health* 57:11 (1967): 2000–2008.

Dostoevski, Fëodor. *The House of the Dead.* New York: Dell, 1967.

Eliot, T. S. *The Complete Poems and Plays 1909–1950.* New York: Harcourt, Brace, Jovanovich, 1962.

The Encyclopedia of Mental Health. Philadelphia: Franklin, 1968.

Erikson, Erik H. *Identity: Youth and Crisis.* New York: W. W. Norton, 1968.

Farb, Peter. *Man's Rise to Civilization.* New York: E. P. Dutton, 1968.

Fenichel, Otto. *The Psychoanalytic Theory of Neurosis.* New York: W. W. Norton, 1945.

Ferlinghetti, Lawrence. *A Coney Island of the Mind.* New York: New Directions, 1968.

Fort, Joel. *The Pleasure Seekers: The Drug Crisis, Youth and Society.* Indianapolis: Bobbs-Merrill, 1969.

———. *Comparison Chart of Mind-Altering Substances.* San Francisco: Fort Center for Solving Special Problems, 1969.

———. "Pot: A Rational Approach." *Playboy* 16:10 (1969): 131–216.

———. "Social Problems of Drug Use and Drug Policies." *California Law Review* 56:1 (1968): 273–291.

Freud, Sigmund. *Basic Writings.* New York: Modern Library, 1938.

———. *Civilization and Its Discontents.* New York: W. W. Norton, 1962.

———. *The Complete Introductory Lectures on Psychoanalysis.* New York: W. W. Norton, 1966.

Friedman, Maurice. *To Deny Our Nothingness.* New York: Delacorte Press, 1967.

Fromm, Erich. *The Heart of Man.* New York: Harper and Row, 1964.

Ginsberg, Allen. *Howl and Other Poems.* San Francisco: City Lights Books, 1956.

Goodman, Louis S., and Gilman, Alfred. *The Pharmacological Basis of Therapeutics.* New York: Macmillan, 1955.

Grier, William H., and Cobbs, Price M. *Black Rage.* New York: Basic Books, 1968.

Hale, Dennis, ed. *The California Dream*. New York: P. F. Collier, 1968.

Hazlitt, William C. *English Proverbs*. Detroit: Gale, 1907.

Hedgepeth, William, and Stock, Dennis. *The Alternative: Communal Life in New America*. New York: Macmillan, 1970.

Heinlein, Robert A. *Stranger in a Strange Land*. New York: G. P. Putnam's Sons, 1961.

Hesse, Hermann. *Steppenwolf*. New York: Modern Library, 1963.

Hippocrates. *Genuine Works*. New York: Dover Publications, 1958.

Hopkins, Jerry, ed. *The Hippie Papers*. New York: Signet Books, 1968.

Huxley, Aldous. *The Doors of Perception*. New York: Harper and Row, 1954.

Jones, Reese. "Myths about Marijuana." Paper read at a drug-abuse conference, September 20, 1970, sponsored by the Department of Continuing Education in Health Sciences, University of California, San Francisco.

Kenniston, Kenneth. *The Uncommitted*. New York: Dell Books, 1957.

Kerouac, Jack. *On the Road*. New York: The Viking Press, 1957.

Kesey, Ken. *One Flew Over the Cuckoo's Nest*. New York: The Viking Press, 1962.

———. *Sometimes a Great Notion*. New York: The Viking Press, 1963.

Koestler, Arthur. *The Act of Creation*. New York: Macmillan, 1964.

Kramer, J.; Fishman, V.; and Littlefield, D. "Amphetamine Abuse: Patterns and Effects in High Doses Taken Intravenously." *Journal of the American Medical Association* 201:5 (1967): 480–484.

Kramer, John C. "New Directions in the Management of Opiate Dependence." *The New Physician* 18:3 (1969): 203–209.

Kramer, J., and Bass, R. A. "Institutionalization Patterns Among Civilly Committed Addicts." *Journal of the American Medical Association* 208:12 (1969): 2297–2301.

Leary, Timothy. *High Priest*. New York: New American Library, 1968.

Leary, Timothy, and Alpert, Richard. *The Psychedelic Experience*. New York: University Books, 1965.

Leary, Timothy, et al. *The Psychedelic Reader*. New York: University Books, 1965.

Lemere, Frederick. "The Danger of Amphetamine Dependency." *American Journal of Psychiatry* 123:5 (1966) 171–178.

Leonard, George. *Education and Ecstasy*. New York: Delacorte, 1969.

Lindesmith, Alfred R. *The Addict and the Law*. Bloomington, Indiana: Indiana University Press, 1965.

Lorenz, Konrad. *On Aggression*. New York: Harcourt, Brace, Jovanovich, 1966.

Luce, John. "A Case of Terminal Euphoria." *Esquire* 72:1 (1969): 65–78.

———. "A Young Doctor's Crusade." *Look* 31:16 (1967): 24–28.

———. "Bill Graham's Fillmore." *San Francisco Magazine* 8:11 (1966): 41–64.

———. "Bill Graham: The P. T. Barnum of Rock and Roll." *Eye* 2:3 (1969): 20–23.

———. "End of the Road." *California Living*. In press.

———. "Jefferson Airplane Loves You." *Look* 31:11 (1967): 52–55.

———. "The Esalen Experience." *San Francisco Magazine* 10:1 (1968): 31–48.

———. "The Hippies and Christianity." *Journal of Psychedelic Drugs* 2:1 (1968): 36–37.

———. "The Incredibles." *Look* (1968): 51–58.

———. "Two Days on the Farm with Kesey." *Confluence* 1:2 (1968): 29–31.

———. "Where Should You Touch." *Eye* 1:8 (1968): 30–34.

———. "Whither the Hippies." *San Francisco Magazine* 9:5 (1967): 39–45.

McCary, James L. *Human Sexuality.* New York: Van Nostrand Reinhold, 1968.

McLuhan, Marshall. *Understanding Media.* New York: McGraw-Hill, 1964.

Mailer, Norman. "The White Negro." *Dissent,* 1957. Reprinted by City Lights Books, 1961.

Manheimer, D. I.; Mellinger, G.; and Balter, M. B. "Psychotherapeutic Drugs: Use Among Adults in California." *California Medicine* 109:12 (1968): 445–451.

Marcuse, Herbert. *Eros and Civilization.* New York: Random House, 1955.

Marlowe, Christopher. *Doctor Faustus.* Cambridge, Massachusetts: Harvard University Press, 1966.

Maslow, Abraham. *Towards a Psychology of Being.* New York: Van Nostrand Reinhold, 1968.

Menninger, Karl. *The Crime of Punishment.* New York: The Viking Press, 1968.

———. *Man Against Himself.* New York: Harcourt, Brace, Jovanovich, 1940.

Meyers, Frederick H.; Jawetz, Ernest; and Goldfein, Alan. *Review of Medical Pharmacology.* Los Altos, California: Lange Medical Publications, 1968.

Meyers, Frederick H., and Smith, D. E. "Drug Abuse: Recommendations for California Treatment and Research Facilities." The First Annual Report of the Drug Abuse Information Project. *California Medicine* 109:12 (1968): 191–197.

Morris, Desmond. *The Human Zoo.* New York: McGraw-Hill, 1969.

———. *The Naked Ape.* New York: McGraw-Hill, 1966.

Oremland, Jerome D. "A Skeptical View of LSD as a Therapeutic Agent." Delivered in April, 1963, to the San Francisco Psychological Association.

———. "My Three Hippies." Paper read at "A Psychoanalytic View of the Current Drug Scene," conference sponsored by the Department of Psychiatry, University of Utah Medical School and the San Francisco Psychoanalytic Institute, August, 1969, at Salt Lake City.

Perls, Frederick; Hefferline, Ralph F.; and Goodman, Paul. *Gestalt Therapy.* New York: Julian Press, 1951.

Piaget, Jean. *The Moral Judgment of the Child.* New York: The Free Press, 1966.

Rapaport, David. *Collected Papers.* New York: Basic Books, 1967.

Rigney, Francis J., and Smith, L. Douglas. *The Real Bohemia.* New York: Basic Books, 1961.

Rilke, Rainer Maria. *Letters to a Young Poet.* New York: W. W. Norton, 1954.

Roheim, Geza. *Magic and Schizophrenia.* New York: International Universities Press, 1962.

Roszak, Theodore. *The Making of a Counter Culture.* New York: Doubleday, 1968.

Schoenfeld, Eugene. *Dear Dr. Hip Pocrates.* New York: Grove Press, 1969.

Schutz, William C. *Joy.* New York: Grove Press, 1967.

Shakespeare, William. *The Merchant of Venice.* New Haven: Yale University Press, 1950.

Shick, J. F. E.; Smith, D. E.; and Meyers, F. H. "Use of Amphetamine in the Haight-Ashbury." *Journal of Psychedelic Drugs* 2:1 (1968): 139–171.

———. "Use of Marijuana in the Haight-Ashbury." *Journal of Psychedelic Drugs* 2:1 (1968): 49–65.

Smith, D. E. "Acid Heads vs. Speed Freaks: A Conflict Between Drug Subcultures." *Clinical Pediatrics* 14:4 (1969): 56–61.

———. "First and Second Annual Report on Drug Abuse to the California Legislature." *Drug Abuse Papers 1969.* Berkeley: University of California Berkeley Extension, 1969.

———. "LSD and the Psychedelic Syndrome." *Clinical Toxicology* 2:1 (1969): 69–73.

Smith, D. E. "LSD, Violence and Radical Religious Beliefs." *Journal of Psychedelic Drugs* 3:1 (1970): 38–41.

———. "Runaways and Their Health Problems in Haight-Ashbury during the Summer of 1967." *American Journal of Public Health* 59:11 (1969): 181–186.

———. "The Characteristics of Dependence in High-Dose Methamphetamine Abuse." *The International Journal of Addictions* 4:3 (1969): 453–459.

———. "The New Generation and the New Drugs." *California Health* 25:8 (1968): 7–11.

———. "The Trip: There and Back." *Emergency Medicine* 12:8 (1969): 48–55.

Smith, D. E., and Bentel, D. "Third Annual Report to the California Legislature." Unpublished manuscript. San Francisco: Department of Pharmacology, University of California Medical Center, December, 1969.

Smith, D.E.; Luce, J.; and Dernburg, E. "The Health of Haight-Ashbury." *Transaction* 7:6 (1970): 35–45.

Smith, D. E., and Mehl, C. "An Analysis of Marijuana Toxicity." *The New Social Drug: Medical, Legal, and Cultural Perspectives on Marijuana.* Englewood Cliffs, New Jersey: Prentice-Hall, 1970: 63–77.

Smith, D. E., and Rose, A. J. "The Group Marriage Commune: A Case Study." *Journal of Psychedelic Drugs.* 3:1 (1970): 115–119.

Smith, D. E., and Sternfield, J. "Natural Childbirth and Cooperative Childbearing in Psychedelic Communes." *Journal of Psychedelic Drugs.* 3:1 (1970): 120–124.

Smith, D. E., and Sturges, C. S. "The Semantics of the San Francisco Drug Scene." *ETC* 26:2 (1969): 168–175.

Smith, D. E.; Wesson, D.; and Lannon, L. "New Developments in Barbiturate Abuse." *Drug Abuse Papers, 1969.* Berkeley: University of California Berkeley Extension, 1969.

Smith, Roger. *The Marketplace of Speed.* San Francisco, 1969. Unpublished manuscript.

———. "The World of the Haight-Ashbury Speed Freak." *Journal of Psychedelic Drugs* 2:2 (1969): 172–188.

Solomon, David, ed. *The Marijuana Papers.* Indianapolis: Bobbs-Merrill, 1966.

Stekel, Wilhelm. *Compulsion and Doubt.* New York: Washington Square Press, 1965.

———. *Patterns of Psychosexual Infantilism.* New York: Washington Square Press, 1966.

Thompson, Hunter S. *The Hell's Angels.* New York: Ballantine Books, 1967.

Tolkien, J. R. R. *The Lord of the Rings.* Boston: Houghton Mifflin, 1967.

Von Hoffman, Nicholas. *We Are the People Our Parents Warned Us Against.* New York: Dell, 1968.

Watts, Alan W. *Psychotherapy East and West.* New York: Pantheon Books, 1961.

———. *The Joyous Cosmology.* New York: Pantheon Books, 1962.

Weil, Andrew T.; Zinberg, Norman E.; and Nelsen, Judith M. "Clinical and Psychological Effects of Marijuana in Man." *Science* 162 (1968): 12:34–42. Also appears in *The New Social Drug*. David M. Smith, M.D., ed. Englewood Cliffs, New Jersey: Prentice-Hall, 1970.

Weinraub, Michael, Laura and Simon. *Summer 1969, A Diary of Visits to Communes in Oregon and Northern California*. San Francisco, (1969). Unpublished manuscript.

Wilmer, Harry A. *Social Psychiatry in Action: A Therapeutic Community*. Springfield, Illinois: Thomas, 1958.

Wolf, Leonard, ed. *Voices from the Love Generation*. Boston. Little, Brown, 1968.

Wolfe, Burton H. *The Hippies*. New York: New American Library, 1968.

Wolfe, Tom. *The Electric Kool-Aid Acid Test*. New York: Farrar, Straus and Giroux, 1968.

Yablonsky, Lewis. *The Hippie Trip*. New York. Pegasus, 1968.

———. *Synanon: The Tunnel Back*. New York: Macmillan, 1965.

Yeats, William Butler. *Collected Poems*. New York: Macmillan, 1955.

Yoors, Jan. *The Gypsies*. New York: Simon and Schuster, 1967.

II. Journals and Pamphlets Associated with the Haight-Ashbury Free Medical Clinic

Smith, D. E., ed. "The Contemporary Heroin Scene." *Journal of Psychedelic Drugs*. In press.

———, ed. "Current Marijuana Issues." *Journal of Psychedelic Drugs* 2:1 (1968).

———. *Drug Abuse Papers 1969*. Berkeley: University of California Berkeley Extension, 1969.

———. "LSD: The Psychedelic Experience and Beyond." *Journal of Psychedelic Drugs*. In press.

———. "Psychedelic Drugs and the Law." *Journal of Psychedelic Drugs* 1:1 (1967).

———. "Psychedelic Drugs and Religion." *Journal of Psychedelic Drugs* 1:2 (1968).

———. "Speed Kills: A Review of Amphetamine Abuse." *Journal of Psychedelic Drugs* 2:2 (1969).

III. Books Associated with the Haight-Ashbury Free Medical Clinic

Frykman, J. *A New Connection: An Approach to the Compulsive Drug User*. San Francisco: C/J Press, 1970.

Smith, D. E., ed. *The New Social Drug: Medical, Legal and Cultural Perspectives on Marijuana*. Englewood Cliffs, New Jersey: Prentice-Hall, 1970.

IV. Films Associated with the Haight-Ashbury Free Medical Clinic.

Community Approaches to Drug Abuse. Guidance Associates, Pleasantville, New York.

Darkness, Darkness. Nolan, Wilton, and Wootten, Inc. Palo Alto, California.

Escape to Nowhere. Professional Arts, San Mateo, California.

Marijuana: What Can You Believe? Guidance Associates, Pleasantville, New York.

The Alienated Generation. Guidance Associates, Pleasantville, New York.

The Speedscene. Bailley Films, Los Angeles, California.

You Can't Grow a Green Plant in a Closet. Zeal Productions, Mill Valley, California.

GLOSSARY

The following is a listing of the drug slang and the psychiatric terms used in **Love Needs Care.** The psychiatric definitions are adapted from those in **The Encyclopedia of Mental Health.**

A

A	Lysergic acid diethylamide, or LSD.
ACAPULCO GOLD	A superior grade of marijuana which is somewhat gold in color and is supposedly grown in the vicinity of Acapulco, Mexico.
ACID	LSD.
ACID HEAD	An LSD user.
AMBIVALENCE	The coexistence of two opposing emotions, such as love and hate.
AMP	Ampule.
AMPED	Wired on crystal or methedrine.
ANACLITIC	Leaning on; in psychoanalysis the word denotes the dependence of an infant on his mother or her surrogates.
ANACLITIC DEPRESSION	An acute and striking impairment of an infant's development which usually occurs following a sudden separation from a mothering person.
ANXIETY	Apprehension, tension and/or uneasiness which stems from the anticipation of danger, the source of which is largely unknown or unrecognized. Anxiety is primarily of intrapsychic origin, while fear is the emotional response to a consciously recognized threat or danger.

B

BAG	(1) About one ounce of marijuana (see also **lid**). (2) In connection with powdered drugs, a small square of paper folded into a rectangle in order to hold the drug. (3) Small plastic coin collectors' bag used for powdered drugs. (4) A category or classification, particularly a rut or habit (e.g., to be in the same bag).
BAG OF BUNK	A bag containing sugar without heroin.
BALL	To have sexual intercourse.
BALLOON	Container for heroin.

BARBS	Barbiturates.
BEANS	Benzedrine.
BEAT	Bohemian.
BEATNIK	A term used by the media to describe a bohemian.
BENNIES	Benzedrine in tablet form.
BERNICE	Cocaine.
BIKER	A motorcycle rider.
BLACK MOTE	Marijuana that has been cured in sugar or honey and then buried for a period of time to lengthen its effects.
BLOW THE MIND	To dazzle or astonish and/or disturb.
BLOW THE VEIN	To use too much pressure on a weak or sclerose vein, causing it to rupture.
BLUE BULLETS	Amytal sodium.
BLUE DEVILS	Amytal sodium.
BLUE DOLLS	Amytal sodium.
BLUE HEAVEN	Amytal sodium or morphine.
BLUE AND REDS	Tuinal: 50 percent Amytal sodium, 50 percent secobarbital (Blue Tips).
BLUES	Sodium Pentothal.
BOOST	To steal, shoplift.
BOOT-AND-SHOE HYPE	A poor hustler and/or heroin addict.
BREAD	Money.
BREW	Beer.
BUMMER	A bad experience.
BUM TRIP	A bad experience.
BURN	To sell impure drugs.
BUSH	Marijuana.
BUST	To arrest.
BUSINESSMAN'S TRIP	The experience of taking DMT, a short-acting hallucinogen.

C

C	Cocaine.
CALM CENTER	A quiet, dimly-lit room used to detoxify and talk down people using drugs, especially hallucinogens.
CAN	About one ounce of marijuana; a Prince Albert tobacco can (one to one and three-quarter ounces).
CANDY	Cocaine.
CANDYMAN	Dealer of cocaine.
CAP	(1) Number-five gelatin capsule used to package drugs. (2) The head. (3) To put down.
CARGA	Spanish for heroin.
CARTWHEELS	Benzedrine.
CATTLE RUSTLERS	People who shoplift and/or steal food which they then resell for profit on the black market.
CHANGES	The changes one goes through in life.
CHICAGO GREEN	Dark-green marijuana said to be popular in Chicago.
CHICK	A girl or woman.
CHIP	To use drugs occasionally, especially heroin.

380

CHOPPER	Motorcycle.
CHRISTMAS TREE	Green and white time spansule containing a stimulant and a barbiturate or meprobamate.
CLAP	Gonorrhea.
COKE	Cocaine.
COKE FREAK	Someone who abuses cocaine.
COLD TURKEY	A condition of heroin withdrawal; immediate withdrawal without the benefit of medication.
COLUMBUS BLACK	Marijuana.
COMMUNE	Group living arrangement.
COME DOWN	To return to normal consciousness after being high.
COMPULSION	A persistent behavior that cannot be ceased by logic or reasoning.
CONNECTION	Drug dealer, especially of heroin.
COOK	To concoct chemically; one who produces drugs.
COOL	Calm, tranquil, unassertive; self-control.
COP	To acquire, snatch, steal.
COP OUT	To give up, to sell out, particularly to the Establishment.
CORAL	Chloral hydrate.
COUNT	The amount of purity of a drug.
CRABS	Pediculosis or scabies.
CRANK	Methamphetamine in powdered form.
CRANK BUGS	Imaginary insects which drug users may feel crawling over or under their skin.
CRASH	To sleep, to come down from a drug high.
CRASH PAD	Temporary sleeping quarters.
CRINK	Methamphetamine in powdered form.
CRIS	Methamphetamine in powdered form.
CRISTINA	Methamphetamine in powdered form.
CROSS-TOPS	Benzedrine.
CRUTCH	The holder used to smoke a roach down short without burning the fingertips.
CRYSTAL	Methamphetamine in powdered form, or cocaine crystals.
CRYSTAL PALACE	A residence of amphetamine abusers.
CUNT	An area of vein favored for injection.

D

DEFENSE MECHANISMS	Intrapsychic defense processes, operating unconsciously, which are employed to seek resolution of emotional conflict and freedom from anxiety.
DELUSION	A false belief maintained against logic.
DEPRESSION	Psychiatrically, a morbid sadness, dejection or melancholy to be differentiated from grief which is appropriate to that which is lost. Depression may be neurotic or psychotic in intensity.
DEX	Dextroamphetamine tablets or capsules.
DEXIES	Dextroamphetamine tablets or capsules.
DICE	Desoxyn, methamphetamine.
DIG	To understand or enjoy.

DIGGERS	A group of hippies deriving their name from an English society which practiced utopian communism.
DILLIES	Dialalidid, dihydromorphinone.
DIME	Ten dollars.
DIME BAG	A bag of drugs costing ten dollars.
DITCH	The inside of the elbow, which has two large veins.
DO YOUR THING	To engage in whatever you want to do, especially in the face of opposition and/or convention.
DOLLAR	One hundred dollars.
DOPE	Marijuana.
DOPE FIEND	Term used by drug users to parody society's view of them.
DOPER	Drug user.
DOWNER	Sedatives.
DOWNS	Sedatives.
DOUBLE TROUBLE	Tuinal.
DRIPPER	Eyedropper.
DROP	To ingest orally (e.g., to drop acid).
DROP A DIME	To call the police to cause a raid or arrests.
DUST	Cocaine.

E

EARTH MOTHER	A maternal person; one who nurtures and is close to nature.
EGO	From the Latin I am; refers to that part of the psyche which possesses consciousness, maintains its identity, and recognizes and tests reality.
EGO BOUNDARY	The perceptive process through which the ego recognizes its identity and distinguishes between subjective phenomena and those which originate in the outside world.
EGO FUNCTIONS	Various actions of consciousness, such as speech and reality testing, through which the ego manifests itself. Freud wrote in **An Outline of Psychoanalysis** that the ego controls voluntary movement and the instinct of self-preservation by becoming aware of stimuli from within and without, by storing up experience, by avoiding excessive stimuli and by learning to bring about appropriate modifications in the external world to its own advantage.
EUPSYCHIC	Pertaining to the release of psychic impulses for purposes which are alleged to be beneficial to man and society.

F

FAR OUT	An all-purpose word meaning great or that which defies understanding.
FIFTEEN CENTS	Fifteen dollars.
FIT	Paraphernalia for injection.
FIX	Intravenous injection.

FLAKE	Cocaine.
FLASH	The intense orgasmlike euphoria experienced immediately after an intravenous injection.
FLATFOOT HUSTLER	One who can hustle in a variety of ways.
FLIGHT OF IDEAS	Verbal skipping from one idea to another before the last one has been concluded.
FLIP CHICK	Crazy girl.
FLOWER CHILDREN	A term applied to the hippies by the media.
FOURS	Empirin compound with codeine.
FREAK	(1) To become afraid, and/or temporarily deranged, especially from drugs. (2) Wild sex. (3) A person who identifies himself as crazy, unconventional, bizarre and/or degenerate in the eyes of society.
FUZZ	Police.

G

GANG BANG	A group sexual experience or rape.
GARBAGE	To scavenge food from garbage cans.
GARBAGE JUNKIE	An addict who will use almost any drug.
GASKET	Anything that can be placed on the small end of an eyedropper to prevent air from leaking between the dropper and the needle.
GEE	Intravenous injection.
GET ONE'S HEAD TOGETHER	To compose oneself; to achieve tranquillity, sometimes after the continued abuse of hallucinogens and/or other drugs.
GIG	A job, profession, or musical engagement.
GOING UP	The opposite of coming down; becoming high on drugs.
GOLD	Marijuana.
GOOFERS	Sedatives; more properly, glutethimide.
GOOF BALLS	Sedatives.
GRAPES	Wine.
GRASS	Marijuana.
GROK	From Robert Heinlein's **Stranger in a Strange Land**; to understand telepathically, to empathize and more . . .
GROOVE	A pleasurable experience.
GROOVY	Pleasurable.
GUIDE	One who leads you through a hallucinogenic experience.
GURU	A wise person, usually male, who may have had many hallucinogenic experiences.

H

H	Heroin.
HABIT	Addiction.
HALLUCINATION	A false sensory perception in the absence of an actual external stimulus.
HANG-UP	Psychological problem.
HARRY	Heroin.
HASSLE	An intrusion; or, to intrude upon.

HAY	Marijuana.
HEAD	A regular user of something, probably a drug.
HEADQUARTERS	Stores selling items of interest to acid heads.
HEAT	(1) Police. (2) A gun.
HEAVY	That which is emotionally imposing.
HEMP	Marijuana.
HEP	Hepatitis.
HEROIN	Diacetylmorphine, a derivative of morphine.
H.I.P.	Haight Independent Proprietors, an organization of the new community.
HIP	To be in the know, particularly about the drug underground.
HIPPIE	A derivation of Norman Mailer's term "hipster" which was and is favored by the media.
HIPPIE MODALITY	A term coined by Dr. Ernest Dernburg to describe the personality characteristics and modes of perception common among hippies.
HIT	A single dose.
HOG	Benactyzine, a sedative-hynotic-general anesthestic.
HOLD	To possess drugs.
HOODIE	A term coined by Dr. Ernest Dernburg to describe a psychopath.
HORSE HEARTS	Dexedrine.
HOT	Stolen.
HUSTLE	To pursue women, money and/or drugs.
HYKE	Hycodan, dioxycodinone hydrochloride.
HYPE	Someone who injects drugs.
HYSTERICAL PERSONALITY	A personality type distinguished by shifting feelings, susceptibility to suggestions and impulsive behavior.

I

IN VIVO	In life.

J

JACKED UP	Wired or stimulated.
JACKING OFF THE SPIKE	Releasing pressure on the pacifier before all of the liquid has gone into the vein, allowing blood to reenter the outfit. This is sometimes repeated several times to wash all of the drug into the blood and to heighten its orgasmic effects.
JD	Juvenile delinquent.
JIVE	Marijuana.
JOINT	(1) Marijuana cigarette. (2) Prison. (3) Penis.
JOY POWDER	Heroin.
JUG	Ampule or multidose vial of liquid drugs.
JUICE	Hard liquor.
JUNK	Heroin.
JUNKIE	(1) Someone who uses heroin. (2) Oftentimes one drug user will call another whom he feels is worse off than himself a "junkie."

384

K

KARMA	Fate, from Buddhism and Hinduism.
KEY	Kilogram or 2.2 pounds of marijuana.
KICK THE HABIT	To terminate addiction.
KNICK-KNACK	To finger and/or steal objects.

L

LID	About one ounce of marijuana.
LIKE	An essentially meaningless expletive, usually used as a substitute for "that is to say."
LLESCA	Spanish word for marijuana.

M

MAGIC MUSHROOM	Psilocybin.
MAINLINE	To inject a drug, particularly heroin, intravenously.
MAINTAIN	To control one's behavior and/or cope with life.
MAN, THE	(1) The police. (2) One's connection. (3) White people
MARYJANE	Marijuana.
MDA	2, 3-methylenedioxyamphetamine, a psychotomimetic amphetamine.
METH	Methedrine or methamphetamine.
METH FREAK	Person who likes to use methamphetamine.
METH HEAD	Person who likes to use methamphetamine.
MEXICAN BROWN	Brown marijuana from Mexico.
MISS	When the tip of the needle slips out of the vein or goes through the vein and the drug is injected into the tissue surrounding the vein.
MISS EMMA	Morphine.
MODALITY	A sense department or category, such as speech.
MOOD ELEVATORS	Antidepressants.
MOTA	Mexican word for good marijuana.
MOTOR	That which pertains to motorcycle-riding and/or gangs.
M.S.	Morphine sulfate.
MUSCLE	To inject the drug intramuscularly because of inability to find a good vein, to conceal the needle mark or to lengthen the effects of the drug.

N

NABS	Police.
NARC	Narcotic agent.
NARCISSISM	Self-love; in a broader sense, a degree of self-interest which is normal to early childhood but pathological when seen to a similar degree in adulthood.
NARCOS	Narcotic agents.
NEEDLE FLASH	A short high that might come between the time the needle enters the tissue and the drug enters the blood stream.
NEEDLE FREAK	One who gets a thrill out of using the needle.
NEMBIES	Nembutal, pentobarbital sodium.
NEUROSIS	An emotional maladaption due to unresolved instinctual conflicts.

NICKEL	Five dollars.
NICKLE BAG	A bag, or drugs costing five dollars.
NOD OUT	To lose consciousness while high on heroin.
NOW-NESS	The present; living therein.

O

O	Opium.
OBSESSION	A persistent idea or impulse that cannot be eliminated by logic or reasoning.
OD	Overdose.
OLD LADY	One's female lover, wife, or mother.
OLD MAN	One's male lover, husband, or father.
OP	Opium.
OUTFIT	Paraphernalia for injections.
OUTLAW	A motorcycle rider and/or Club member who does not belong to an Establishment riders' organization.
OUT OF SIGHT	Superb; too wonderful to be described.
OVERAMP	To become acutely toxic on speed; the equivalent of overdosage.
OVER THE HIGH SIDE	To ride a motorcycle off a turn.

P

PAD	Bohemian term for residence.
PANAMA RED	Marijuana.
PAPER	A small square of paper folded into a rectangle to contain powdered drugs.
PAPER BOY	A dealer of heroin.
PARANOIA	An acute or chronic disorder which is characterized by intricate and internally logical systems of persecutory and/or grandiose delusions.
PARANOID	Overly suspicious but perhaps not delusional.
PARENT SURROGATE	One who is related to as if she or he stood in place of a mother or father.
PEACE PILL	PCP or phencyclidine, a sedative-hypnotic-general anesthetic used primarily in the practice of veterinary anesthesia.
PER	Prescription.
P.G.	Paregoric.
PHENNIES	Phenobarbital.
PIECE	(1) One ounce. (2) A gun, especially a pistol. (3) A girl.
PIECE OF STUFF	One ounce of heroin.
PILES	Hemorrhoids.
PILL FREAK	Someone who likes to take a lot of pills.
PILL HEAD	Someone who likes to get high on pills.
PINKS	Seconal sodium.
PIPE	Large vein.
POINT	Hypodermic needle.
POPPERS	Amyl nitrite.

386

POT	Marijuana.
POT HEAD	Someone who likes to get high on marijuana.
POWDER	Amphetamine in powdered form.
PRIDE	A hairstyle favored by some blacks.
PROJECTION	A defense mechanism through which that which is emotionally unacceptable to the self is unconsciously rejected and attributed to others.
PROTOPLASMIC CONSCIOUSNESS	A state without ego boundaries in which one feels contiguous with the external world.
PSYCHEDELIC	Hallucinogenic; that which blows one's mind.
PSYCHOPATH	Or sociopath; a person whose behavior is predominantly antisocial yet not psychotic and is characterized by impulsive actions satisfying immediate and narcissistic interests.
PSYCHOSIS	A severe emotional disorder in which there is a departure from normal patterns of thinking, feeling and acting, which is commonly characterized by loss of contact from reality, distortion of perception, diminished control of impulses and abnormal mental content, including delusions and hallucinations.
PSYCHOTOMIMETIC	Mind-altering.

R

RAINBOWS	Tuinal.
RAP	To discuss, particularly to talk excitedly without concern for one's companions.
RAT	(1) To inform. (2) An informer.
RED BIRDS	Seconal sodium.
RED BULLETS	Seconal sodium.
RED DEVILS	Seconal sodium.
RED DOLLS	Seconal sodium.
REDS	Seconal sodium.
REEFER	Marijuana.
REGISTER	When blood appears in the outfit, indicating the vein has been punctured.
REGRESSION	The readoption, partially or symbolically, of more infantile ways of gratification.
RIG	Paraphernalia for injections.
RIGHTEOUS	Pharmacologically pure; of good intent.
RIP OFF	To rob.
ROACH	The butt of a marijuana cigarette.
ROD	Gun, especially a pistol.
ROLLER	A vein that will not stay still for an injection.
ROPE	Marijuana.
ROWDY	Anyone who is uncool.
RUN	A drug binge.
RUNS	Diarrhea.
RUSH	The intense orgasmlike euphoria experienced immediately after an intravenous injection.

S

SATORI	From Zen Buddhism; a state of enlightenment and serenity.
SCENE	A place where something is happening.
SCHIZOPHRENIA	A severe emotional disorder of psychotic depth which is manifested by retreat from reality with delusions, hallucinations and regressive behavior.
SCHMECK	Heroin, diacetylmorphine.
SCORE	(1) to obtain drugs, sex or other supplies. (2) When blood appears in the eyedropper.
SCRIPT	Prescription.
SCRIPTWRITER	(1) Sympathetic doctor. (2) Someone who forges prescriptions.
SECCY	Seconal sodium.
SEGGY	Seconal sodium.
SELL OUT	To relinquish one's individuality or compromise one's integrity for financial profit or because of the opposition of society.
SHACK UP	To sleep and/or live with one's lover.
SHIT	(1) Heroin, diacetylmorphine. (2) Sometimes marijuana.
SHOOT	To make an injection.
SHOOTING GALLERY	A place where people are injecting drugs.
SHRINK	Psychiatrist.
SIDEWALK COMMANDO	A hustler and/or psychopath.
SILVER BIKE	Syringe with chrome fittings, or a chrome hypodermic needle.
SIMPLE SIMON	Psilocybin.
SYPH	Syphillis.
SKAG	Heroin.
SKIN POP	To inject drugs immediately under the skin.
SMACK	Heroin.
SMACK FREAK	Someone who likes or is addicted to heroin.
SMACK HEAD	Someone who likes or is addicted to heroin.
SMOKE	Marijuana.
SNITCH	Informer.
SNIVEL OVER USED COTTONS	To acquire the cottons used to strain impurities from drugs and extract the contents for one's own use.
SNOW	(1) Cocaine. (2) White heroin.
SNOWBIRD	Cocaine user.
SOUL	A state of exuberance and strong feeling allegedly possessed by blacks.
SPACED-OUT	Disoriented, either on a temporary or a permanent basis, and often because of the abuse of drugs.
SPEED	Any central nervous system stimulant, especially methamphetamine.
SPEEDBALL	(1) To inject a stimulant mixed with an opiate. (2) To use stimulants and opiates together. (3) A combination of stimulants and opiates.

388

SPEED DEMON	Someone who abuses stimulants.
SPEED FREAK	Someone who abuses stimulants.
SPEEDSTER	A stimulant user.
SPIKE	Hypodermic needle.
SPLASH	Methamphetamine.
SPLIT	To leave, evacuate, or run away.
SPOON	A spoon used to melt drug crystals; a quantity of drugs, especially heroin.
SQUARE	Conventional, conforming, bourgeois.
STONED	Drunk or high.
STP	DOM or 2,5-dimethoxy-4-methylamphetamine, a psychotomimetic amphetamine.
STRAIGHT	The opposite of hip; square, conventional, conforming.
STREET PEOPLE	People who eat, sleep, live or make their living on the street.
STREET-WISE	Knowledgeable about the underground; criminally experienced.
STRUNG-OUT	Upset and/or disoriented, especially because of habitual use of a drug.
STUFF	Heroin.
SUDS	Beer.
SUPEREGO	In Freudian theory that part of the psyche which has unconsciously identified with important people from early life, particularly parents. The supposed or actual wishes of these people are taken over as parts of one's personal standards and help form the conscience.

T

TEA	Marijuana.
TEXAS TEA	Marijuana.
THC	Tetrahydrocannabinol, the active ingredient in marijuana.
TICKET	Drug used to provide a hallucinogenic trip.
TICKET AGENT	Dealer of hallucinogenic drugs.
TIE	Anything that is used to tie off the vein for an injection.
TOO MUCH	Another general term referring to those things which beggar description.
TOXIC PSYCHOSIS	A psychosis or major psychological break with reality induced by a toxic chemical.
TRACK	(1) The mark left from an injection. (2) The mark from repeated injections.
TRANK	Tranquilizer.
TRIBE	A group of hippies.
TURN OFF	To deaden or disrupt a pleasant experience.
TURNOUT	A torture, in the name of punishment, by one's peers.

U

UNCOOL	Displeasing, unaware, overly conservative.
UPPERS	Stimulants, especially Benzedrine or Dexedrine.
UPS	Stimulants, especially Benzedrine or Dexedrine.

UPTIGHT	Anxious, distressed.
UNCONSCIOUS	In Freudian thought, that part of the psyche which is only rarely subject to consciousness.

V

VALLEY	The inside of the elbow, which has two large veins.
VIBRATION or VIBES	The sensations that are allegedly given off by others and enter a mind "sensitized" by drugs.

W

WEED	Marijuana.
WINO	Someone who drinks wine.
WITCH DOCTOR	An underground healer who may prescribe toxic drugs.
WITHDRAWAL	A pattern of action, induced by persistent frustration, in which a person removes himself from the realm of conflict and obtains satisfaction through such acts as daydreaming.
WORKS	Paraphernalia for injections.
WORK THE MEATRACK	To engage in prostitution.

Y

YATA	Mexican slang word for someone who is crazy.
YELLOW BULLETS	Nembutal, pentobarbital sodium.
YELLOW DOLLS	Nembutal sodium.
YELLOW JACKETS	Nembutal sodium.
YELLOWS	Nembutal sodium.

APPENDIX I

The following list contains many of the drugs discussed in *Love Needs Care.* In most cases, the chemical and generic or trade name of these compounds are given, along with their formulas.

Central Nervous System Stimulants

Dextroamphetamine (Dexedrine)

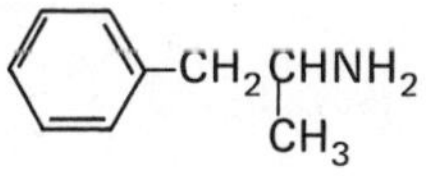

Methamphetamine (Methedrine)

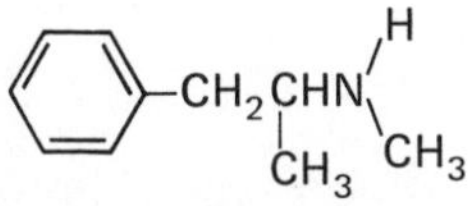

Methylphenidate (Ritalin)

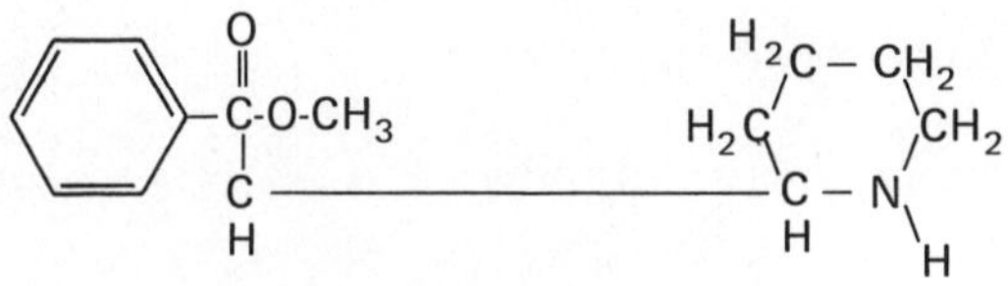

Cocaine (benzoylmethylecgonine)

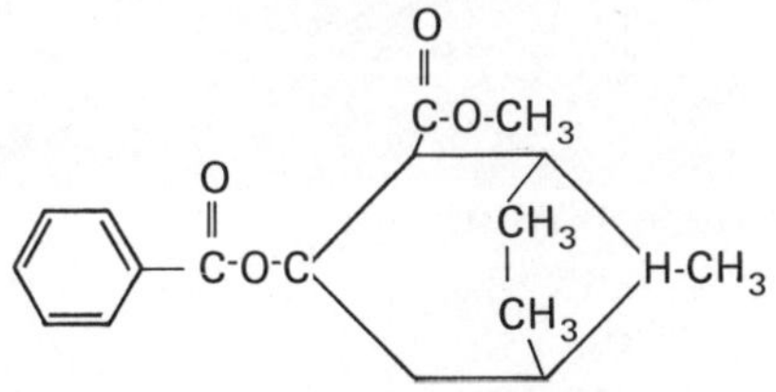

Sedative-Hypnotic-General Anesthetics

Ethyl alcohol

C_2H_5OH
or
H_3C-CH_2-OH

Barbiturates and barbituratelike drugs

Secobarbital (Seconal)

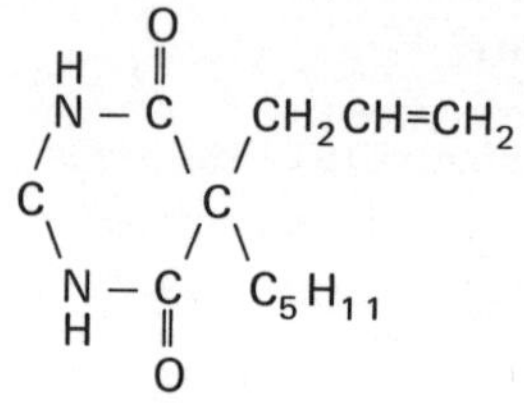

Phenobarbital

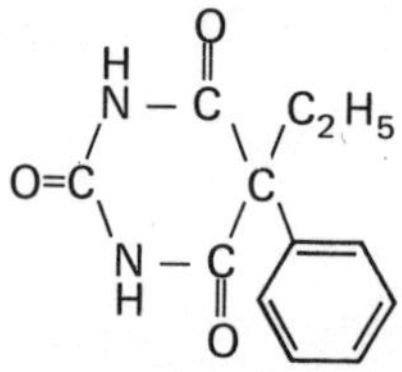

Chlordiazepoxide (Librium)

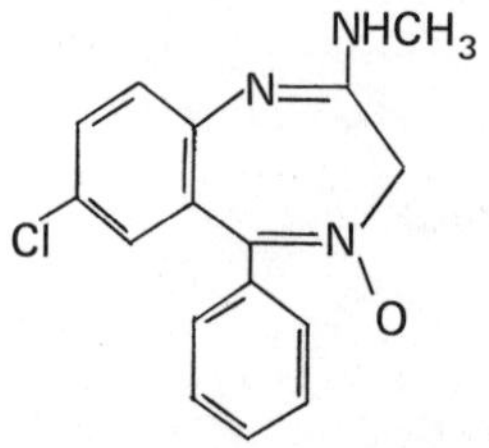

Tetrahydrocannabinol (THC)

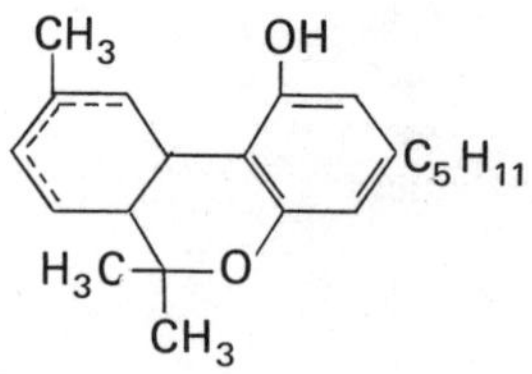

Volatile Hydrocarbons (carbon tetrachloride, toluene)

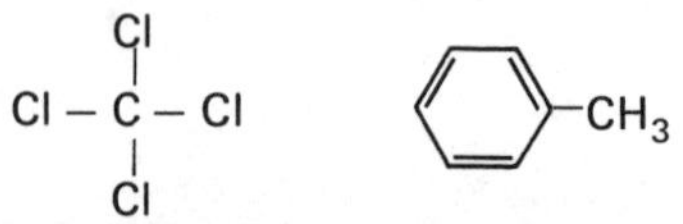

PCP — Phencyclidine

(Sernyl) (1-(1-Phenylcyclohexyl) piperidine monohydrochloride)

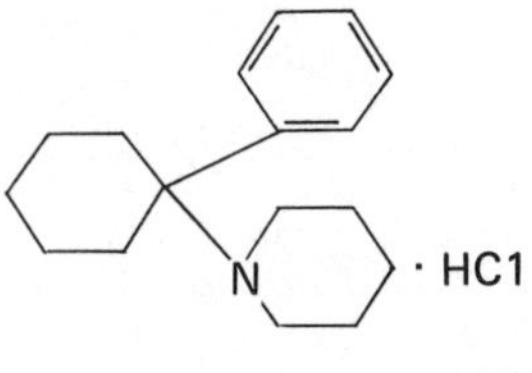

Hallucinogens

Lysergic acid diethylamide (LSD)

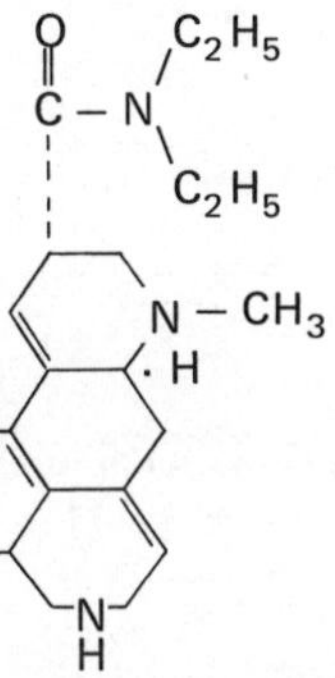

Mescaline (3,4,5-trimethoxyamphetamine)

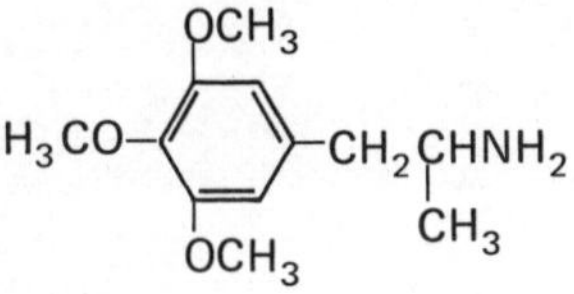

Psilocybin

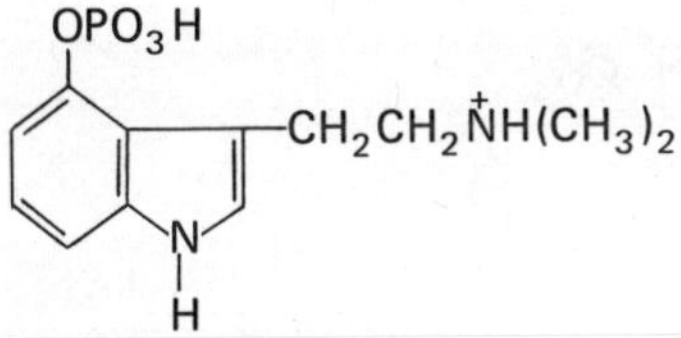

Dimethyltryptamine (DMT)

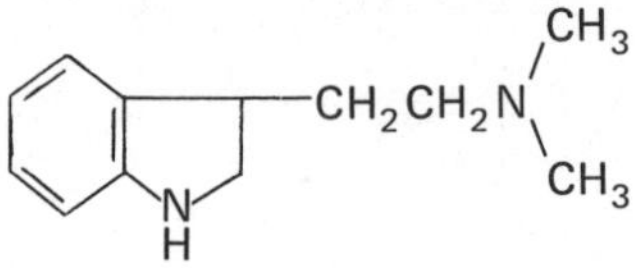

Psychotomimetic Amphetamines

MDA (2,3-methylenedioxyamphetamine)

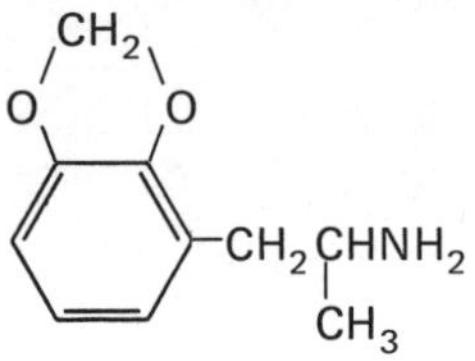

STP (DOM, 2,5-dimethoxy-4-methylamphetamine)

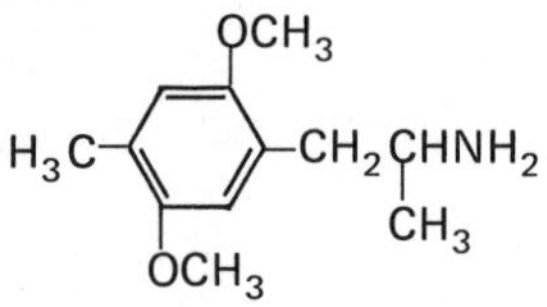

Narcotics

Morphine

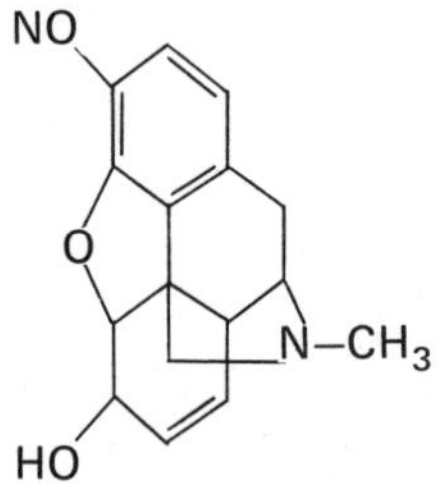

Heroin (diacetylmorphine)

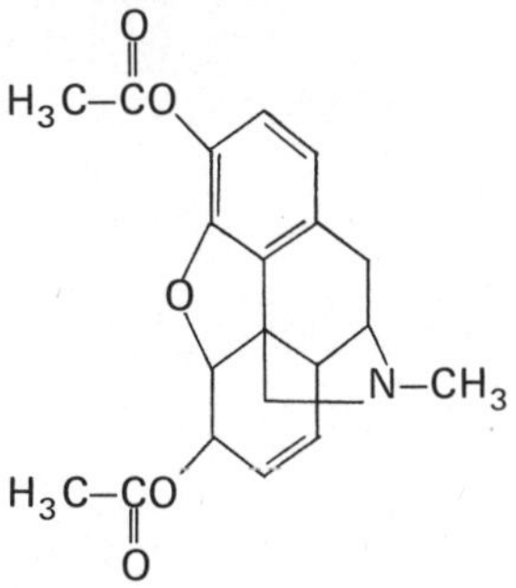

Methadone (dl-4,4-diphenyl-6-dimethylamine-3-heptanone)

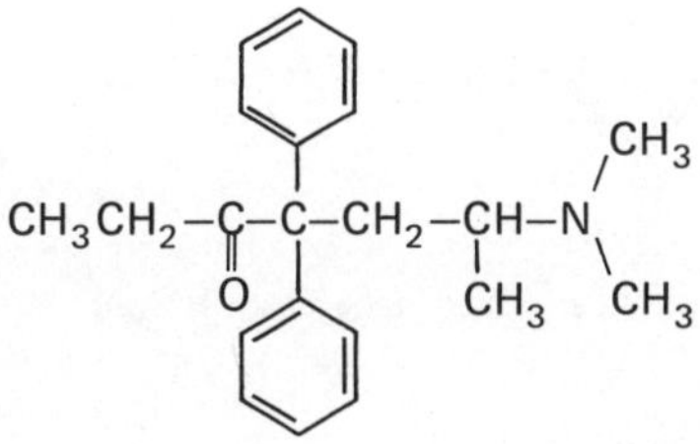

Miscellaneous

Parasympatholytic Agents

Atropine (dl-hyoscyamine)

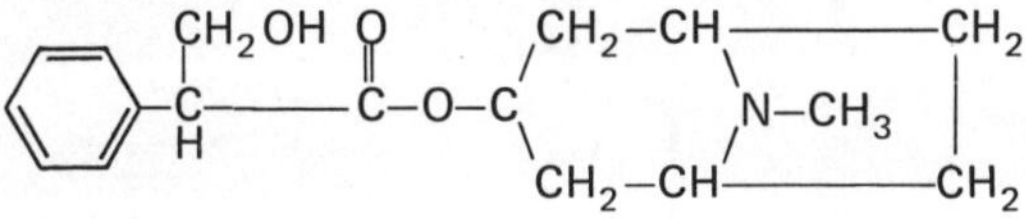

Scopolamine (l-hyoscine)

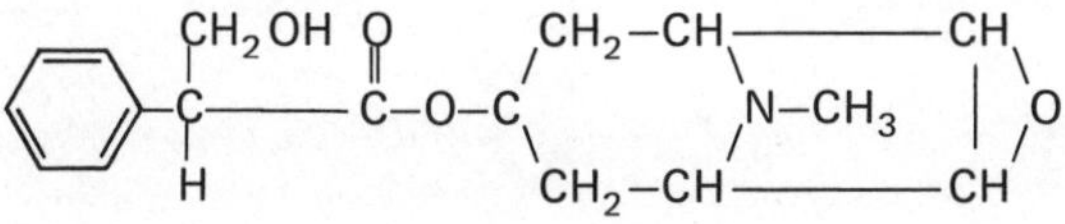

Major Tranquilizers

Chlorpromazine (Thorazine)

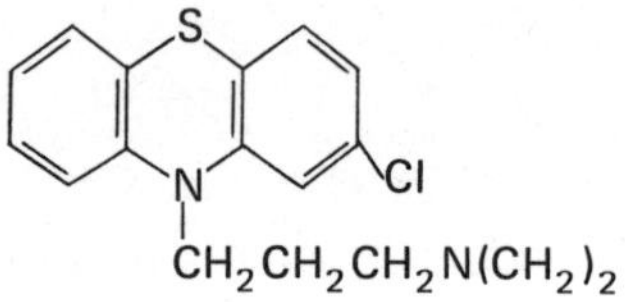

$CH_2CH_2CH_2N(CH_2)_2$

Benactyzine

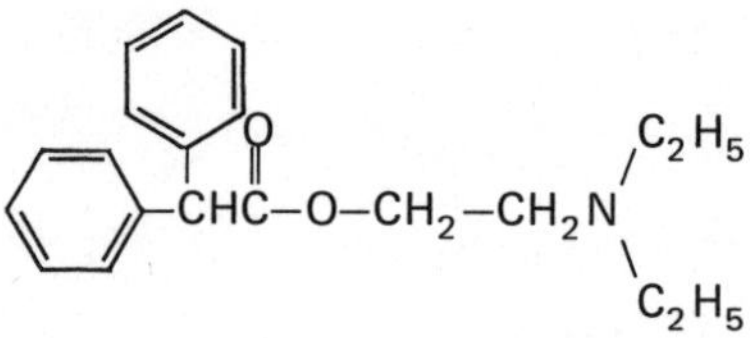

$-CHC-O-CH_2-CH_2N\begin{smallmatrix}C_2H_5\\C_2H_5\end{smallmatrix}$

Amyl nitrite (a coronary vasodilator)

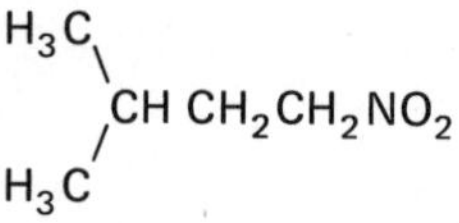

$\begin{smallmatrix}H_3C\\H_3C\end{smallmatrix}CH\ CH_2CH_2NO_2$

Reprinted are several of the forms and handouts used by the Haight-Ashbury Free Medical Clinic.

PEOPLE ARE COMING TOGETHER:

A COMMUNITY
MEETING
TO RAP ABOUT HEALTH, NUTRITION, ETC.

HAIGHT FREE CLINIC PEOPLE, BLACKMAN'S CLINIC PEOPLE, BROTHERS AND SISTERS FROM THE COMMUNES, FROM THE STREETS, MAMAS FROM LA LECHE LEAGUE ARE COMING . . . . .

YOU ARE NEEDED SO WE CAN ALL GET IT TOGETHER

WHAT ARE OUR HEALTH NEEDS?

WHAT CAN WE DO ABOUT THEM? ARE YOU INTERESTED IN STARTING PROJECTS IN THE STREET, ON YOUR BLOCK? HOW CAN WE GET MEDICAL SUPPLIES AND INFORMATION INTO THE COMMUNITY?

HOW CAN THE CLINICS BETTER SERVE THE COMMUNITY?

TIME: THURSDAY, MARCH 5 at 8:00 P.M.

PLACE: FREE CITY U. COFFEE HOUSE
(Howard Church) OAK and BAKER streets

HEROIN WITHDRAWAL PROJECT

Date ——————————————

Name ———————————————— Age ——— Sex ——— Race ——————

Address ———————————————— Haight ( )   City ( )   Out of Town ( )

Family Status: (Circle) M S W D CH SEP No. of Dependent Children ——————

Habit: Size ———————————————— Where Hooked ——————————

First Used Heroin: Age ———————————— First Hooked: Age ——————————

Time Since Last Clean: ————————————————————————

Previous Withdrawal History: Times 0 ( ) 1 ( ) 2 ( ) 3 ( ) 4 ( ) up ( )

How Withdrawn: "Cold" ( ), Methadone ( ), Self-Med ( ), M.D. Med ( )

Symptoms: Runny Nose ( ), Abd. Cramps ( ), Muscle Cramps ( ),

Joint Pains ( ), Jittery ( ), Nausea and Vomiting ( ),

Diarrhea ( ), Sleepless ( ), Muscle Twitches ( ),

Other ————————————————————

————————————————————

Reason for Withdrawal: No More Money ( ), Got Busted ( ), Family ( )

Other ————————————————————————————

Other Drugs: (dates) (experimental, reg. user, compulsive, abuser, etc.)

GRASS: ————————————————————————

————————————————————————————

ACID: ————————————————————————

SPEED: ————————————————————————

BARBS: ————————————————————————

ALCOHOL: ——————————————————————

Regular Job? Yes ( ) No ( ) Lost job because of habit? Yes ( ) No ( )

Trained for a job? ——————————————————————

Aftercare: 409 ( ) Other ( ) MD's Est. of Motivation ——————————

Symptoms (grade from 0-3) _____

Restless, Jittery _____

Sleeplessness _____

Nausea and Vomiting _____

Diarrhea _____

Abd. Cramps _____

Muscle Cramps — back _____

                legs _____

                other _____

Headache _____

Joint Pain _____

Runny Nose _____

Sweats and Chills _____

Other (specify) _____

Medication _____

For Sleep _____

                Chloral Hydrate _____

                Noludar _____

                Other _____

For Sedation _____

                Phenobarb _____

                Valium _____

                Other _____

For GI _____

                Bel Phen _____

                Bentyl w/PB _____

                Antrenyl w/PB _____

                Compazine _____

                Other _____

Pain _____

                Talwin _____

                Darvon _____

                Other _____

Other Meds: _____

HAIGHT - ASHBURY MEDICAL CLINIC

NAME _____ AGE _____ IF UNDER 21 GET
      LAST   FIRST   ADMIN. O.K. 1st.

BIRTH DATE ___/___/___ HAS PATIENT BEEN TREATED HERE BEFORE?_____

PATIENT'S ADDRESS _____ PHONE _____
                                        CITY

NAME OF CLOSE FRIEND OR RELATIVE _____ PHONE _____

ADDRESS _____
                                   CITY   STATE

DRUG ALLERGIES: IF UNDER 21: SELF SUPP. _____FOR _____

                           MARRIED_____ PREG. _____ GI _____

I HEREBY AUTHORIZE TREATMENT:

_____

     PATIENT'S SIGNATURE

****

LOG #	DATE / /	CHIEF COMPLAINT (SYMPTOMS), HISTORY AND EXAMINATION

HAIGHT - ASHBURY MEDICAL CLINIC
DRUG TREATMENT PROGRAM
San Francisco, California

REFERRAL FOR SERVICE

Referred to _____

Address _____

Re: _____
       last   first   middle

Reason for Referral _____

_____

_____

_____

_____

Referred by: JOHN H. FRYKMAN/ _____ Phone _____

I give my consent for release of information to the Drug Treatment Program on myself.

_____
                                  Patient

****

Please send us information concerning your treatment of the above patient. We appreciate your help with this case.

                                  John H. Frykman
                                  Director

TREATMENT RECORD

DRUG TREATMENT PROGRAM
San Francisco, California
John H. Frykman, Director

Name _____ Date _____

              Last   First   Middle

Address _____Phone _____

Birth date _____/ _____/ _____   Birthplace _____

Education Level (Circle one) Less than 8, 9, 10, 11, 12, 13, 14, 15, 16

Race _____   How Long in Area? _____

How Long at Present Address? _____

Who Referred You to Us? _____

Address _____Phone _____

Welfare? _____ Worker _____ Medi-Cal No. _____

Medical History (Hepatitis, Heart, Lung, Epilepsy, etc.) _____

_____

_____

General Physical Appearance _____

_____

Psychiatric History _____

_____

Previous Medical Treatment, Current Treatment (What, Where, and When)

_____

History of Drug Use: Chronology (When, Types, Frequency, & Amounts)

1st Drug	2nd Drug	3rd Drug	4th Drug	5th Drug	6th Drug

History of Present Problem: Type _____ Frequency _____ Amount _____

Main Complaints _____

_____

_____ Interviewer _____

RESIDENCE AGREEMENT
Group Living Houses
DRUG TREATMENT PROGRAM
San Francisco, California

Name _____ Date _____ Rent _____

Room Assignment _____ Occupation _____

Friend or relative for reference _____
                                                                name

_____
            relationship   address

This is a treatment program facility. Because of this and the fact that the house could be closed for improper operation, we need to have you make a few simple agreements with us:

1. There will be no use, holding, or trafficking of dangerous drugs, narcotics, paraphernalia, or anything else that you might suspect to be illegal.
2. Weapons will not be permitted. This is a house of peace and healing, a sanctuary, not a place of destruction and violence.
3. Crashers and friends are not to be allowed to stay overnight in the house and are to visit only with the permission of the Drug Treatment Program coordinator.
4. No one is to sit around the house all day. You will be required to work, to be in a school or training program, or to be looking for work or training.
5. The privacy of the house will be upheld — no one will be allowed to visit or intrude without the permission of the community, the coordinator, and the director of the Drug Treatment Program.
6. Living expenses such as rent, food, cleaning supplies, household items, etc., will be shared by the entire community.
7. Responsibilities for maintaining the house (cooking, cleaning, housework, etc.) will also be shared.
8. Encounter sessions will take place once weekly. Community meetings will also take place at least once weekly (to assign responsibilities, take care of housekeeping matters, etc.).
9. The respect of personal property will be upheld at all times.
10. Both couples and single individuals will be allowed to live in the house. When it is possible, a couple will be allowed to share the same room together.
11. Any changes in this agreement will be worked out by the community, the coordinator, and the program director.

We are here to help you change your style of life, to give you a chance to turn on to happiness and security without the use of drugs. We are only helpers; the main job is up to you. We ask your full cooperation. Anyone not living up to this agreement may be expelled from the Group Living House immediately. Any instances of breaking the agreement will be reviewed at the community meetings. Ultimate responsibility will rest with the coordinator and the director of the Drug Treatment Program.

Signed _____

Date _____

APPLICATION TO VOLUNTEER

DRUG TREATMENT PROGRAM
San Francisco, California
John H. Frykman, Director

This information is for our confidential files only.

Name _____
                 Last   First   Middle

Address _____Phone _____

Age _____ Education (Circle one) High School 1 2 3 4 College 1 2 3 4

Do you type? _____ WPM _____   Major_____

Would you have time for treatment-oriented activities and outings? _____

Would you have an available car? _____

What kinds of activities are you most interested in? _____

_____

How would you describe your own drug experience, if any.

Describe any experience you have had with nursing, social work, drug-abuse treatment, alcohol-abuse treatment, social problems, counseling, or encounter groups.

What are your feelings on drug abuse; how would you define drug abuse; and how does that relate to you volunteering your services to our program?

Drug Treatment Program
Haight-Ashbury Medical Clinic
San Francisco, California

GUIDELINES FOR CENTER OPERATIONS

1. A sign should be posted in the Drug Treatment Center stating: NO HOLDING, USING, OR DEALING. ANY OF THESE COULD CLOSE OUR PROGRAM.

2. A biographical sketch should be kept on all employees and staff people, including letters of recommendation, if appropriate. One copy would be kept in the files, another sent to Youth Projects, Inc.

3. When and if the facilities of the program are overtaxed, reasonable limits should be set as to the number of people receiving treatment. In advance of the establishment of residential programs, the number of people to be admitted will be determined.

4. An advisory committee will be established to evaluate and make suggestions concerning the operation of the program. These people should include professionals, former drug users, volunteers, members of the community, and staff. There shall be at least one liaison person representing the program to Youth Projects, Inc.

5. A position paper with respect to the program's philosophy and plan of treatment shall be kept on file in each center. This would also include the standard forms used by the program for medical histories, referrals, volunteer applications, etc.

6. The staff will communicate through its relationship with those who come into the office that the center is not a place for lounging, loitering, or rapping. Outside of the framework of actually working with people who have come for help, this kind of activity is disruptive to the objectives of the program.

7. Volunteers should be screened as to their ability in working with the program. Before taking on responsibilities, they will have to participate in our groups and attend at least one training session. Volunteers need to be stable, mature people, able to respond to the crises that come our way.

8. When the office opens, a staff person should be present to assume ultimate responsibility for what takes place. Except in the evening and unusual situations, the office should not be left totally in the care of a volunteer.

9. Emergency procedures, which are clearly defined for volunteers, will be kept continuously up-to-date.

10. Regular training sessions will be set up for volunteers: to train new volunteers, to keep continuing volunteers up-to-date, and to give volunteers a chance to share their insights with the staff.